'THE CRUEL MADNESS OF LOVE'
SEX, SYPHILIS AND PSYCHIATRY
IN SCOTLAND, 1880–1930

THE WELLCOME SERIES
IN THE HISTORY OF MEDICINE

Forthcoming Titles:

The Imperial Laboratory:
Experimental Physiology and Clinical Medicine
in Post-Crimean Russia

Galina Kichigina

Permeable Walls:
Historical Perspectives on Hospital and Asylum Visiting

Edited by Graham Mooney
and Jonathan Reinarz

The Wellcome Series in the History of Medicine series editors are
V. Nutton, M. Neve, and R. Cooter.
Please send all queries regarding the series to Michael Laycock,
The Wellcome Trust Centre for the History of Medicine at UCL,
183 Euston Road, London NW1 2BE, UK.

'THE CRUEL MADNESS OF LOVE'
SEX, SYPHILIS AND PSYCHIATRY
IN SCOTLAND, 1880–1930

Gayle Davis

Amsterdam – New York, NY 2008

First published in 2008
by Editions Rodopi B.V., Amsterdam – New York, NY 2008.

Editions Rodopi B.V. © 2008

Design and Typesetting by Michael Laycock,
The Wellcome Trust Centre for the History of Medicine at UCL.
Printed and bound in The Netherlands by Editions Rodopi B.V.,
Amsterdam – New York, NY 2008.

Index by Rosemary Anderson.

British Library Cataloguing in Publication Data
A catalogue record for this book is available from the British Library

ISBN 978-90-420-2463-2

'"The Cruel Madness of Love":
Sex, Syphilis and Psychiatry in Scotland, 1880–1930' –
Amsterdam – New York, NY:
Rodopi. – ill.
(Clio Medica 85 / ISSN 0045-7183;
The Wellcome Series in the History of Medicine)

Front cover:

Alexander Morison's portrait of a man in the final stage of general paralysis,
*c.*1840, courtesy of the Royal College of Physicians of Edinburgh;
nineteenth-century map of Scotland, courtesy of the Wellcome Library, London.

© Editions Rodopi B.V., Amsterdam – New York, NY 2008
Printed in The Netherlands

All titles in the Clio Medica series (from 1999 onwards) are available to
download from the IngentaConnect website: http://www.ingentaconnect.co.uk

Contents

Abbreviations

CSF	Cerebrospinal Fluid
EUL	Edinburgh University Library
Gartnavel	Glasgow Royal Asylum
GP	General Paralysis (of the insane)
GPI	General Paralysis of the Insane
HP	Hereditary Propensity
ID	Primary Key (unique identifier)
KI	Potassium Iodide
LHB	Lothian Health Board
LHSA	Lothian Health Services Archive
MPA	Medico-Psychological Association
MRC	Medical Research Council
NHSA	Northern Health Services Archives
NHSGGCA	NHS Greater Glasgow and Clyde Archives
PA	Previous Attack
PHS	Public Health Service
PRO	Public Record Office
REA	Royal Edinburgh Asylum
Rosslynlee	Midlothian and Peebles District Asylum
SAPS	Scottish Asylums' Pathological Scheme
'606'	Salvarsan
SWARI	Scottish Western Asylums' Research Institute
TNA	The National Archives
Woodilee	Barony Parochial Asylum

List of Figures

List of Tables

List of Images

List of Images

Acknowledgements

It may come as no surprise to hear how much enthusiasm you are met with when your topic of research is sex and madness. I would like to record my sincere gratitude to the many people who have helped me in the preparation of this book. This project was made possible through the financial support of the Economic and Social Research Council, for which I am most grateful. I wish also to thank Mike Laycock at *Clio Medica* for efficiently answering my *many* queries as I prepared the final manuscript, and the editors and two anonymous referees for their supportive and constructive comments.

I am indebted to a number of archivists for facilitating access to their clinical records and for mesmerising me on a daily basis with their incredible knowledge of the riches that they hold. In particular, the staff of both the Lothian Health Services Archive and the NHS Greater Glasgow and Clyde Archives (particularly Alistair Tough) assisted me on a daily basis for several years, and their expertise has proved extremely valuable to this project. I am grateful to Fiona Watson (Northern Health Services Archives) for enticing me out of lowland Scotland – albeit briefly – to visit her wonderful collections in Aberdeen and Inverness; and to Morag Williams (NHS archivist for Dumfries and Galloway) for fruitful discussions relating to her superb archival collection for the Crichton Royal Hospital. I would also like to thank the staffs of Edinburgh and Glasgow University Library Special Collections, Edinburgh Central Library, the Mitchell Library, the National Archives (PRO), the National Archives of Scotland, the National Library of Scotland, the Royal College of Physicians of Edinburgh (particularly Iain Milne), the Royal College of Physicians and Surgeons of Glasgow (particularly James Beaton and Carol Parry), and the Wellcome Library (particularly Lesley Hall), for their help in assisting my research. Thanks, above all, to Helen Zealley (formerly Director of Public Health for Lothian Health Board) and Harry Burns (Chief Medical Officer for Scotland, formerly Director of Public Health for Greater Glasgow Health Board) for allowing me access to the clinical records of the Edinburgh and Glasgow institutions respectively.

I owe a great debt to the shared expertise of a number of scholars, including Mike Anderson, Jonathan Andrews, Helen Coyle, Anne Crowther, Marguerite Dupree, Matt Egan, Emma Halliday, Jen Harrison,

Anne Kerr, Emese Lafferton, Chris Lawrence, Susan Lemar, Sharon Mathews, Francis McKee, Bob Morris, Alison Nuttall, Maureen Park, Frank Rice, Martin Rorke, and Donald Spaeth. Indeed, it was Anne Crowther and Marguerite Dupree who enticed me into the social history of medicine in the first place – like the proverbial child-catcher – and who have consistently supported my work ever since, for which I am incredibly grateful. I wish to thank Roy Porter and Steve Sturdy for their invaluable comments on an earlier draft of this work. Most grateful thanks, also, to Malcolm Nicolson for toughening me up at an early stage with his sharply insightful constructive criticisms and for his long-term support of this work.

In addition, I would like to thank those clinicians and clinician–historians who generously shared their expertise with me on various aspects of neurosyphilis, past and present: Jeanne Bell, Dale Garbutt, Dugald Gardner, Alex Gordon, Juliet Hurn, Colin Smith, and Iain Smith. Particular thanks must go to Allan Beveridge for sharing his considerable knowledge of Thomas Clouston and Victorian Edinburgh, and for his generally soothing psychiatric presence throughout this project.

I owe a special debt of gratitude to two colleagues at the University of Edinburgh who have played a major role in the completion of this book. Roger Davidson first introduced himself to me as 'the VD man', but in fact his expertise on the social history of venereal disease is only one strand of the intellectual and other benefits that I have gleaned from a decade spent in the shelter of his wings. An unparalleled mentor and nurturer, I am blessed to have had such a thorough academic apprenticeship in his care. As both Lothian Health Services archivist and historian of psychiatry, Mike Barfoot has furnished me with a (seemingly) never-ending array of archival material, a rich stream of interpretative ideas (usually over scampi lunches), and considered criticisms of my work from start to finish. In both cases, their intellectual expertise, practical help and friendship have meant more to me than I – a person rarely short of words – can ever say or repay. If my own sanity has remained intact through the completion of this project (if), it is due mostly to their consistent support, guidance and wonderful humour.

More generally, I would like to express my gratitude to those who have fostered my love of history through their talented and dedicated teaching, especially those who good-heartedly urged me to do something else with my life, thereby fuelling my determination to go as far as possible with the discipline! Indeed, it has been asserted – by someone named in these acknowledgements – that historians of psychiatry are not easy people to spend time with (!) so, finally, I would like to thank my family and friends for their support and patience, particularly my mother. I dedicate the book to my wonderful maternal grandparents for everything they gave me and for,

Acknowledgements

in the final years of my gran's life, teaching me – with dignity, courage and humour – more about dementia than I could ever learn from books.

For Gran and Poppy

And most of all would I flee from the cruel madness of love,
The honey of poison-flowers and all the measureless ill

A. Tennyson, *Maud*

1

Introduction

During the early nineteenth century, general paralysis of the insane (GPI) emerged as a new and devastating form of insanity. Characterised by severe mental and physical symptoms, it inflicted the suffering of degenerative dementia upon its victims in tandem with developing bodily paralysis. There was no cure for this condition, the diagnosis therefore conferring an almost certain death sentence upon its victims. Nor was this 'most terrible of all brain diseases' a rare condition,[1] for by the late-nineteenth century as many as twenty per cent of British male asylum admissions received this diagnosis.[2] The chronic and fatally progressive nature of GPI, and the intensive nursing care which it therefore required, caused it to take up a disproportionate amount of asylum resources. Furthermore, since most of those diagnosed were middle-aged males in the prime of their working lives, the socio–economic implications of the disease were a further source of considerable worry. While various efforts were made to gain better understanding of this complex and feared condition, and to find an effective treatment, it was not until penicillin's arrival in the 1940s that a sharp decline was reported in its incidence. With this successful treatment now finally available, GPI soon appeared to have become a mercifully rare disease.

This is a study primarily of the history of GPI, a disease for which physicians and historians have made boldly 'Whiggish' claims but for which a detailed published study has not previously been undertaken. The study also constitutes a wider history of the developing epistemological relationship between syphilis and insanity. While the cause of GPI was probably its least understood element during the nineteenth century, it became clear by the early twentieth century that syphilis was a central factor in its aetiology. Such a discovery allowed psychiatrists – or alienists, as this study will refer to them for the sake of historical accuracy – to begin to diagnose the disease more accurately with the help of newly developed laboratory tests for syphilis.

In the light of developing medical understandings of syphilis and its sequelae, early twentieth-century physicians reconceptualised syphilis as a chronic relapsing disease that could go into hiding after the initial sores had disappeared, only to reassert itself as it began a damaging spread through the internal organs, and able to induce gastrointestinal pain, blindness, deafness, paralysis and insanity. GPI was simultaneously reclassified as a disease of late, or tertiary, syphilis which followed on from the primary and then secondary stages of syphilitic infection. Indeed, by the 1920s, GPI formed the core of a new wider disease category, neurosyphilis, an umbrella term which grouped together those diseases held to be late manifestations of syphilis that had infiltrated the nervous system, including tabes dorsalis, syphilitic insanity and cerebral syphilis.

This study focuses particularly upon the years between 1880 and 1930, the critical period not only in the medical understanding of both syphilis and GPI, but also in the shaping of neurosyphilis as a disease group. During this period, *Treponema pallidum*, the spirochaete responsible for syphilis, was discovered. Serological tests, including the Wassermann reaction, soon became available to detect syphilis in the blood and cerebrospinal fluid (CSF). Meanwhile, physicians also developed a number of innovative therapies to treat GPI and its related disorders, including one of the first somatic therapies to be used within psychiatry, malarial therapy. In terms of causation, diagnosis and treatment, this half century was therefore crucial in the historical development of GPI and the relationship between syphilis, insanity and psychiatry.

In order to provide a detailed and archivally rich investigation of GPI and neurosyphilis, a geographically localised approach has been taken. Four asylums from central Scotland have been selected which are deemed to be broadly representative of the region as a whole, two from the West and two from the east of the country. Two of these institutions, the Royal Edinburgh Asylum (east) and Glasgow Royal Asylum (west), were among the earliest and most prestigious of the Scottish asylums. The remaining institutions, Midlothian and Peebles District Asylum (east) and Barony Parochial Asylum (west), epitomise the other level of asylum care then operating in Scotland, intended to serve pauper patients within their designated district. These four institutions were felt to reflect the range of institutional provision for the insane in Scotland during the late nineteenth and early twentieth centuries. Furthermore, and indeed crucially, a complete run of admission registers and case notes exist for each of these institutions during this period, furnishing an exceptionally rich set of insights into the social background and medical experience of these patients.

A number of historians have extolled the value of local and regional studies as a means of exploring a particular medical theme. Virginia Berridge, and Gayle Davis and Roger Davidson have, for example, stressed the importance of the local state and medical culture in the formation and implementation of central government policy with respect to AIDS and abortion.[3] John Pickstone has argued that detailed local research can both augment and amend claims made within the existing secondary literature, and allow one the opportunity to connect the different features of medicine that tend to be separated in national or international studies.[4] At the same time, however, such historians stress the importance of placing local studies within an explicitly comparative structure in order to highlight patterns of convergence and divergence, and to tease out broader implications. This detailed empirical study of Scottish asylumdom, its staff and neurosyphilitic patient populations, will therefore be contextualised within a broader British and European framework. Such an approach will reveal how the Scottish situation forms part of a larger story, and is intended to make the study of much wider relevance.

Historiographical overview

The history of psychiatry has become an exciting and sophisticated field of research over the past three decades. Much work has focused around the dramatic rise of the asylum as a response to insanity during the nineteenth century, the consequently emerging psychiatric profession which assumed control of inmates, and wider shifting relations between patient, doctor and state. All of these themes developed from Andrew Scull's seminal work, *Museums of Madness*,[5] a wide-ranging historico–sociological interpretation which has provoked a generation of scholars to interrogate a broader array of primary sources at the micro-level in order to provide more subtle and tightly-focused analysis.[6] This historiographic pre-occupation with the lunatic asylum has led to some excellent studies of individual British institutions,[7] which have served also to alert historians to the complex history of madness that underpinned the coming of the asylum.[8]

Scull has discussed the importance of 'social, political, economic, and cultural phenomena' to his work.[9] It is arguable that the absence within this list of 'clinical' indicates a lacuna within the historiography of psychiatry more generally. Despite the offerings of individual institutional histories, there is still much to be said on the practicalities of asylumdom, particularly the day-to-day clinical and diagnostic activities of these institutions. Little more has been written on psychiatric therapeutics, and what alienists could do and did do to their patients in the name of treatment.[10] By focusing within the clinical context upon the ways in which psychiatric diagnoses were made and disease classifications shaped, and then by placing such themes within their wider social context, this study attempts to bridge the gap between clinical and social histories of psychiatry.[11]

The distinctive trajectory of nineteenth-century psychiatry in Scotland has attracted some notable scholarly attention. Jonathan Andrews has done much to elucidate the developing culture of Scottish asylumdom, and the pre-occupations and theories of Scottish alienists, with particular regard to the 'Glasgow school' during the nineteenth century.[12] The clinician–historian Allan Beveridge has also contributed much to our understanding of the 'Edinburgh school' of psychiatry during the Victorian era.[13] However, the Scottish historiography has focused almost entirely upon the chartered (royal) institutions to date, and therefore neglects the provision of district and parochial asylums from the 1870s onwards.[14]

Taking the vibrant historiography of British psychiatry as a whole, patient populations tend to be considered collectively within their institutional context, rather than in terms of specific diagnostic categories. Where individual studies do focus upon disease categories, there appears to be a preference for categories that remain prominent, in one form or another, within modern medicine. Thus we have, for example, work on the history of senile dementia,[15] schizophrenia,[16] depression,[17] and post-traumatic stress disorder.[18] The fact that neurosyphilitic disorders are only rarely diagnosed in the post-antibiotic era perhaps explains their relative absence within this body of literature. Moreover, much of this work tends to be either 'clinical' or 'social' in focus, rather than providing a broader overview of the socio–medical shaping of a disease entity, which is the intention of this study.

There are three notable exceptions. Berrios and Porter's *A History of Clinical Psychiatry* provides a short but valuable introduction to the clinical and social construction of a wide range of psychiatric diagnostic categories.[19] Each disease entity is considered in two separate sections – 'clinical' then 'social' – which ensures that both aspects of the disorder's history are considered, but epitomises, rather than transcends, the historiographical divide between these two perspectives.[20] Mark Micale and Hilary Marland more fulsomely explore the clinical and social history of one particular disorder in their respective works on hysteria and puerperal insanity, the insanity of childbirth.[21] Indeed, Micale strongly criticises 'the sociologising impulse' that has pushed scholars to pursue the social, political and economic determinants of past medical thinking and practice to the neglectful detriment of 'other crucial factors, especially clinical and cognitive ones'.[22] Micale's *Approaching Hysteria* is intended not as a history of the disease category 'hysteria', but as a history of its definition as both disease and cultural metaphor, an aim achieved by focusing upon both the medical and cultural historiography of hysteria – medico–scientific texts, fictional writings, and social and political criticisms – this dual focus intending to overcome the 'stubborn and unproductive' medico–cultural dichotomy.

Nonetheless, the historiography of psychiatry contains little substantial work that relates directly to syphilis or to the neurosyphilitic diseases, despite the importance ascribed by historians to GPI and the fact that its history has resonances for a range of debates within the social history of both psychiatry and medicine more generally. The only neurosyphilitic disease to be addressed by historians to date has been GPI. This is found most prominently in the work of Edward Hare, Margaret Thompson, and Juliet Hurn. Hare, himself a clinician–historian and epidemiologist, provides a most useful historical and epidemiological overview of GPI's spread through Europe between the early nineteenth and mid-twentieth centuries.[23] He posits that the disease arose from a mutation in the syphilitic virus towards the end of the eighteenth century, and raises some interesting issues, not least the confidence in each generation of psychiatrists to diagnose GPI but their eagerness to doubt the validity and accuracy of their predecessors.

Thompson explores GPI within the wider context of the relationship between alcohol, sexuality, vice and madness; and in relation to an individual asylum and its patients, by focusing upon the records of the Royal Edinburgh Asylum during Thomas Clouston's period as Physician-Superintendent (1873–1908).[24] Hurn provides a much more comprehensive history of the disease within the British context, though in fact using mostly English records, and offers an interesting account of the relationship of GPI to the development of the psychiatric profession.[25] However, such a broad study, in terms both of its geographical and chronological foci, allows that author little space for detailed work at the level of the individual patient record, or what we might call the 'daily realities' of clinical practice within the asylum.

This concentration on GPI is understandable, given the statistical importance of this disease to British asylum admissions, but neglects entirely those other neurosyphilitic disorders – cerebral syphilis, syphilitic insanity and tabes dorsalis – diagnosed and treated within British asylums. A disproportionate amount of historiographic attention has also been given to one particular treatment for GPI, malarial therapy. Widely regarded as the most successful, not to mention most bizarre, form of therapy for this disorder prior to the availability of penicillin, a number of articles on this subject might be described simply as non-analytical, triumphalist histories that describe the 'incalculable contribution' the therapy's inventor, Julius von Wagner-Jauregg, made 'towards the amelioration of human suffering'.[26] Indeed, Wagner-Jauregg has been the subject of an interesting biography which considers in some detail the Austrian alienist's development of malaria therapy, although in fact the author's prime concern seems to be to eulogise her subject, with very little consideration of the wider reception and application of Wagner-Jauregg's work.[27]

However another, more sophisticated, strand of historiography on this subject has considered the practicalities, ethics and successes of malarial therapy within the wider historical context of those physical therapies that alienists began to embrace enthusiastically in the first half of the twentieth century, including electroconvulsive therapy and psychosurgery.[28] Joel

Braslow, in particular, has used malarial therapy as a case study in order to examine the physician–patient encounter, and to consider how biological treatments might affect physicians' perceptions of patients, or enhance a physician's ability to empathise with a patient's suffering.[29] Significantly, his research does not take at face value the contemporary published assertions that this treatment furnished an effective cure.

Those historians who have discussed GPI more generally within their work have tended to adopt a relatively narrow range of historiographical approaches. These have included a decidedly heroic, Whiggish approach to diagnosis;[30] the triumph of laboratory methods in refining and objectifying psychiatric diagnosis;[31] GPI as an example of a stable and paradigmatic disorder within the development of psychiatric taxonomies;[32] GPI as proving the organic basis of insanity through the clinching of the syphilitic aetiology;[33] and GPI in relation to a range of social dysfunctions, illustrative in particular of concerns over 'degeneration'.[34] Such work has particularly tended towards the positivist tradition in depicting a sharp opposition between enlightened scientific progressivists who supported a syphilitic cause and traditionalists who opposed the syphilitic hypothesis.[35] The making of this link between GPI and syphilis has not been considered in any depth by historians, but merely mentioned in passing in most general accounts which appear to believe it unnecessary to analyse this 'correct' belief in the syphilitic theory, only feeling it necessary to trivialise previous 'erroneous' beliefs.

In addition, the existing historiography is based on a fairly narrow source base, and has neglected clinical records almost entirely.[36] The majority of this work has concentrated upon contemporary medical literature, particularly psychiatric textbooks and the publications of key physicians. Those more detailed studies of GPI have tended to combine this medical literature with administrative medical records, especially the annual reports of either specific asylums or the General Board of Commissioners in Lunacy.[37]

The historiography of venereal disease even more rarely explores the relationship between syphilis and insanity, or indeed the sequelae of syphilis more generally, tending to focus instead upon initial infection.[38] Nonetheless, this body of literature does provide insight into the complex interaction between medicine, morality, sexuality and venereal disease.[39] The issues of control and moral regulation with which these scholars relate sexuality to the medical profession can arguably be extended to the later stages of syphilis. The interpretative frameworks of gender, generation, class and race, employed by historians to interpret more fully the responses to syphilis, will also be considered as possible ways to interpret the tertiary form of the disease.

Synopsis

This book will begin with a contextual and broadly narrative chapter, to place the detailed Scottish case study that is offered subsequently within a useful wider context. Chapter 2 examines those forms of institutional provision that existed in Scotland for the insane during the nineteenth and early twentieth centuries. These years witnessed the development of the system of asylumdom in Scotland, particularly through the impact of the Lunacy (Scotland) Act of 1857 which, amongst other things, stimulated the development of a much more comprehensive system of care for the insane poor than had previously existed.[40] The four Scottish asylums forming the institutional focus of this study – the Glasgow Royal Asylum (Gartnavel), Royal Edinburgh Asylum (REA), Barony Parochial Asylum (Woodilee), and Midlothian and Peebles District Asylum (Rosslynlee) – are then described in some depth, particularly their patient populations and key medical personnel. Such information is particularly important for the parochial institutions of Rosslynlee and Woodilee given the dearth of previous historiographical discussion on this type of asylum.

The remaining chapters then shift the study to a more detailed empirical basis. Each explores one theme – clinical diagnosis, laboratory diagnosis, treatment, aetiology – through detailed analysis of a variety of primary sources, and comparatively across the four asylums. Chapter 3 examines the clinical diagnosis of GPI in the pre-laboratory era. The main symptoms are outlined, mental, physical and physiognomonic, within a wider discussion of the pronounced complexities of diagnosing GPI at this time. It is also considered to what extent GPI had a coherent and stable identity by the early twentieth century, just prior to laboratory methods being exploited in order to aid the diagnosis of this disorder.

Chapter 4 then assesses the impact laboratory techniques made upon diagnosis in the second and third decades of the twentieth century, utilising the application of the Wassermann test to the diagnosis of GPI within the four Scottish asylums as a case study.[41] A brief history is provided of the establishment and workings of the two asylum laboratories that were founded in Scotland, established in 1897 and 1909 in Edinburgh and Glasgow respectively. Much has been written on the interface between clinical medicine and laboratory science in the late nineteenth and early twentieth centuries, although outside the psychiatric context.[42] The Wassermann test provides an excellent means of studying the interaction between laboratory and clinical psychiatry, and the ways in which both professional groups – that is, pathologists and alienists – produced and negotiated medical knowledge with specific regard to the diagnosis and identity of GPI.

Chapter 5 explores the treatment of the neurosyphilis disease group prior to the application of penicillin in the 1940s. A comprehensive overview is provided of the therapies employed in the Scottish asylums from 1880 to 1930, which ranged from the traditional anti-syphilitic mercury treatment, through the arsenical therapies, to the rather less orthodox malarial therapy of the 1920s. The ways in which alienists implemented these therapies, and with what degree of success, are considered.

The epistemologies of causation in relation to GPI over the nineteenth and twentieth centuries are explored in Chapter 6. The recognition of syphilis as a cause of GPI was scant during the nineteenth century, during which time the disease was depicted as a broad and multi-causal concept which related largely to the destructive influences of the urban environment, and particularly to the excesses of alcohol, tobacco and sex. This chapter is therefore contextualised within the wider social concerns and sexual politics of the *fin-de-siècle* period. The decade after 1900 has been portrayed as crucial to the growing acceptance of the 'syphilitic hypothesis'. The extent to which Scottish alienists embraced the mounting scientific evidence of the importance of syphilis as a causal factor in GPI is therefore examined.

Chapter 7 draws the threads of the study together with regard to the socio–medical shaping of the neurosyphilis disease family during the years between 1880 and 1930. Conclusions are drawn on what are seen to be the most significant features of the study, in particular those relating to the diagnosis, treatment, epidemiology and aetiology of GPI, and to the professional position of alienists more generally. Finally, although clinicians have charted a dramatic decline in the incidence of GPI and other forms of neurosyphilis in the second half of the twentieth century, a decline that they attribute almost entirely to penicillin, some aspects of modern medical debate are provided which suggest that this diagnostic label should not be confined to history just yet.

Sources

This study will move between two types of archival material – the published medical writings and the clinical case notes – in an attempt to compare and contrast the published and unpublished, and in some respects public and private, views of Scottish alienists, and thereby to gain deeper insight into medical conceptions and constructions of this diagnostic group.[43] At the published level, the major medical and psychiatric journals have been trawled as they were an important forum for physicians to discuss their work. It must be remembered, however, that such journals subjected medical writings to editorial control, and were often aimed at a particular audience or intended to reflect the opinion of the body that they were created to serve, be it an institution or professional group. Psychiatric textbooks and pamphlets, which tended to be journal article off-prints, provide a further source of the published views of alienists. Scottish alienists and pathologists published widely during this period, particularly the Physician-Superintendents of the royal asylums, thereby providing useful insights into contemporary psychiatric thought.

Annual reports also fall within this category of sources. The General Board of Commissioners in Lunacy in Scotland furnished a comprehensive annual report on psychiatry in Scotland, based upon biannual asylum visitations, which related both to each individual asylum and to the national picture. These appear to have constituted the only regularly printed source of systematic national information on mental health services prior to the mid-twentieth century. The annual reports of the four asylums selected as the basis for this study provide much further useful contextual information on their total patient populations and upon the major concerns and professed achievements of each institution. However, this source has two major weaknesses: firstly, its format is inconsistent both over time and between institutions, thus making comparisons problematic; secondly, these reports were intended to both inform and encourage subscribers, and thus statistics might be subject to some manipulation to make circumstances appear more favourable than they actually were. As a result, their printed figures do not always tally with the clinical sources. Even the most detailed studies of GPI to date have tended to focus upon such published and administrative source materials, leaving much of the clinical domain still to be explored.

A detailed exploration of asylum case notes will form the second level of this study. The archives of both the royal and parochial asylums of central Scotland for the period covered by this study are substantial and available to scholars. A number of the parochial institutions have only recently closed, allowing the release of clinical records that have been catalogued by archivists but have yet to be exploited in any depth by historians. Despite some significant interpretative studies,[44] clinical records remain a rich but neglected source amongst historians of medicine. The confidential nature of patient records, the sheer volume of some collections,[45] and the technical complexity of some of the information they contain, have acted as disincentives to their use for historical research.

There is, furthermore, a wide spectrum of opinion within the historiography on how robust case notes are as an historical source. At one extreme, Nicol and Sheppard argue that hospital clinical records 'tell you what was really done to patients, and from this is to be derived the most trustworthy and complete assessment of what doctors believed and thought at any given time, and how their minds were working'.[46] At the other, Petrie and McIntyre deem medical records to be merely 'chaotic repositories of information'.[47] This study will demonstrate that, while both viewpoints have some merit, clinical records offer much potential to the historian for they provide fascinating insights into medical epistemology, bring together information from numerous sources on individual patients, and contain unique information unobtainable elsewhere. In particular, historical case notes can be a valuable source concerning everyday clinical practice, allowing insight into contemporary concepts of disease and therapeutic strategies, since it is arguably in these records that the theory, discourse and practice of medicine converge. We are thereby able to heed Erwin Ackerknecht's plea for a behaviourist approach to the history of medicine, that is, to analyse 'what doctors *did* in addition to what they *thought* and *wrote*'.[48]

A survey of those historians who have exploited case notes within their research reveals that the history of psychiatry is very much over-represented, and outlines the variety of uses to which case notes can be put. Some scholars have used case notes in order to provide a richer and more detailed account of life within an individual asylum than had been possible using purely administrative records.[49] Others, in attempting to explore the history of 'madness' as well as the history of 'psychiatry', have combined the qualitative material contained in case notes with patient letters, autobiographical writings and even patient artwork, in order to explore both the individual and collective experience of insanity.[50] A further group have used case notes to explore the doctor–patient relationship, and the wider interaction and negotiations in the triangular relationship between asylum, patient and family/friends.[51] Yet others have used case notes within their studies of gender and psychiatry, and to interrogate more fully Elaine Showalter's historiographical assertions with regard to madness being a 'female malady'.[52]

It is hoped that this study will draw further attention to the intellectual richness of case notes for those who remain to be converted. Nonetheless, these records come with a range of methodological and interpretative issues that must first be overcome before they can be used profitably. The case notes used here were almost exclusively bound volumes, rather than the individual case folders which most institutions had switched to by the mid-twentieth century.[53] This brief discussion of issues surrounding the construction and interpretation of these documents will therefore limit itself to the bound variety, notwithstanding more recent innovation in medical record design. There was, in fact, no formal legal requirement for Scottish asylums to keep case books during the period of this study, but only to keep a General Register of Admissions under the Lunacy (Scotland) Act of 1857. However, better records may have been equated with better patient care, thus ensuring that these institutions *did* keep such records. Moreover, as Andrews asserts, no Scottish equivalent was needed for the 1845 Lunacy Act, which made it compulsory for English asylums to keep case books, because by this time case notes were already in use in each of the Scottish Royal asylums.[54]

Methods of clinical data collection appear to have been, to some extent, idiosyncratic and inconsistent, having developed as much by tradition and in response to *ad hoc* demands as by any logical approach to the satisfaction of data needs. After about 1880, hospitals began to take advantage of printed forms, which were produced by commercial suppliers, in order to achieve regularity and uniformity in the recording and presentation of information. Before the introduction of this pro forma, information was noted down in straight prose. The actual information recorded remained largely the same after printed forms were introduced, but it could be said to have inadvertently become more user-friendly as an historical source, particularly in making this source amenable to database analysis and other computer manipulations. **Image 1.1, overleaf, gives** an example of a typical pro forma layout. The pro forma has had both supporters and opponents. Supporters claim that the criteria of thoroughness and reliability could not be satisfied by records which were open-ended or of a variable format; while opponents claim that an individualistic approach to medicine was inhibited, that such forms may provide misleading indicators that a particular test or examination has been carried out, or that they might induce stereotypic written responses to complicated and diverse medical observations.

Certainly, despite the introduction of the pro forma in the REA in 1874, in Woodilee in 1900, and in Gartnavel not until the 1920s, patient records are frequently incomplete due, presumably, to a combination of the inability or unwillingness of patients and their relatives to provide information, the failure of staff to record information, and the failure of clerks to copy information from other sources. Physicians may have depended more on memory for clinical facts, particularly if they were fairly familiar with that particular patient, with some perhaps viewing such records principally as an *aide mémoire*. There is also a clear class element to such record completion, in that records of pauper patients tend to be less detailed than those of fee-payers. Institutions may have been safeguarding themselves against legal action here since fee-paying patients were more likely to complain about their treatment than paupers. In short, as Harold Garfinkel has noted, there are often '"good" organisational reasons for "bad" clinic records'.[55]

Yet case notes have generally become fuller and bulkier as new types of document are generated, as more tests are carried out on patients, and as the fear of legal action makes doctors reluctant to discard documentation. Case notes thereby provide the most consistent and clearly recorded examples of functions and techniques being integrated into the hospital, including the work of the asylum laboratories which forms the basis of Chapter 4 of this book. However, in the period when the Scottish asylums lacked a designated

Image 1.1

Sample Pages from the Royal Edinburgh Asylum Case Notes, c.1881.

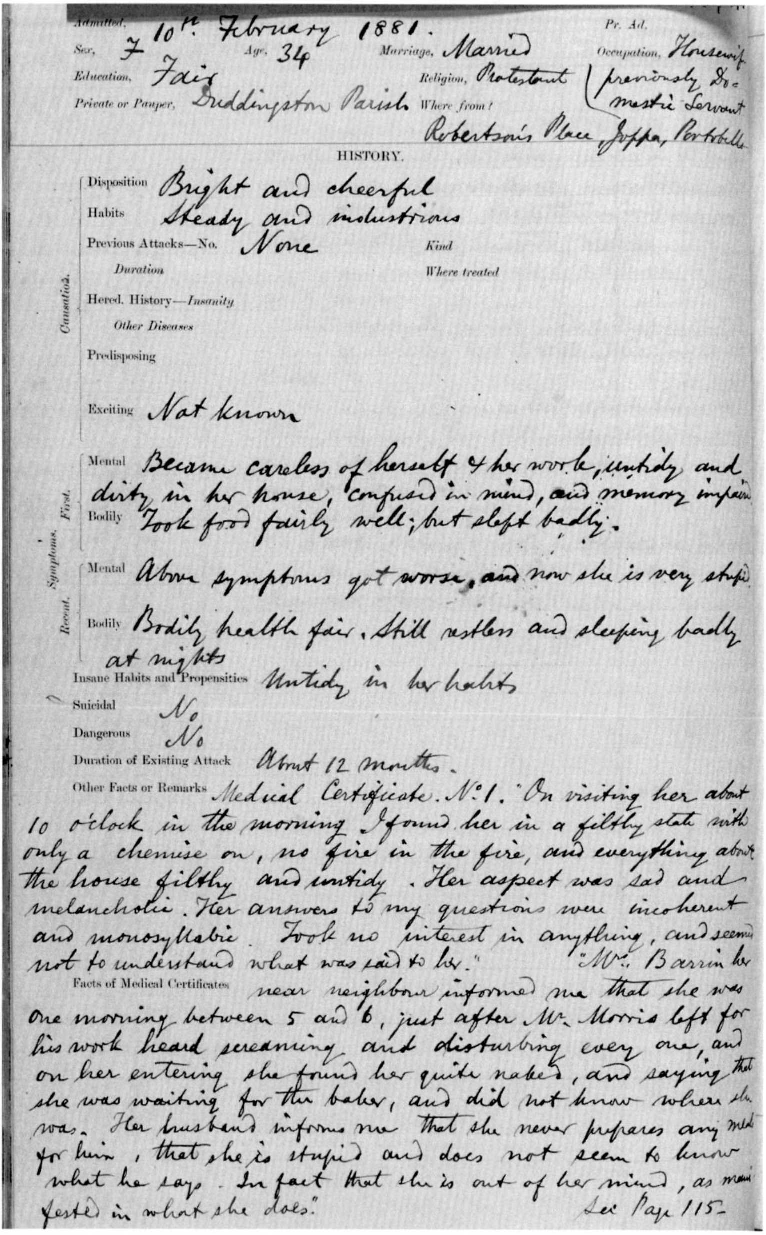

Admitted, 10th February 1881. Pr. Ad.
Sex, F Age, 34 Marriage, Married Occupation, Housewife (previously Domestic Servant)
Education, Fair Religion, Protestant
Private or Pauper, Duddingston Parish Where from? Robertson's Place, Joppa, Portobello

HISTORY.

Causation.
Disposition Bright and cheerful
Habits Steady and industrious
Previous Attacks—No. None Kind
Duration Where treated
Hered. History—Insanity
Other Diseases
Predisposing
Exciting Not known

Symptoms. First.
Mental Became careless of herself & her work, untidy and dirty in her house, confused in mind, and memory impaired
Bodily Took food fairly well; but slept badly.

Symptoms. Recent.
Mental Above symptoms got worse, and now she is very stupid
Bodily Bodily health fair. Still restless and sleeping badly at nights

Insane Habits and Propensities Untidy in her habits
Suicidal No
Dangerous No
Duration of Existing Attack About 12 months.
Other Facts or Remarks Medical Certificate. No. 1. "On visiting her about 10 o'clock in the morning I found her in a filthy state with only a chemise on, no fire in the fire, and everything about the house filthy and untidy. Her aspect was sad and melancholic. Her answers to my questions were incoherent and monosyllabic. Took no interest in anything, and seemed not to understand what was said to her." "Mrs. Barrin her
Facts of Medical Certificates near neighbour informed me that she was one morning between 5 and 6, just after Mr. Morris left for his work heard screaming and disturbing every one, and on her entering she found her quite naked, and saying that she was waiting for the baker, and did not know where she was. Her husband informs me that she never prepares any meals for him, that she is stupid and does not seem to know what he says. In fact that she is out of her mind, as manifested in what she does." See Page 115.

STATE ON ADMISSION.

Exaltation Have Some, of a quiet kind, exaggerated feeling of bien-être

Depression None

Excitement None at time of admission. Said to be restless and noisy at times

Enfeeblement Great — is quite stupid & silly

Memory Much Impaired — e.g., cannot tell how long she has been married

Coherence Incoherent *Can answer questions?* Only in a very stupid confused way —

Delusions No definite delusions expressed at time of admission

Other Abnormalities

Appearance A fairly nourished, but very stupid-looking woman

Skin Clean **Hair** Dark, mixed with a little grey

Eyes Light-brown **Pupils** Right larger than left

Muscularity Fair **Fatness** Average

Nervous System—Motor Articulation impaired. Pupils unequal. Tongue tremulous

Sensory Blunted

Reflex Action **Special Senses** Apparently healthy

Retina

Lungs Healthy

Heart Healthy

Tongue Moist, clean, very tremulous **Bowels** Regular

Other Organs, Abnormalities, Bruises, &c. Small sore on left Index finger

Appetite Fair

Urine

Menstruation

Pulse 84, regular, but rather weak. **Temp.** 98.6°

Height **Weight** 8:11

Disease General Paralysis **Skae's Classification**

General Bodily Health and Condition Weak. Articulation impaired. Small sore on left Index finger. Slight bruises on arms and legs

PREDOMINANT FEATURES.

A Acute Delirium and Incoherence.	B Simple Excitement.	C Simple Depression.	D Stupor.	E H; pochondria.	F Strong Suicidal Impulses.	G Remittency, or Intermittency.	H Choreic Movements.	I Hallucinations.	J Enfeeblement.

case folder for each patient, personal and professional correspondence would simply be inserted between the case-note pages, rather than the information being transposed onto the case note itself, thus introducing the potential risk of loss over time, a variable that we have no way of gauging. In addition, those patients who supplied an unusually rich history, or lived long enough to 'outgrow' the standard four-page pro forma allocated to them, would have further information scattered on available pages later in that, or subsequent, case-note volumes. Researchers must steer a meaningful course between these two extremes, identifying then questioning the comprehensiveness and quality of that case-note data available to them.

The case notes of an asylum patient were multi-authored and compiled from a number of different sources that were brought together in order to give quickly accessible information about the patient whilst they were resident in that institution. This information was elicited from the patient, his or her relatives, and/or family doctor, and then within the asylum the physicians, pathologist, and any special diagnostic departments involved. In this sense, case notes are themselves a form of information linkage, for they bring together a variety of admission data on each patient, which is transposed into the volume by a clerk, with progress reports then filled in directly by the asylum physicians.

Indeed, some historians have utilised case notes as a gateway to the 'patient perspective' with respect to both insanity and committal.[56] However, it is to be noted with caution that patient testimony is only really found in those letters written by the patient and retained in their case notes, an activity heavily policed by the asylum authorities.[57] Patients appear only rarely to have been consulted within the general admissions process, and such testimony – or fragmentary narratives – that are inserted into their case notes as supposedly direct quotes may have been taken out of context or edited to fit the pro forma. The physicians and clerks are no less the teller of these tales, for they act as a filter within the recording process. Thus, patient records contain built-in interpretation and evaluation. The same could be said for the testimony of the patient's family and friends. Whilst this group tended to provide much of the admitting information, and were indeed often the instigator for asylum committal,[58] their information is taken from its original context and fitted into a medical record-keeping framework which they would not necessarily understand. Furthermore, families might also be averse to providing such information, or exhibit a tendency to be 'creative' with the answers they gave for reasons of sensitivity and stigma, and particularly where issues surrounding 'hereditary propensity' might taint themselves. Thus, I would argue that case notes provide observations about the insane rather than any kind of straightforward access to the insane themselves, and that this source in fact provides as much, or perhaps more, information about those *recording* the information than it does the patients.

The first page of the case notes, including medical certificates detailing the reasons for admission, was filled in primarily on the basis of family testimony. This included an account of the patient's illness, the facts of his background, and the significant events of his life, in order to gain some understanding of formative experiences, attitudes and symptoms. The history was concerned with symptoms conceived to be subjective, which patients had noted for themselves or recalled through specific questioning. This was distinct from the physical examination noted on the second page, which addressed signs that were thought to be objective as noted by the examining physician. These first two pages (see Image 1.1) were probably compiled from other sources and transcribed by a clerk into the case notes, raising the possibility of transcription errors. The progress reports were then filled in by individual physicians directly on to the subsequent blank pages. These pages are intended to provide a chronological record of the patient's progress throughout the duration of their institutional care. However, the quality and regularity of entries could vary widely amongst patients, depending upon the length of stay and how interesting physicians deemed the case to be: some had weeks, or even months, between entries if their condition was perceived to be chronic and stable.[59]

The medical background to diagnostic and therapeutic decisions is not always supplied within these documents. It was not always documented exactly when a patient received laboratory tests or a specific treatment. Indeed, we cannot assume that every instance of testing or treatment was documented, not least if the progress notes were written in haste. Furthermore, it is generally impossible to tell at which point during their stay a patient was assigned to a specific diagnostic category. Indeed, while Physician-Superintendents appear only rarely to have assumed the time-consuming task of filling in the case notes themselves, during Thomas Clouston's period as Physician-Superintendent of the REA (1873–1908), he reserved the exclusive right to complete the 'diagnosis' section of the case notes, so that each diagnosis is in his handwriting and was almost certainly not filled in immediately upon the patient's admission. However, annual reports and contemporary medical publications can profitably supplement case-note material in such instances, and allow us to piece together more thoroughly medical epistemologies and behaviours.

In short, researchers have to be willing to invest a significant amount of time and energy into understanding and analysing case notes systematically in order to reap the rewards from them. They are certainly not an unproblematic source able to provide simple and privileged access to 'clinical reality'. However, it is believed that the findings of this study more than justify this labour-intensive project as a way to more profitably and systematically explore the relationship between clinical ideas and behaviour.

Methodology

In analysing the shaping of GPI as a diagnostic category, clinically, pathologically and socially, this study draws upon a 'framing' methodology.[60] This theoretical concept, which treats the boundaries between science, medicine and society as porous, has enabled scholars to acknowledge the biological dimension of illness but also to engage with the social and cultural perceptions that surround and shape representations of disease.[61] One of the most influential proponents of the 'framing' concept, Charles Rosenberg, has argued that disease is 'a good deal more complex' than 'simply a less than optimum physiological state', for 'explaining sickness is too significant – socially and emotionally – for it to be a value-free enterprise'.[62] Rosenberg instead stresses the historical and cultural contingency of disease, defining it as 'at once a biological event, a generation-specific repertoire of verbal constructs... [and] a sanction for cultural values'.[63] Such a theory, which holds epistemology to be central and allows both the clinical and cultural profile of the neurosyphilitic disorders to be explored, will provide the 'intellectual' methodology for this study.[64]

It could be argued that use of the term 'neurosyphilis' is somewhat anachronistic prior to the 1920s, the decade in which it entered medical parlance once the common syphilitic aetiology of this range of disorders had been thoroughly established. However, the term 'neurosyphilis' is used nominally throughout this study as a convenient way to refer collectively to all forms of insanity understood by 1930 to be caused by the syphilitic spirochaete – GPI, tabes dorsalis, syphilitic insanity and cerebral syphilis – rather than as a means of retrospective diagnosis. Indeed, this group of diseases had been acknowledged to have some sort of relationship, both to syphilis and to each other, decades before this umbrella term was coined.

Various practical techniques have also been employed in order to make this study manageable yet rigorous. First, the patient population had to be defined carefully. All patients admitted to the four Scottish asylums between January 1880 and December 1930 with some form of the neurosyphilitic disease group as their final diagnosis were located within the asylum records. The notion of 'final diagnosis' is important here because, in some cases, GPI was not diagnosed formally until post mortem. Indeed, the diagnostic process appears to have been composed of three parts – patients were diagnosed upon admission (a preliminary diagnosis recorded in the admission registers),[65] during their asylum stay (recorded in the case notes, and which might revise their admission diagnosis),[66] and upon death (in the post-mortem registers, but often recorded in the case notes also).[67] Thus diagnosis was not a static process, but ever-changing as the patient progressed through their asylum stay, a process taken account of in this study.

Since the case books were voluminous and the number of neurosyphilitics fairly high, it was felt necessary to resort to sampling for two of the asylums. The main objective was to be able to make statistically justifiable statements about each institution, and to obtain as far as possible consistent and unbiased estimates of the patient population. Systematic sampling, the selection of every *n*th case, is particularly useful when a large number of cases are recorded in an orderly manner in registers and lists, so this was employed where a diagnostic category was relatively large. Such a system allowed a fairly even distribution of patients over the entire period under study.

However, systematic sampling is potentially disadvantageous where a population contains a periodic type of variation or subgroup that is small enough to be missed entirely from the selection of every *n*th case. Whilst GPI cases constituted by far the majority of neurosyphilitics residing in British asylums in this period, this fact must not be allowed to obscure those more unusual diagnoses of the neurosyphilitic family of diseases. In order to ensure that those few cases of juvenile GPI, tabes dorsalis and cerebral syphilis were included in the study, a 100 per cent sample of each was taken. This method is known as disproportionate stratified sampling, because each group (or diagnostic label) is separated out (stratified), and those smaller groups are sampled in a way that is disproportionate to the larger groups.

In the case of the Royal Edinburgh Asylum, every fifth patient of the 1,416 GPI cases found was selected, and every second of the 87 syphilitic insanity cases, providing a 20 per cent and 50 per cent sample respectively. Since only 38 cases of post-mortem GPI were found, each of these was retained, providing a total patient population for this institution of 363, or 24 per cent of all neurosyphilitic cases. For Barony Parochial Asylum, every fourth case of GPI and post-mortem GPI was selected from the 701 and 120 patients discovered respectively, providing a 25 per cent sample. Only 7 cases of juvenile GPI were found, so that all of these were retained. This provided a total patient population for this institution of 212, or 26 per cent of all neurosyphilitic cases. The remaining two asylums, Glasgow Royal Asylum and Midlothian and Peebles District Asylum, were more straightforward. A sample was not felt to be necessary since the total number of neurosyphilitic patients resident over this fifty-year period, according to the admission registers and case notes, was only 160 and 176 patients respectively. Table 1.1, overleaf, provides a clear breakdown of these patient populations defined for each of the four Scottish asylums.

Table 1.1

Scottish Neurosyphilitic Patients Included in Study Sample

	Royal Edinburgh Asylum	Barony Parochial Asylum	Glasgow Royal Asylum	Midlothian and Peebles District Asylum
GPI	281 (20%)	175 (25%)	149 (100%)	45 (100%)
Post-mortem GPI	38 (100%)	30 (25%)	9 (100%)	131 (100%)
Juvenile GPI	0 -	7 (100%)	0 -	0 -
Syphilitic Insanity	44 (50%)	0 -	0 -	0 -
Tabes Dorsalis	0 -	0 -	1 (100%)	0 -
Cerebral Syphilis	0 -	0 -	1 (100%)	0 -
Total per asylum	363 (24%)	212 (26%)	160 (100%)	176 (100%)

n=911

Source: *Glasgow Royal Asylum Register of Lunatics*, 1871–1963, NHSGGCA13/ 6/78–80; *Glasgow Royal Asylum Case Books*, 1880–1930, NHSGGCA13/5/62–194; *Register of Discharges and Removals*, 1874–1942, LHSA LHB33/5/1–2; *Rosslynlee Case Books*, 1880–1930, LHSA LHB33/12/5–36; *Barony Parochial Asylum Registers of Admissions*, 1875–1957, NHSGGCA30/10/1–4; *Barony Parochial Asylum Case Books*, 1880–1930, NHSGGCA30/4/1–63 and NHSGGCA30/5/1–61.

It is possible that some patients will have been missed through this methodology, since the 'diagnosis' part of admission registers and case notes was not always filled in, and some patients did not die in the asylum, thereby preventing a post-mortem diagnosis from being recorded. These problems are particularly acute for Midlothian and Peebles District Asylum, whose case notes did not formally record a diagnosis ('form of disorder') until 1922. Until this time, if the general register either did not record a diagnosis, or recorded a disorder other than a form of neurosyphilis and the post-mortem diagnosis was not recorded, it was felt too subjective as well as time-consuming to read through all case notes and make a retrospective diagnosis. This explains why the post-mortem GPI patients far outnumber the GPI patients in this particular institution. Furthermore, there is the issue of patients admitted to the four Scottish asylums with 'syphilis' as their suspected cause of insanity. Since the insane could, like those in the outside world, suffer from syphilis without it progressing to the tertiary stage, such patients were not included in this study unless their diagnosis was one of the neurosyphilitic group of disorders. While the patient sample is unlikely to be entirely comprehensive, what is crucial is that all of the cases included were deemed by the asylum physicians of the period to be neurosyphilitic.

Once issues of sampling had been resolved, the computer was employed in order to help with the processing and analysis of the resulting information. In order to count, compare and contrast the considerable amount of data which the case notes contain on the 911 selected patients and to link such information to other medical records – principally the admission registers – an Access relational database was constructed for each of the four asylums.[68] Within this computation process, while the basic integrity of the documents was maintained as fully as possible, some entries had to be standardised in order to allow a more meaningful analysis. However, the original information was always retained within the database as well, so as not to prematurely collapse the data while coding systems were being constructed.

Appendix 1 outlines the table contents of the largest database, that of the Royal Edinburgh Asylum, and denotes derived variables – that is, where information was coded, standardised or altered in any way from its original form – with an asterix.[69] Each patient was ascribed a unique 'ID number' that allowed them to be linked between each table within the database, and a 'foreign key' that allowed them to be linked to each of their symptoms, treatments and other data of a variable nature. Those case notes which contain a pro forma were semi-structured and thus more amenable to database insertion, whereas the pre-pro forma patient records and the running prose of the progress notes were more problematic. Thus, although this study has employed specially constructed databases for each asylum, qualitative methods were also used when this was the more practical option, particularly with respect to the progress notes.

Finally, while each patient was ascribed a unique identifying number within the databases for ease of linkage between database tables and different asylum sources, this study will refer to individual patients by their name in order to make the study more 'human'. It should be stressed, however, that all patient names have been altered systematically and then abbreviated in order to protect the privacy of named individuals.

Notes

1. T. Clouston, 'How the Scientific Way of Looking at Things Helps Us in our Work', 1908, Lothian Health Services Archive (LHSA), LHB7/14/8, 9.
2. J. Hurn, 'The Changing Fortunes of the General Paralytic', *Wellcome History*, 4 (1997), 5–6: 5.
3. V. Berridge, *AIDS in the UK: The Making of Policy, 1981–1994* (Oxford: Oxford University Press, 1986) 287; G. Davis and R. Davidson, '"The Fifth Freedom" or "Hideous Atheistic Expediency": The Medical Community and Abortion Law Reform in Scotland, *c.*1960–75', *Medical History*, 50 (2006), 29–48.
4. J. Pickstone, 'Medicine in Industrial Britain: The Uses of Local Studies', *Social History of Medicine*, 2 (1989), 197–203.
5. A. Scull, *Museums of Madness: The Social Organization of Insanity in Nineteenth-Century England* (London: Allen Lane, 1979). Scull's early work was itself inspired, in part, by Foucault's wide-ranging speculations on madness and the pretensions of modern science. See M. Foucault, *Madness and Civilization: A History of Insanity in the Age of Reason* (London: Routledge, 1995).
6. See, for example, J. Melling and B. Forsythe (eds), *Insanity, Institutions and Society, 1800–1914: A Social History of Madness in Comparative Perspective* (London: Routledge, 1999); R. Porter and D. Wright (eds), *The Confinement of the Insane: International Perspectives, 1800–1965* (Cambridge: Cambridge University Press, 2003).
7. See, for example, A. Digby, *Madness, Morality and Medicine: A Study of the York Retreat, 1796–1914* (Cambridge: Cambridge University Press, 1985); C. MacKenzie, *Psychiatry for the Rich: A History of Ticehurst Private Asylum, 1792–1917* (London: Routledge, 1992); J. Andrews *et al.*, *The History of Bethlem* (London: Routledge, 1997).
8. See, for instance, R. Porter, *Mind-Forg'd Manacles: A History of Madness in England from the Restoration to the Regency* (London: Athlone Press, 1987); P. Bartlett and D. Wright, *Outside the Walls of the Asylum: The History of Care in the Community 1750–2000* (London: Athlone, 1999); A. Suzuki, *Madness at Home: The Psychiatrist, the Patient, and the Family in England, 1820–1860* (Berkeley: University of California Press, 2006).
9. A. Scull, *The Insanity of Place, The Place of Insanity: Essays on the History of Psychiatry* (London: Routledge, 2006), 5.
10. What has been written has focused, in the main, on the array of 'desperate' somatic remedies – including electric shock and lobotomies – embraced by alienists in the early twentieth century, as will be discussed below.
11. Scull has attributed this divide to the professional or disciplinary 'schism' between those clinician–historians and social historians working in the field.

12. See, for example, J. Andrews and I. Smith, 'The Evolution of Psychiatry in Glasgow During the Nineteenth and Early Twentieth Centuries', in H. Freeman and G. Berrios (eds), *150 Years of British Psychiatry, Volume II: The Aftermath* (London: Athlone, 1996), 309–38; J. Andrews, 'A Failure to Flourish?: David Yellowlees and the Glasgow School of Psychiatry', Parts 1 and 2, *History of Psychiatry*, 8 (1997), 177–212 & 333–60; J. Andrews, *'They're in the Trade… of Lunacy, They "Cannot Interfere"– They Say': The Scottish Lunacy Commissioners and Lunacy Reform in Nineteenth-Century Scotland* (London: Wellcome Institute for the History of Medicine, 1998); J. Andrews, 'Raising the Tone of Asylumdom: Maintaining and Expelling Pauper Lunatics at the Glasgow Royal Asylum in the Nineteenth Century', in Melling and Forsythe (eds), *op. cit.* (note 6).

13. See, especially, A. Beveridge, 'Thomas Clouston and the Edinburgh School of Psychiatry', in G. Berrios and H. Freeman (eds), *150 Years of British Psychiatry, 1841–1991* (London: Gaskell, 1991), 359–88; A. Beveridge, 'Madness in Victorian Edinburgh: A Study of Patients Admitted to the Royal Edinburgh Asylum under Thomas Clouston, 1873–1908', Parts 1 and 2, *History of Psychiatry*, 6 (1995), 21–54 and 133–56.

14. Two exceptions are H. Sturdy, 'Boarding Out the Insane, 1857–1913: A Study of the Scottish System', PhD thesis, University of Glasgow (1996); G. Doody, A. Beveridge and E. Johnstone, 'Poor and Mad: A Study of Patients Admitted to the Fife and Kinross District Asylum between 1874 and 1899', *Psychological Medicine*, 26 (1996), 887–97.

15. See, for example, T. Beach, 'The History of Alzheimer's Disease: Three Debates', *Journal of the History of Medicine and Allied Sciences*, 42 (1987), 327–49; G. Berrios, 'Memory and the Cognitive Paradigm of Dementia During the Nineteenth Century: A Conceptual History', in R. Murray and T. Turner (eds), *Lectures on the History of Psychiatry: The Squibb Series* (London: Gaskell, 1990), 194–211.

16. Known previously as 'dementia praecox'. See, for instance, M. Boyle, 'Is Schizophrenia What it Was? A Re-Analysis of Kraepelin's and Bleuler's Population', *Journal of the History of the Behavioral Sciences*, 26 (1990), 323–33; R. Ion and M. Beer, 'The British Reaction to Dementia Praecox, 1893–1913', Parts 1 and 2, *History of Psychiatry*, 13 (2002), 285–304 and 419–31.

17. See, for example, J. Oppenheim, *"Shattered Nerves": Doctors, Patients, and Depression in Victorian England* (Oxford: Oxford University Press, 1991); C. Callahan and G. Berrios, *Reinventing Depression: A History of the Treatment of Depression in Primary Care, 1940–2004* (Oxford: Oxford University Press, 2005); A. Horwitz and J. Wakefield, *The Loss of Sadness: How Psychiatry Transformed Normal Sorrow into Depressive Disorder* (Oxford: Oxford University Press, 2007).

18. Much has been written specifically on 'shell shock', in addition to the more general, and rapidly growing, literature exploring the physical and psychological costs of war. See, for instance, M. Stone, 'Shellshock and the Psychologists', in W. Bynum, R. Porter, and M. Shepherd (eds), *The Anatomy of Madness: Institutions and Society*, Vol. II (London: Routledge, 1985), 242–71; B. Shepherd, *A War of Nerves* (London: Jonathan Cape, 2000); P. Leese, *Shell Shock: Traumatic Neurosis and the British Soldiers of the First World War* (Basingstoke: Palgrave Macmillan, 2002).

19. G. Berrios and R. Porter (eds), *A History of Clinical Psychiatry: The Origin and History of Psychiatric Disorders* (London: Athlone, 1995). Over forty historians and clinician–historians have contributed to this work, which covers a whole range of disorders, divided between three sections: neuropsychiatric disorders, functional psychoses, and neuroses and personality disorders.

20. We are also left to contemplate why a small number of these clinical constructs, including multiple sclerosis, have no corresponding 'social' section.

21. M. Micale, *Approaching Hysteria: Disease and its Interpretations* (Princeton: Princeton University Press, 1995); H. Marland, *Dangerous Motherhood: Insanity and Childbirth in Victorian Britain* (Basingstoke: Palgrave Macmillan, 2004).

22. Micale, *op. cit.* (note 21), 132.

23. E. Hare, 'The Origin and Spread of Dementia Paralytica', *Journal of Mental Science*, 105 (1959), 594–626.

24. M. Thompson, 'The Mad, the Bad and the Sad: Psychiatric Care in the Royal Edinburgh Asylum (Morningside), 1813–1894', PhD thesis, Boston University Graduate School (1984); M. Thompson, 'The Wages of Sin: The Problem of Alcoholism and General Paralysis in Nineteenth-Century Edinburgh', in W. Bynum, R. Porter and M. Shepherd, *The Anatomy of Madness: The Asylum and Psychiatry*, Vol. III (London: Routledge, 1988), 316–340.

25. J. Hurn, 'The History of General Paralysis of the Insane in Britain, 1830 to 1950', PhD thesis, University of London (1998).

26. H. Rollin, 'The Horton Malaria Laboratory, Epsom, Surrey (1925–1975)', *Journal of Medical Biography*, 2 (1994), 94–7: 94.

27. M. Whitrow, *Julius Wagner-Jauregg, 1857–1940* (London: Smith-Gordon, 1993).

28. See, especially, E. Valenstein, *Great and Desperate Cures: The Rise and Decline of Psychosurgery and Other Radical Treatments for Mental Illness* (New York: Basic Books, 1986); J. Braslow, *Mental Ills and Bodily Cures: Psychiatric Treatment in the First Half of the Twentieth Century* (Berkeley: University of California Press, 1997). See, also, A. Scull, 'Somatic Treatments and the

Historiography of Psychiatry', *History of Psychiatry*, 5 (1994), 1–12, and an equally provocative retort from H. Merskey, 'Somatic Treatments, Ignorance, and the Historiography of Psychiatry', *History of Psychiatry*, 5 (1994), 387–91.

29. J. Braslow, 'Effect of Therapeutic Innovation on Perception of Disease and the Doctor–Patient Relationship: A History of General Paralysis of the Insane and Malarial Fever Therapy, 1910–1950', *American Journal of Psychiatry*, 152 (1995), 660–5, analyses the language of medical records from a Southern California Asylum and contrasts pre-malaria descriptions of neurosyphilitic patients as 'hopeless' and 'immoral' with more positive and empathetic post-malaria verdicts on these patients.

30. See, for example, W. Nicol, 'General Paralysis of the Insane', *British Journal of Venereology*, 32 (1956), 9–16; T. Rosebury, *Microbes and Morals: The Strange Story of Venereal Disease* (London: Secker and Warburg, 1972).

31. See, for instance, J. Oriel, *The Scars of Venus: A History of Venereology* (London: Springer-Verlag, 1994).

32. See for example, Thompson, 'The Mad, the Bad and the Sad', *op. cit.* (note 24); E. Engstrom, *Clinical Psychiatry in Imperial Germany: A History of Psychiatric Practice* (Ithaca: Cornell University Press, 2003), 107-10. For a refutation of this claim, see G. Berrios, '"Depressive Pseudodementia" or "Melancholic Dementia": A Nineteenth Century View', *Journal of Neurology, Neurosurgery, and Psychiatry*, 48 (1985), 393–400. Berrios disputes the monolithic nature of the GPI diagnosis, citing as evidence wide nineteenth-century disagreements concerning the clinical domain, course and histopathology of GPI.

33. See, for instance, G. Zilboorg and W. Henry, *A History of Medical Psychology* (New York: Norton, 1941), Ch.13; E. Ackerknecht, *Medicine at the Paris Hospital, 1794–1848* (Baltimore: The Johns Hopkins Press, 1967), 170–1.

34. See, for example, E. Showalter, *The Female Malady: Women, Madness and English Culture, 1830–1980* (London: Virago, 1996), 111–12.

35. See, for instance, Zilboorg and Henry, *A History of Medical Psychology*, 538–46; C. Quétel, *History of Syphilis* (Cambridge: Polity Press, 1990), 162–4; D. Leigh in C. Thompson (ed.), *The Origins of Modern Psychiatry* (Chicester: John Wiley and Sons, 1987), 218–21. Leigh states: 'An etiological and therapeutic ignorance, as has been so often the case in medicine, led to some astonishing statements from even the most respected physician.' (219)

36. The sole exception to this appears to be Braslow, *op. cit.* (note 29).

37. See, for example, Thompson, 'The Wages of Sin', *op. cit.* (note 24); Hare, *op. cit.* (note 23).

38. It is not entirely clear why there has been this historiographic pre-occupation with infection and the primary stage of syphilis. It might be connected to

the fact that the statutory legislation relating to venereal disease has concentrated on infection, leading historians to do the same. It may also reflect the more immediate public concern over contracting such a disease, and thus the wish to understand and master it more thoroughly than the later stages of syphilis, which a patient might take twenty years to reach or never reach at all.

39. See, for example, A. Brandt, 'Sexually Transmitted Diseases', in W. Bynum and R. Porter (eds), *Companion Encyclopedia of the History of Medicine*, Vol. I (London: Routledge, 1993), 562–84; R. Davidson, *Dangerous Liaisons: A Social History of Venereal Disease in Twentieth-Century Scotland* (Amsterdam: Rodopi, 2001); R. Davidson and L. Hall (eds), *Sex, Sin and Suffering: Venereal Disease and European Society since 1870* (London: Routledge, 2001).

40. The history of psychiatry should not, of course, be equated with the history of confinement. Excellent studies in recent years have begun to shift our focus to the levels of care and control exercised over the insane outside these institutions, and to the permeability of the asylum walls. See, for example, Bartlett and Wright, *op. cit.* (note 8).

41. Other diagnostic tests were also available for GPI before 1930, including Lange's colloidal gold, which was introduced in 1912 but not employed within the Scottish asylums until the early 1920s, and even then only sparingly.

42. See L. Jacyna, 'The Laboratory and the Clinic: The Impact of Pathology on Surgical Diagnosis in the Glasgow Western Infirmary, 1875–1910', *Bulletin of the History of Medicine,* 62 (1988), 384–406 for an influential early study of this interaction. For further interesting interpretations of the contentious place of the laboratory within British clinical medicine, see, for example, A. Cunningham and P. Williams (eds), *The Laboratory Revolution in Medicine* (Cambridge: Cambridge University Press, 1992); S. Sturdy and R. Cooter, 'Science, Scientific Management, and the Transformation of Medicine in Britain, *c.*1870–1950', *History of Science*, 36 (1998), 421–66; C. Lawrence, 'A Tale of Two Sciences: Bedside and Bench in Twentieth-Century Britain', *Medical History*, 43 (1999), 421–49; R. Wall, 'Using Bacteriology in the Hospital and Society: England, 1880–1939', PhD thesis, Imperial College London (2007); A. Hull, 'Teamwork, Clinical Research, and the Development of Scientific Medicines in Interwar Britain: The "Glasgow School" Revisited', *Bulletin of the History of Medicine*, 81 (2007), 569–93.

43. It might be noted that these categories are not entirely dichotomous since annual reports and published articles were compiled, to some extent, from case notes and other clinical data.

44. See, especially, G. Risse and J. Warner, 'Reconstructing Clinical Activities: Patient Records in Medical History', *Social History of Medicine*, 5 (1992), 183–205; and J. Andrews, 'Case Notes, Case Histories, and the Patient's

Experience of Insanity at Gartnavel Royal Asylum, Glasgow, in the Nineteenth Century', *Social History of Medicine*, 11 (1998), 255–81, which also analyses the interesting relationship between case notes and case histories.

45. Indeed, a deadly combination of bulk, inadequate resources and lack of contemporary medical insight into the potential utility and importance of these documents for historical, medical and epidemiological research has led to the 'wholesale destruction' of these records in certain quarters, particularly south of the Border. See E. Higgs and J. Melling, 'Chasing the Ambulance: The Emerging Crisis in the Preservation of Modern Health Records', *Social History of Medicine*, 10 (1997), 127–36.

46. A. Nicol and J. Sheppard, 'Why Keep Hospital Clinical Records?', *British Medical Journal*, 290 (1985), 263–4: 264.

47. J. Petrie and N. McIntyre (eds), *The Problem Oriented Medical Record: Its Use in Hospitals, General Practice and Medical Education* (Edinburgh: Churchill Livingstone, 1979), 2.

48. E. Ackerknecht, 'A Plea for a "Behaviorist" Approach in Writing the History of Medicine', *Journal of the History of Medicine and Allied Sciences*, 22 (1967), 211–14: 214. Ackerknecht's plea seemed to grow from his irritation with scholars like Michel Foucault who 'thought that language – terminology – constituted reality', whereas medicine must 'be considered in terms of acts, not simply extrapolated from the language that rationalised and categorised those acts'. See C. Rosenberg, 'Erwin H. Ackerknecht, Social Medicine, and the History of Medicine', *Bulletin of the History of Medicine*, 81 (2007), 511–32: 528.

49. See, for example, Digby, *op. cit.* (note 7); C. MacKenzie, 'Social Factors in the Admission, Discharge, and Continuing Stay of Patients at Ticehurst Asylum, 1845–1917', in Bynum, Porter and Shepherd, *op. cit.* (note 18); Beveridge, 'Madness in Victorian Edinburgh', *op. cit.* (note 13).

50. See, for instance, R. Porter, *A Social History of Madness: Stories of the Insane* (London: Weidenfeld and Nicolson, 1987); M. Barfoot and A. Beveridge, 'Madness at the Crossroads: John Home's Letters from the Royal Edinburgh Asylum, 1886–87', *Psychological Medicine*, 20 (1990), 263–84; M. Barfoot and A. Beveridge, "Our Most Notable Inmate': John Willis Mason at the Royal Edinburgh Asylum, 1864–1901', *History of Psychiatry*, 4 (1993), 159–208; A. Beveridge and M. Williams, 'Inside "The Lunatic Manufacturing Company": The Persecuted World of John Gilmour', *History of Psychiatry*, 13 (2002), 19–49.

51. See, for example, A. Suzuki, 'Framing Psychiatric Subjectivity: Doctor, Patient and Record-Keeping at Bethlem in the Nineteenth Century', in Melling and Forsythe (eds), *op. cit.* (note 6), 115–36; C. Coleborne, 'Families, Patients and Emotions: Asylums for the Insane in Colonial

39

Australia and New Zealand, *c.*1880–1910', *Social History of Medicine*, 19 (2006), 425–42.

52. See, for example, K. Davies, "'Sexing the Mind?": Women, Gender and Madness in Nineteenth Century Welsh Asylums', *Llafur*, 7:1 (1996), 29–40; P. McCandless, 'A Female Malady?: Women at the South Carolina Lunatic Asylum, 1828–1915', *Journal of the History of Medicine and Allied Sciences*, 54 (1999), 543–71; Marland, *op. cit.* (note 21).

53. Gartnavel switched to case folders shortly before 1930, so these have been included in order to form a complete run of patient admissions. While a complete run of bound case-note volumes were located for the REA and a patient sample worked out accordingly, a series of case folders were subsequently discovered at the Royal Edinburgh Hospital during the course of this research. The exact purpose of these folders remains a mystery, as they tend to replicate patient information already noted within the bound volumes, with extra information or paperwork added only on occasion. Since they provide little additional data and, more importantly, are not available for the patient population as a whole, it was decided to concentrate exclusively upon the bound volumes for the purposes of this study.

54. Andrews, *op. cit.* (note 44), 258.

55. H. Garfinkel, *Studies in Ethnomethodology* (New Jersey: Prentice-Hall, 1967), 186.

56. See, for example, Andrews, *op. cit.* (note 44), 255; F. Condrau, 'The Patient's View Meets the Clinical Gaze', *Social History of Medicine*, 20 (2007), 525–40: 525.

57. Medical staff were permitted to open all patient correspondence in order to prevent any letters being sent which were deemed 'unsuitable'; for example, if it was felt that the letter might offend the addressee. In addition, we are unable to gauge what proportion or type of patient letters were retained in the case notes, but these outpourings are unlikely to constitute a balanced range of patient testimony. See A. Beveridge, 'Life in the Asylum: Patients' Letters from Morningside, 1873–1908', *History of Psychiatry*, 9 (1998), 431–69.

58. David Wright has been particularly influential in attempting to shift the patient's family to the forefront in terms of asylum confinement. See, especially, D. Wright, 'Getting Out of the Asylum: Understanding the Confinement of the Insane in the Nineteenth Century', *Social History of Medicine*, 10 (1997), 137–55.

59. The rules on the front cover of the REA case-note volumes state: 'In all recent acute and interesting cases, very frequent if not daily entries are to be made at first.' All other cases were to be reviewed on the first day of January, April, July and October, although most cases were in fact reviewed more frequently.

60. Jacalyn Duffin provides a highly readable introduction to this subject for the non-specialist reader, in which she explores how disease concepts are constructed and infused with cultural meanings. See J. Duffin, *Lovers and Livers: Disease Concepts in History* (Toronto: Toronto University Press, 2005).

61. While comprising part of a wider 'social constructivist' school of thought, the concept of 'framing' is generally held to be less programmatically charged and – crucially for the purposes of this study – more flexible in allowing one to acknowledge and engage with the biological dimensions of disease without any implication that disease concepts are purely 'socially' constructed.

62. C. Rosenberg, 'Framing Disease: Illness, Society, and History', in C. Rosenberg and J. Golden (eds), *Framing Disease: Studies in Cultural History* (New Brunswick: Rutgers University Press, 1992), xiii, xiv.

63. *Ibid.*, xiii. Rosenberg's work in this sphere goes back much further than the widely influential *Framing Disease*. His 1962 book, *The Cholera Years: The United States in 1832, 1849, and 1866* (Chicago: Chicago University Press, 1962), employed the nineteenth-century cholera epidemics as a lens through which to view American society. Rosenberg has recently paid homage to those who influenced him most in this area, and to whom he dedicated *Framing Disease*: Erwin Ackerknecht – who stressed that disease was defined not simply by a biological event, but by the society in which it occurred – and Owsei Temkin – who argued that disease should be understood as a time- and place-specific aggregate of behaviours, practices, ideas and experiences. See Rosenberg, *op. cit.* (note 48); C. Rosenberg, 'What is Disease? In Memory of Owsei Temkin', *Bulletin of the History of Medicine*, 77 (2003), 491–505.

64. George Rousseau, *et al.* have taken the 'framing' of disease in a consciously different direction from *Framing Disease*, by focusing not upon historical periods and social factors but upon private voices – poets, novelists, philosophers and diarists – and their literary embodiments, and by exploring 'the range of narrative modes sought by those eager to express their thought about states of health or illness'. See G. Rousseau, *et al.* (eds), *Framing and Imagining Disease in Cultural History* (Basingstoke: Palgrave Macmillan, 2003), 12.

65. The admission registers record the name, age, gender and marital status of each patient, as well as an initial cause and form of insanity.

66. Although this diagnosis was noted on the 'admission' part of the case notes, we cannot be sure at which point the case-note diagnosis was made during the patient's stay in the asylum. It is unlikely that it was filled in immediately upon the patient's admission, since it can differ from the admission register diagnosis.

67. A post-mortem diagnosis was not recorded for all patients who died in the asylum, but is a useful indicator of the difficulties of diagnosing the neurosyphilis diseases since, in some cases, the case-note and post-mortem diagnoses differ. However, it should be noted that, in some cases, physicians may have long thought such patients to be neurosyphilitic but not wished to record this until pathological proof could be obtained at post mortem.

68. An Access relational, rather than flatfile, database was favoured because it holds information more efficiently where the amount of data varies from patient to patient. This is particularly true of the number of treatments a patient received, or the range of symptoms noted for each patient.

69. The other three databases are similar in structure, only varying slightly to reflect minor differences in each institution's case-note format.

2

Scottish Institutional Provision for the Insane

We shall now explore Scottish segregative responses to the insane during the nineteenth and early twentieth centuries. Four asylums – the Royal Edinburgh Asylum (REA), Glasgow Royal Asylum (Gartnavel), Midlothian and Peebles District Asylum (Rosslynlee), and Barony Parochial Asylum (Woodilee) – will be explored in detail, including information on the population they served and a biographical account of their key personnel, the Physician-Superintendents who were generally responsible for diagnosing inmates. Such information is particularly important for the latter two institutions, Rosslynlee and Woodilee, as the historiography of Scottish psychiatry has hitherto focused heavily upon the chartered asylums and neglected the parochial asylums almost entirely.

Prior to the mid-nineteenth century, the insane could be placed into a number of non-specialised institutions within Scotland.[1] The Royal Infirmary of Edinburgh opened in 1741 with purpose-built lunatic wards. At this time, prisons housed both the dangerous and criminally insane. In addition, the fee-paying and, in some cases, parish-supported patients could seek help in one of the private institutions in existence and it is probably safe to assume that there were some further private houses offering a rudimentary service in at least Edinburgh and Glasgow by the end of the eighteenth century. A further potential receptacle for the insane at this time was the lunatic wards of some poorhouses. By 1857, there were seventeen such poorhouses – the equivalent of the English workhouses – which accommodated over eight hundred patients. The poorhouse in Glasgow, the Towns Hospital in Clyde Street, opened in 1732; while in Edinburgh, the poorhouse was located in Teviot Row and opened in 1743. It was, in fact, principally because of the conditions pertaining in these poorhouses that the chartered or 'royal' asylums came into existence, completing the so-called 'mixed economy' of care for the insane in the nineteenth century.[2] The chartered asylums differed from the other services then available because they were purpose-built institutions for the insane, and accepted, in principle at least, both private (fee-paying) and public (parish-supported) patients.

The chartered asylums

Although there was no statutory requirement in Scotland to provide institutional care for the insane, eight royal asylums with philanthropic origins were founded between 1781 and 1839 (see Table 2.1). In England, public-subscription asylums subsequently gave way to the county asylum provided for under legislation of 1808 and 1845, while the charitable institution remained predominant in Scotland. The involvement of the Scottish urban middle class was crucial to their development in a way that was less apparent in the case of the English asylums. Only the Crichton Royal and James Murray asylums were endowed by individual philanthropists. The royal asylums in Aberdeen, Dundee, Edinburgh, Glasgow and Montrose were all reliant upon the support of the public in both a financial and organisational capacity. Their annual reports had a wide readership and were vital in encouraging subscriptions and public interest in these institutions.[3]

As charitable foundations, the royal asylums had, as an early ideal, the provision of aid to the needy and less well off. However, in practice, all seven institutions diversified into providing this service to the middle-class insane for a fee, making them in part resemble the private, commercialised system dominant in England, although the 'free trade' in lunacy was never practised on such a scale as in England and Wales.[4] With less enthusiasm, they also contracted with the local parochial authorities to receive many of their pauper insane, in a period before district and parochial asylums were widespread. These chartered asylums thus offered a dual, class-demarcated service: on the one hand, there was the 'private' fee-paying service, which was itself rigorously divided into expensive provision for the upper classes and a much less costly option for the 'middling sort'; and on the other, the pauper service where the board and maintenance of rate-aided patients were paid by the local authority. The quality and type of service inevitably differed with the fee. Thus, very comfortable havens were created for the middle class in co-existence with the practice of 'psychiatry for the poor'. Hence the class division noted in so much of the organisation of insanity in Victorian Britain was readily seen in the main Scottish cities.

Geographically the chartered asylums were well situated to serve the needs of town dwellers. Lanarkshire, a thriving industrial region for manufacturing, mining and agricultural activity, contained nearly a quarter of the population of Scotland. It was well provided with institutional accommodation, particularly Glasgow, which had seven institutions wholly or in part for the insane at this time – a royal asylum, three poorhouses and three private madhouses – as well as boarding-out provisions. However, by the mid-nineteenth century, the greatest concentration of institutions was in

Table 2.1

The Chartered Asylums of Scotland

These asylums, constituted by Royal Charter and Act of Parliament, were established in the following chronological order:

Year	Original Title
1781	Montrose Lunatic Asylum
1800	Aberdeen Lunatic Asylum
1813	Edinburgh Lunatic Asylum
1814	Glasgow Asylum for Lunatics
1820	Dundee Asylum for Lunatics
1827	James Murray's Asylum for Lunatics (Perth)
1839	Crichton Institution for Lunatics

the Edinburgh area, where there was one royal asylum, three poorhouses, fifteen private madhouses and a school for idiots.

The Parochial Asylums

The passing of two pieces of legislation added a further dimension to Scottish provision for the insane: the Poor Law Amendment (Scotland) Act of 1845 and the Lunacy (Scotland) Act of 1857. While previously, local government had been structured primarily on geographical grounds, with burghs and parishes operating according to the number and needs of population, the 1845 Poor Law legislation established directly elected bodies – parochial boards – to deal with the problem of pauperism, under the control of an external and central authority, the Board of Supervision. Hence, although the old burghal structures remained, a new one emerged. The line of demarcation was to be pauperism, with those falling below that line coming under the purview of the parochial boards and those above having their civic needs catered for by the burghal institutions.

As far as Edinburgh and Glasgow were concerned, the new post-1845 parochial boards operated more or less within the same geographical areas as the pre-1845 parishes. Thus, in Edinburgh, the result was the establishment of the Canongate, St Cuthberts and City parishes, while in Glasgow the four traditional parishes of City, Barony, Gorbals and Govan became the sites of four separate parochial boards. With respect to health care, the importance of these developments was that the new parochial boards were legally required to build poorhouses within their area of jurisdiction, both to

45

provide shelter for paupers, including insane paupers, and to offer a modicum of medical care.

The Scottish Lunacy Commission enquiry of 1855–7, which highlighted the deplorable situation in which many pauper lunatics were kept, encouraged legislative action. The primary outcome was the Lunacy (Scotland) Act, 1857. Broadly speaking, this legislation had three major effects: it tightened up the certification of insane patients, created a General Board of Commissioners in Lunacy for Scotland, and divided the country into 'lunacy' districts which were to assume responsibility for their own insane through the provision of parochial or district asylums.

In terms of certification, whereas previously only one certificate from a medical man had been required for committal, two medical certificates were now required following the 1857 Act. Two physicians had to examine the patient separately and received a fee for their service. Also required was a petition, which in the case of pauper patients was completed by the Inspector of the Poor, and for private patients was completed by a relative. Both medical certificates and petition were sent to the Sheriff who decided if the petition should be granted. There were legal differences here between Scotland and England in several respects. Firstly, the decision whether to grant the order was a legal one and was made by the Sheriff. Secondly, in Scotland the procedure for certification was essentially the same for private and pauper patients, whereas in England the two classes were treated differently. Thirdly, the English system placed no limit on the length of detention, whereas in Scotland the order expired after three years. Finally, the Superintendent had the power to discharge immediately any patient considered to be sane without having to go through any cumbersome administrative channels.[5]

The 1857 Act also created a General Board of Commissioners in Lunacy (Lunacy Board) for Scotland.[6] Previously, the Shrievalty had held the major responsibility for provision for the insane in Scotland. Membership of the new Board of Commissioners was small, consisting initially of an unpaid Chairman – generally an experienced politician with no real experience of lunacy administration – two paid Medical Commissioners and not more than three other unpaid Legal Commissioners. Its composition was therefore an occasionally uncomfortable partnership of medical men, lawyers and administrators. Its powers included the management and regulation of all matters arising in relation to lunatics, wherever they resided, and the regulation of a system of visitation and inspection to all asylums, houses and other buildings containing lunatics, to be made twice yearly by the paid commissioners.[7] In 1858, there were ten officials supervising a total of approximately 10,000 patients.[8] Scotland's peripatetic Commissioners in Lunacy therefore covered the length and breadth of the land, investigating every royal, district and private asylum, and every 'cottage' dwelling in which an insane person was housed. The Lunacy Board retained the same structure for fifty-six years, until it was replaced in 1913 by the Board of Control.[9]

Finally, the 1857 Act provided for the division of the country into lunacy districts in which district asylums were, if need be, to be built for the reception of pauper patients. Scotland was divided into twenty-seven such districts, which comprised groups of counties, single counties or single parishes, and their officials were to assume responsibility for the care of all insane persons residing within their district. The only public asylum in existence before 1857, in Elgin, received recognition as a district asylum, and similar institutions were subsequently opened in Lochgilphead, Argyll, Perth, Inverness, Banff, Fife, Haddington, Ayr and Stirling. These district asylums became the Scottish equivalent of the English county asylums. The 1857 Act was intended to replace the previously random and haphazard methods of provision for the insane with a national, rationalised structure, and the legislation certainly led to marked growth in asylum provision on a scale similar to that implemented over a decade earlier in England and Wales. While poorhouses were granted licenses from the Lunacy Board for the reception of harmless patients not amenable to curative treatment, the Board viewed them with disfavour and regarded them as of merely temporary utility until district asylums were erected and able to accommodate all insane pauper patients. Royal asylums were thereby intended to reduce their pauper patients in order to develop their private élite service.

Despite this compulsory requirement of the Act, many Scottish local authorities remained unwilling to foot the bill well into the late nineteenth century and continued to shunt their pauper insane from one institution to another in search of the cheapest rates. In the west of Scotland, most local authorities did not begin to establish their own asylums until after 1870, six parochial and district asylums being established in the area during the period from 1873 to 1897. Indeed, district asylums were not established in Aberdeen, Dundee, Edinburgh, Paisley or Renfrew until the early twentieth century. Sixteen poorhouses with lunatic wards were still functioning in 1901, and the number of insane cared for domestically remained high, being 17.57 per cent of the total as late as 1901.[10] Nonetheless, by 1913, less than a fifteenth of patients registered with the Lunacy Board were in poorhouses or private asylums, whereas at mid-century the proportion had been nearly half.[11] By then, there were seven royal asylums, twenty-two district asylums, three private madhouses, and fourteen poorhouses licensed to receive lunatics in Scotland.

In addition, it should be recognised that not all provision for the insane was institution-based.[12] A pioneering policy of boarding out harmless, chronic insane patients in the community was formally introduced in the year following the passage of the 1857 Act. Up to twenty-five per cent of registered pauper and private patients – particularly congenitally weak-minded idiots and imbeciles – were soon boarded out, normally to live with relatives. As the system developed, an increasing number of patients who suffered from acquired forms of insanity, having reached a quiescent stage, were discharged 'unrecovered' from asylums to such private dwellings, mainly under the care of strangers. This practice was to become well established in Scotland, and was one of the unique features of Scottish lunacy provisions, particularly the degree of formal, centralised control exercised by the Commissioners over this system. Nonetheless, it never became a feasible alternative to institutional confinement for the majority of Scotland's insane and the asylum populations continued to grow. It should also be noted that no cases of the neurosyphilis disease group appear to have been boarded out during the period from 1880 to 1930, at least from my sample of patients, almost certainly due to the fact that these patients tended to be quite advanced in their incapacity, mentally and/or physically.

The majority of all patients were certified and compulsorily detained under the Scottish Lunacy Act, and their admission to the asylums involved an often protracted bureaucratic admission process which could prove distressing to patients and their relatives. Only twenty-six neurosyphilitic patients of the 911 in my sample were voluntary admissions.[13] Such admissions were not formally sanctioned by lunacy legislation until 1862, but within a few decades the principle was being strongly encouraged by the Lunacy Board. The Commissioners, asylum Directors and Medical Officers interpreted the growth of voluntary admissions optimistically as a sign of the growing confidence of the community in the asylum and in the benefits of early treatment. Indeed, in 1923, David Henderson, Physician-Superintendent of Gartnavel, announced proudly that the number of voluntary patients admitted to his institution in that year was approximately half of total admissions.[14] In England, on the other hand, voluntary admission to a public mental hospital was not fully sanctioned by law until 1930.[15]

Royal Edinburgh Asylum

The chartered asylum in Edinburgh was opened in 1813, its foundation reputedly triggered by the death in Bedlam of the young poet, Robert Ferguson.[16] Erected out of voluntary public contributions, the asylum was originally intended to provide for all classes of society, but for the first three decades of its existence, due to lack of funds, it accepted only paying patients at one guinea per week. This was said to be to the great annoyance of many local citizens and indeed to the concern of the asylum Managers. Eventually,

Image 2.1

Royal Edinburgh Asylum, West House, undated.
Courtesy of Lothian Health Services Archive.

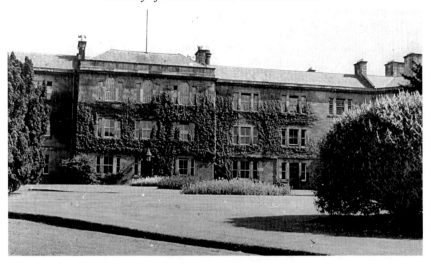

in 1842, the institution opened its 'West House' to accommodate up to five hundred pauper insane (see Image 2.1). This structure was intended to complement its 'East House' where only the private fee-payers resided and which could house up to sixty such patients.

The last quarter of the nineteenth century witnessed increasing battles between the parish boards, who insisted on their right to send all their pauper lunatics to the REA, and the Managers of the asylum, who tried to limit the numbers in order to enable them to admit more middle-class patients of limited means. Throughout his tenure as Physician-Superintendent from 1873 until 1908, Thomas Clouston juggled a variety of conflicting social and economic pressures. He feared that the REA would become a dumping ground for the ever-increasing number of ageing paupers, many of whom were considered incurable, debilitated and malnourished and consequently in need of costly nursing care and better diet.[17] Clouston thus pressed for more pauper insane facilities elsewhere, such as the boarding out of suitable patients and the erection of a new district asylum nearby.[18] This would allow him to create a more attractive environment for private paying patients, who had to be attracted from comfortable homes by convincing relatives of the superiority of his medical regime. This wish to woo more wealthy inmates was largely responsible for

Image 2.2

Craig House, Royal Edinburgh Asylum, c.1900.
Courtesy of Lothian Health Services Archive.

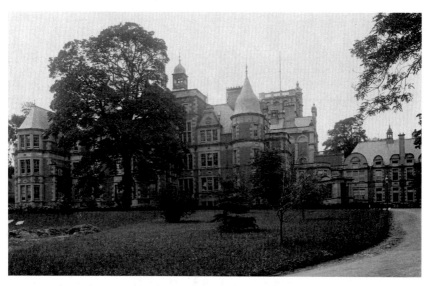

the conception and building of Craig House in 1894 (see Images 2.2 and 2.3). The REA thereafter consisted of two divisions: West House for the rate-aided patients and Craig House for the private patients.[19]

The REA was thus a public institution which reflected the Scottish class system and all of its social inequalities. The divisions between private and pauper patients in Victorian asylums like the REA was a reflection of the outside world, rather than something peculiar to asylumdom. Segregation by class was advocated not only by officials and administrators but by many patients and their families, although predictably most often by those of private means rather than by those on parish rates. Accommodating the genteel in inferior situations and exposing them to the bad habits of the pauper ranks would, it was believed, offend their own feelings and those of their families and thereby retard their recovery. There was, therefore, a strict class demarcation in the facilities offered by the REA. The asylum's extensive Gheel model, which emulated the best features of the famous and controversial Belgian village where the insane were cared for in a home-like atmosphere, comprised elegant homes and villas exclusively for the wealthy private patients. The patients were also divided by gender and by the severity of their mental disorder.

Image 2.3

Main Hall, Craig House, c.1900.
Courtesy of Lothian Health Services Archive.

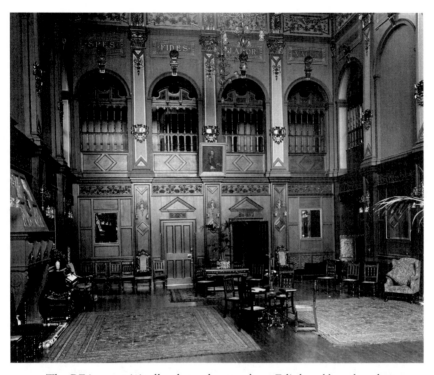

The REA was originally planned not only as Edinburgh's asylum but as a national institution, 'open to patients from every part of Scotland'.[20] However, in practice, this role proved to be more of an ideal than a reality. The vast majority of pauper admissions were from within a twenty-mile radius of the capital, since Scottish Lunacy and Poor Laws forced indigent individuals back to their parish of birth for support. A mere handful of patients were born in England, Ireland or Wales, as well as some foreign inmates from, for example, Spain and Russia, who caused considerable consternation due principally to language difficulties. On the other hand, private patients came from a much wider geographic distribution, with only twenty-six per cent being Edinburgh-born in the decade between 1884 and 1894.[21] Furthermore, the REA contracted to receive the insane of the Orkney Islands.[22]

The asylum day followed a predictable timetable of early rising, eating, exercise and early to bed. Great stress was also laid upon the therapeutic benefits of physical labour, with Clouston's strong belief that it would 'divert the mind from morbid thoughts' and cultivate 'tidiness of dress'.[23] The idea of work as effective treatment was far from new, of course, having been advocated from at least the end of the eighteenth century.[24] In Scotland, work had been used as a form of therapy in the Charity Workhouse 'Bedlam' from the 1830s. The Commissioners in Lunacy strongly advocated its importance to asylum authorities. Their 1853 Report condemned the:

> [U]nnecessary expense of laying out airing courts, levelling off rough ground, formation of slopes... before the asylum is completed, when all these operations... can be far more usefully and effectively undertaken after the asylum has been for some time opened... by male patients, whose own almost unassisted labour may carry out and complete them at much smaller expense.[25]

As Arthur Mitchell, Commissioner in Lunacy, stated in 1881: 'It is scarcely possible to over-estimate the value of work as a means of treatment.'[26] By this year, seventy-four per cent of pauper patients in Scotland were regularly engaged in useful work.

Asylum inmates appear to have worked the hours that they would have normally worked outside. William McKinnon, the first Physician-Superintendent of the REA, serving between 1839 and 1846, encouraged patients to pursue the occupation they had prior to their admission. Male patients thus stoked boilers, baked bread, made clothes and shoes or helped tradesmen maintain the buildings; while female patients cleaned or helped in the stores, kitchen or laundry, where washing tubs were deemed preferable to labour-saving machinery. The surrounding farms and gardens provided further means of employment. Indeed, all seven chartered asylums put their varying acres of land to productive use, and one of the **Lunacy Board's** top priorities, when looking for a site to build new asylums, was enough land for a farm. Clouston believed outdoor labour to be especially valuable in enabling patients to sleep without sedation by tiring them out and discouraging incoherent thought. He also favoured 'sinecures' suitably to encourage these patient endeavours. Payment was usually given in the form of tobacco, sweets or money.[27]

Whilst such manual labour was felt to be extremely useful in the treatment of poorer patients, it was generally deemed inappropriate for private patients. Clouston, in fact, lamented the fact that private patients, by virtue of their class, could not be set to work except voluntarily.[28] Indeed, he occasionally coaxed even the rich male patients into pushing wheelbarrows around the asylum's gardens, but if such an inmate recognised that labour to be inappropriate for a person of his station, such 'therapy' ceased.[29] There is no evidence that this exercise actually improved health, much less promoted recovery, but at the practical day-to-day level, patients' willingness to work seems to have been interpreted by the physicians in terms of how well they were responding to therapy and also how effectively they could be managed and accommodated into the often labour-intensive daily routine of asylum life.[30] Work may have helped patients to accept their new institutionalised lives more easily, as well as aiding the finances of the institution.

Employment was offset somewhat by the participation of both patients and staff in games and social events. Indeed, such 'amusement' was also deemed generally valuable as a therapeutic tool. That is, equally important to Clouston's so-called 'gospel of work' was his 'gospel of play'. REA patients had the opportunity to learn how to dance, play billiards, bowls, cricket, tennis, curling, cards, dominoes, chess and draughts. In addition, community volunteers provided concerts, lectures, poetry readings and balls. Weekly dances were held in the East and West Houses for both sexes. Patients could also relax in their day rooms, with a selection of books, magazines and newspapers to read. The gentlemen depended chiefly on such amusements for their distraction, with board games, billiards, whist and letter-writing constituting their most popular pastimes. Religious worship was also accorded an essential place in the system of 'moral therapy' practised at most asylums,[31] with the REA, like most asylums, having its own Chaplain.

In terms of staffing, the Scottish asylums were initially dominated by lay, rather than medical, influence and control. Six of the seven Royal asylums had no resident physician when first founded, such medical staff as they possessed being appointed in a visiting capacity.[32] Few of the REA Managers were medical men, with the majority drawn from influential sectors of the town's hierarchy, including the Town Council, guilds and church. However, as the nineteenth century wore on, the extent and quality of medical supervision in the royal asylums improved. By 1840, almost all of them had equipped themselves with fully-paid, full-time resident Physician-Superintendents.[33] The first appointment in Scotland appears to have been Alexander Macintosh at Dundee in 1833, followed the next year by W.A.F. Browne at Montrose. In Edinburgh, this major organisational shift occurred in 1839 when William McKinnon was appointed. The strategic appointment of such Physician-Superintendents appears to have been crucial henceforth in shaping the organisation and ideology of the royal asylums.

A full list of REA Physician-Superintendents is provided in Appendix 2. In the period between 1880 and 1930, two personalities dominated the REA, Thomas Clouston and George Robertson. Thomas Clouston (1840–1915) graduated from the University of Edinburgh, where he

Image 2.4

Thomas Clouston, Royal Edinburgh Asylum Physician-Superintendent, 1873–1908. Courtesy of Lothian Health Services Archive.

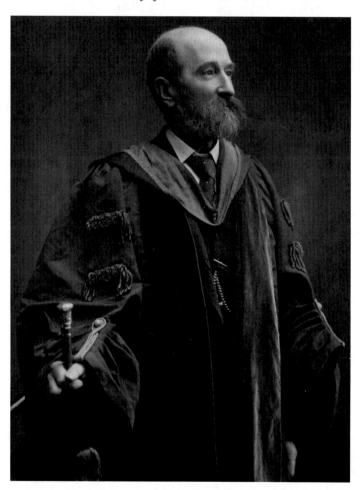

attended the lectures of two men who were to influence him greatly, David Skae and Thomas Laycock. After briefly joining Skae's REA staff as assistant physician, Clouston was appointed Physician-Superintendent of Cumberland and Westmorland Asylum, Carlisle, at the age of twenty-two. He remained there for ten years. Upon Skae's death in 1873, Clouston was recalled to the REA as Physician-Superintendent, where this was to remain his vocation for the next thirty-five years (see Image 2.4). He was also appointed first official Lecturer in Mental Diseases at the University of Edinburgh in 1879, the culmination of a campaign which had begun in the early nineteenth century to achieve academic recognition for the study of insanity.[34] Clouston combined the post of managing Scotland's largest and most prestigious asylum with a career as a prolific writer of clinical textbooks, medical papers and popular articles. Most notably, his *Clinical Lectures on Mental Diseases* went through six editions between 1883 and 1906 and was the recognised textbook on psychiatry for medical students. Clouston became President of the Medico-Psychological Association (MPA) in 1888,[35] and was largely responsible for founding the first Scottish Asylum Laboratory in 1897 – to be discussed in Chapter 4. He retired from the REA in 1908 and a knighthood followed in 1911.

George M. Robertson (1864–1932) graduated from the University of Edinburgh before assisting Clouston in the pathology laboratories of the University. He became Physician-Superintendent of Perth District Asylum in 1892, of Stirling District Asylum in 1899, and finally of the REA in 1908, upon Clouston's retirement (see Image 2.5, overleaf). Robertson proclaimed a wish to 'de-asylumise' such institutions in order to put them on a par with the best general hospitals. During the Great War he asked his REA Board of Managers to establish nursing homes where patients suffering from incipient mental disorders could be watched.[36] The success of the resulting scheme led the Managers to open Jordanburn Nerve Hospital, where patients of all social ranks could be received for examination and treatment in both an in-patient and, more significantly, an out-patient capacity.[37] In 1919, the Managers endowed a chair of psychiatry in the University of Edinburgh – the first such chair in Scotland, which for clinical and teaching purposes was conjoined with the post of Physician-Superintendent of the REA – of which Robertson became the first occupant. He was, furthermore, elected President of the MPA in 1922 and President of the Royal College of Physicians in 1925, before retiring from the REA in 1932.

In fact, the REA produced some of the most prominent and successful of Britain's nineteenth and early twentieth-century alienists. The 'Edinburgh School of Psychiatry' has been portrayed as a thriving site of psychiatric intellect and practice, not only for its teaching innovations and integration of psychiatric teaching into the University Medical Faculty but also for its contributions to nosology and diagnosis.[38] Moreover, even those physicians within the REA who did not advance to the post of Physician-Superintendent often went on to positions of great prominence. Thus, after serving as assistant physician under Skae at the REA, John Sibbald became Physician-Superintendent at Argyll and Bute District Asylum in 1862, Deputy Commissioner in Lunacy in 1870, and Commissioner in Lunacy in 1878. He was knighted in 1899. John MacPherson served as senior assistant

Image 2.5

*George Robertson, Royal Edinburgh Asylum Physician-Superintendent,
1908–32. Courtesy of Lothian Health Services Archive.*

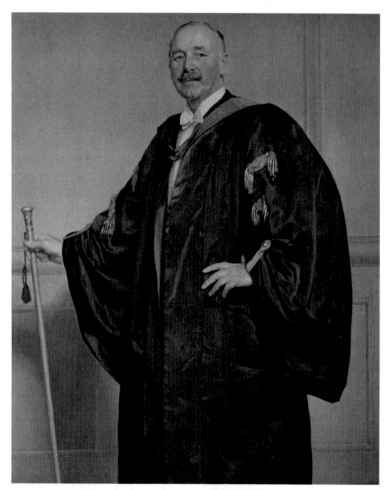

physician at the REA, before becoming Physician-Superintendent at Stirling
District Asylum, then Lecturer on Mental Diseases at the Royal School of
Medicine, Edinburgh. He was appointed Deputy Commissioner in 1900
and then President of the MPA in 1910.

In terms of patient numbers, by the 1880s the asylum had grown in
numbers from its original intake of six patients to an impressive institution
which housed over a thousand. Figure 2.1 charts the total number of

Figure 2.1

Admissions to the REA, 1880–1930

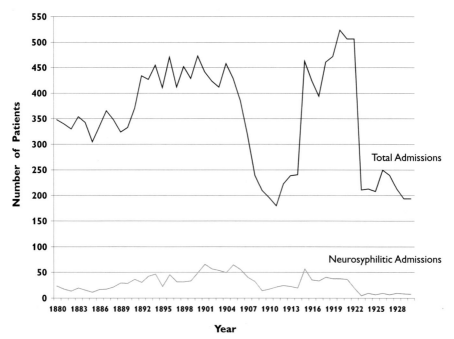

Source: *Royal Edinburgh Asylum Annual Reports*, 1880–1930, LHSA
LHB7/7/8–14.

admissions to the asylum over the period from 1880 to 1930, as well as the
number of specifically neurosyphilitic admissions.[39] Over this fifty-year
period, there was a steady rise in admissions, except in 1907 and 1923 when
admissions dropped dramatically, and 1915 when admissions rose
significantly.[40] The period between 1880 and 1930 saw REA total admissions
fluctuate widely between 179 and 523, and neurosyphilitic admissions
between 4 and 65, with neurosyphilitics constituting an annual average of
eight per cent of total admissions. Of course, since patients could be
diagnosed initially with an alternative disorder, as Chapter 3 will illustrate,
particularly mania and melancholia, the proportion of neurosyphilitics is
likely to have been a little higher than this, as will be true for the other
Scottish asylums.

Glasgow Royal Asylum, Gartnavel

Before 1814 there was no dedicated institution for the insane in Glasgow. The mentally ill of the city were instead housed in cells within its poorhouse, the Town's Hospital, where there was no attempt at treatment. In 1804, one of this institution's directors, Robert McNair of Belvidere, proposed that a hospital be set up specifically for the care of the insane. The asylum was completed in 1814 in Parliamentary Road. It was built to William Stark's panopticon design,[41] which was intended to facilitate the total observation of patients.[42] It opened to wide public interest and acclaim, its site and design inspired by the philosophy of 'moral management' pioneered by the Tukes at the Retreat. The relative speed and financial success with which Glaswegians established their chartered asylum stands in marked contrast to the equivalent Edinburgh venture. Whereas the REA took twenty-one years from conception to completion of the project, Gartnavel took only six years. Glasgow was also more successful in raising funding, attracting £15,541.18.11 in half the time it took Edinburgh to raise £7,500.[43]

In 1843, the asylum relocated to its present site at Gartnavel, by which name it became known (see Image 2.6). The decision to leave Stark's asylum was due mainly to overcrowding and the growth of the City of Glasgow. By now, the asylum was fenced in by other buildings, compromising its potential for expansion. Moreover, since a country setting was held as the ideal in the treatment of the insane, officials decided to move the asylum west to a sixty-six-acre plot of extensive ground, outside the growing urban sprawl.[44] The panopticon model was also considered outdated by now, so that the 'Edinburgh' model was applied to the new site, consisting of an overcrowded and unadorned 'East House' for about 290 paupers and a much smaller 'West House' for the private patients, comparable to a private mansion in its interior features.[45]

Although little difficulty was encountered in raising the substantial funds needed to finance the asylum's initial erection, the prevailing, but misguided, conviction was that the institution would soon become financially self-sufficient. In its early decades, Gartnavel was intermittently in debt, with the Directors repeatedly resorting to raising loans to meet their ambitious building programme, and the asylum's annual reports were full of apologetic and frustrated explanations for building projects delayed or forgone as a result of indebtedness. However, by 1880, the Directors could declare that their debts had been 'extinguished' and the asylum thereafter entered a period of financial prosperity which lasted for the next half century and which allowed a series of ambitious renovation projects.[46] This prosperous state of affairs lasted until the 1930s, at which point the excess of income over expenditure was eroded rapidly.[47]

Image 2.6

Glasgow Royal Asylum, Gartnavel Site, c.1843.
Courtesy of NHS Greater Glasgow and Clyde Archives.

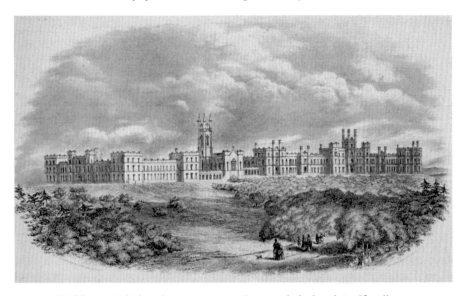

Unlike its Edinburgh counterpart, Gartnavel declared itself willing to accommodate pauper patients from the outset. Paupers from the City of Glasgow were received on a reduced rate of board and constituted a third of the patient population. Yet the institution's catchment area extended much more widely than the City, acting, in effect, as a district asylum for the whole of the west of Scotland, as well as drawing small contingents from the outlying highlands and islands.[48] Thus, parishes as distant as Ayr, Greenock and Campbeltown were making use of its facilities. In relation to the private category, any person in the City of Glasgow or its surrounding settlements who fulfilled the necessary legal and medical criteria could be admitted; although once there, this private patient was confronted with up to eight different fees, the quality of the service offered clearly differing with the price.

However, under David Yellowlees, Physician-Superintendent from 1874 until 1901, asylum officials instituted a policy of discharging all pauper patients and transferring them to the new district asylums, further contributing to the asylum's financial prosperity in these years. Yellowlees argued that his ideal would be a small institution where the medical attendant had individual knowledge of his patients. Moreover, in his view, very few resident pauper patients presented 'any reasonable hope of Recovery' and their presence excluded any 'new and curable cases' from being admitted, thus undermining 'the real usefulness of the asylum as a place of *cure*'.[49] Furthermore, it was argued that the removal of such parish patients would 'raise the social tone of the Institution',[50] although Yellowlees conceded this to be a 'mixed good' since, economically speaking, the useful work done by the parish patients would be lost due to the fact that private patients could not be expected to perform these tasks. In 1889, Gartnavel ceased to admit any further pauper patients.[51]

As in the REA, employment was considered an important part of the therapeutic regime. The early Directors of Gartnavel expressed the view that such occupation prevented the mind from dwelling on its delusions, and considered giving some financial remuneration in return for work undertaken by patients, although the idea was not taken up. Many of the pauper patients worked indoors as domestics or labourers, depending on their gender.[52] In addition, there was plenty of outdoor work for the patients within the grounds of the estate. Patients made roads, landscaped earth, and planted trees and shrubs. The garden also provided soft fruit and vegetables for the asylum. The Directors listed with pride the quantities achieved from their farm each year within their annual reports.

Since such labour was considered degrading for the fee-paying patients, they were instead furnished with distractions such as billiards and carriage rides around the grounds.[53] While Physician-Superintendent Yellowlees accepted that such amusements might usefully 'relieve the monotony of Asylum residence',[54] like Clouston, he argued that employment would be much more valuable to them, for 'neither the sane nor the insane are benefited by a continual round of amusements'.[55] Subsequently, evidence would suggest that Physician-Superintendent David Henderson was responsible for introducing occupation therapy to Scotland at Gartnavel, when he drew on his experiences in the United States. Industrial therapy was formally introduced to the asylum in 1922, the average daily class attendance being approximately ninety-eight. Each class lasted around ninety minutes and involved skills such as simple woodwork, basketry, china painting, metal work and embroidery.

In terms of leisure, bowling was the first sport to be played at Gartnavel, once the bowling green was completed in 1853. Games such as draughts, backgammon and billiards were also soon offered, while a private croquet lawn was provided for the ladies. Iron seats were placed in the grounds, shelters were added for walkers and outdoor sports grew more numerous. Gartnavel even had its own golf course, with the first tee located in front of the West House.[56] In addition, a library was eventually opened, use having previously been made of a travelling version.[57] Further activities included an annual Fancy Dress Ball, theatrical and musical performances by staff and patients, and regular cricket and football fixtures. Divine service was held from 1819 onwards, initially in one of the eight-foot wide galleries of the old asylum and, by 1828, in a purpose-built chapel.

Appendix 2 provides an overview of all Physician-Superintendents serving Gartnavel from its founding until the mid-twentieth century. The asylum had no resident physician when first founded; instead one was appointed in a merely visiting capacity.[58] However, this is not to imply that this task was a trivial one, for among the physician's remits were the admission, examination, treatment and discharge of the patients, the supervision of staff, and the writing and maintenance of a number of reports. The first visiting physicians at Gartnavel were Robert Cleghorn, who served from 1814 to 1819, and John Balmanno, who filled the post between 1819 to 1840. Cleghorn combined his Gartnavel appointment with a thriving private practice and the post of Visiting Physician to the recently opened Glasgow Royal Infirmary. However, the steady growth of the asylum placed increasing demands upon Cleghorn's successor, so that towards the end of his period of office, Balmanno was doing little else but asylum work.[59]

In 1841, the asylum's first full-time resident Physician-Superintendent was appointed. William Hutcheson filled this post for eight years, and oversaw the move to the new site. His successor, Alexander McIntosh, had served previously as a Physician-Superintendent in Dundee. The Physician-Superintendent took on an increasingly omnipotent role as the century unfolded, overtly acknowledged during Oswald's period of office when he became deferentially known as 'The Chief'. In 1915, the post of assistant physician was introduced to replace the medical assistants for which the institution had previously opted. The first person elected to this post was David Henderson, who went on to become Physician-Superintendent of both Gartnavel and the REA.

At Gartnavel, the key Physician-Superintendents for the period under study were David Yellowlees, Landel Oswald and David Henderson. The earliest of these, David Yellowlees (1835–1921), received his MD from the University of Edinburgh in 1857. His first appointment to psychiatry was to assist David Skae at the REA, before going on to become assistant physician and then Superintendent at Glamorgan County Asylum in 1863, then Resident Surgeon and Resident Physician at the Edinburgh Royal Infirmary. Yellowlees was appointed Physician-Superintendent of Gartnavel in 1874 (see Image 2.7, overleaf). He had been partly attracted to Glasgow by the possibility of involvement with formal psychiatric teaching at the University, and in 1880 was appointed as the first Lecturer in Mental Diseases at the University of Glasgow. In 1890, he was elected President of the MPA. Yellowlees continued as Lecturer in Mental Diseases and Physician-

Gayle Davis

Image 2.7

David Yellowlees, Gartnavel Physician-Superintendent, 1874–1901.
Courtesy of NHS Greater Glasgow and Clyde Archives.

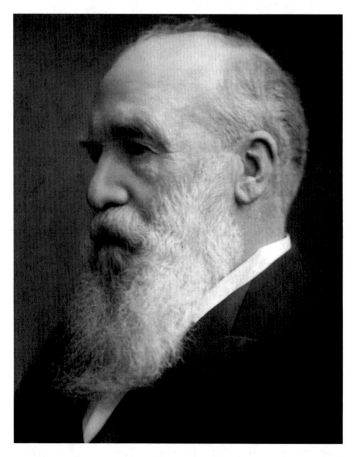

Superintendent of Gartnavel until 1901, when he retired due to failing eyesight.

Upon his graduation from the University of Glasgow, Landel R. Oswald (1861–1928) spent a year as assistant house physician to Sir William Gairdner, who appears to have influenced his choice of psychiatry as a career.[60] Oswald found employment at Gartnavel assisting Yellowlees for five years and then spent a short period travelling in the United States and Germany. In 1895, he was appointed Physician-Superintendent of the newly-built Glasgow District Asylum at Gartloch, where he remained until

Image 2.8

Landel Oswald, Gartnavel Physician-Superintendent, 1901–21.
Courtesy of NHS Greater Glasgow and Clyde Archives.

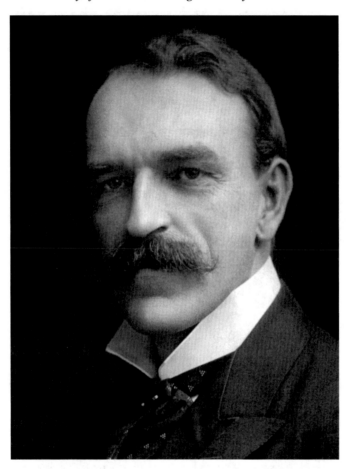

1901, when he returned to Gartnavel to succeed Yellowlees as Physician-Superintendent (see Image 2.8). Oswald also succeeded Yellowlees as the second Lecturer in Insanity at the University of Glasgow in 1904. Oswald was largely responsible for establishing the second Scottish asylum laboratory, the Scottish Western Asylums' Research Institute in 1909 within the grounds of Gartnavel, which Chapter 4 will discuss. Under Oswald, Gartnavel also established the first psychiatric clinic attached to a general hospital in the west of Scotland. In 1910, this psychiatric out-patient clinic

Image 2.9

*David Henderson, Gartnavel Physician-Superintendent, 1921–32.
Courtesy of Lothian Health Services Archive.*

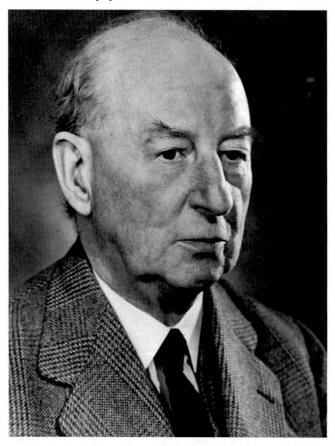

was opened at Glasgow's Western Infirmary, to which Oswald was appointed
Consulting Physician.[61] Oswald resigned on account of ill-health in 1921.

David K. Henderson (1884–1965) was almost certainly the most famous
and successful alienist to be associated with Gartnavel. An Edinburgh
graduate, Henderson decided to specialise in psychiatry and became a
medical officer at the REA under Clouston. He later widened his experience
by undertaking clinical work and postgraduate study at various centres of
excellence in London, Munich, New York and Baltimore. Henderson
worked with the renowned Swiss alienist Adolf Meyer, first at the New York

Psychiatric Institute between 1908 and 1911, and then as Senior Resident Physician at the Henry Phipps Psychiatric Clinic within the Johns Hopkins Hospital in Baltimore.[62] Between these posts, he spent several months in Munich at the Royal Psychiatric Clinic, working under the noted German alienist Emil Kraeplin. Therefore, when Henderson was invited to succeed Oswald as both Gartnavel Physician-Superintendent and Lecturer in Psychiatry at the University of Glasgow, he brought with him extensive knowledge and experience gleaned from his participation in some of the latest initiatives in psychiatric medicine from various centres of excellence. He was also to publish widely on the basis of his varied clinical experience, including the popular textbook *A Textbook of Psychiatry for Students and Practitioners* with R. Gillespie, which extended to ten editions. Henderson left Gartnavel in 1932 to take up the more prestigious post of Physician-Superintendent at the REA and Lecturer in Psychiatry at the University of Edinburgh (Image 2.9). He was knighted in 1947 in recognition of his services to psychiatry.

In 1815, the Glasgow Asylum had six keepers tending some seventy-three patients, a ratio of one to twelve. By 1857, a ratio of just one attendant to every fourteen patients was recorded in the pauper East House, compared to that of one to four in the West House.[63] This institution therefore serves as a prime example of how the issue of overcrowding plagued asylums throughout the nineteenth and early twentieth centuries. The population served by Gartnavel grew at an inordinate rate, increasing by roughly one million in the years between 1841 and 1911.[64] Figure 2.2, overleaf, plots the total number of admissions to the asylum between 1880 and 1930, as well as the number of specifically neurosyphilitic admissions.[65] A slight reduction in total admissions can be noted, due mainly to the rejection of pauper cases, but until 1920 the proportion of neurosyphilitic admissions rose slightly. This fifty-year period saw Gartnavel's total admissions range between 93 and 225, and neurosyphilitic admissions between 1 and 25, with neurosyphilitics constituting an annual average of five per cent of the total admissions.

Barony Parochial Asylum, Woodilee

In 1869, the Barony Parochial Board set up a special committee with responsibility to create adequate provision for the pauper insane of the Barony district, situated to the north-east of Glasgow. The following year, the Committee proposed that an asylum be built which could accommodate four hundred inmates and could be expanded to take six hundred if necessary. They recommended that this be a farm asylum located outside the urban sprawl of Glasgow, within easy reach of a railway and with good drainage and water supplies. The Board approved and set about finding a suitable site, of which Woodilee, Lenzie was the favourite. By March 1871

Figure 2.2

Admissions to Gartnavel, 1880–1930

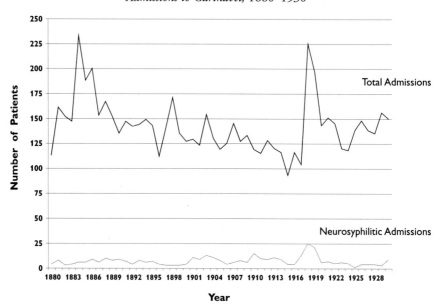

Source: *Glasgow Royal Asylum Annual Reports,* 1814–1940, NHSGGCA 13B/2/221–4.

they had their estate. When the Barony Parochial Asylum opened in 1875 and housed 400 patients, it was the largest parish asylum in Scotland.

In its early years, the asylum was obliged to take anyone whose circumstances brought them within the scope of the Poor Law Acts, including 'state patients' (convicted criminals).[66] In addition, some seventy patients were almost immediately transferred from Gartnavel, although this went only a little way to relieving the overcrowding of that institution. Glasgow had been growing steadily up to the 1870s, but the years that followed saw a more rapid expansion in the city's industrial development and, with it, a population explosion. Thus, forty years after Woodilee asylum opened, it had expanded from four hundred beds to thirteen hundred (see Image 2.10).[67]

The 'parochial' nature of Woodilee made patient segregation by class unnecessary. However, there was quickly a perceived need to separate male and female patients. The Managers thereafter stipulated that no male attendant, servant or patient be permitted in the female wards, nor was any female to enter the male wards except female servants or nurses appointed to

66

Image 2.10

Barony Parochial Asylum, Woodilee, c.1900.
Courtesy of NHS Greater Glasgow and Clyde Archives.

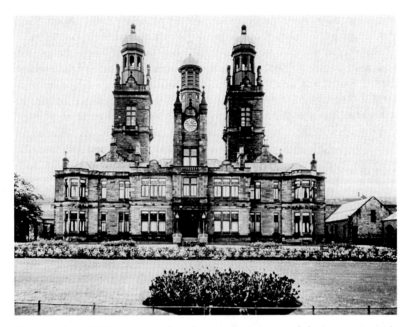

do duty there.[68] Meals were to be taken in the communal dining room, with men sitting on one side and women on the other.

The management of Woodilee distinguished itself in the degree to which its patients, both male and female, were employed in work. By 1881, the Commissioners could proudly report that the number of patients 'actively and profitably employed' at Woodilee was 205 men and 204 women. The remaining 'idle' patients – consisting of 45 men and 32 women – were all judged 'physically incapable of work'.[69] It was argued that such work promoted patient contentment, removed from their minds any sense of imprisonment, and improved their bodily and mental health. Unlike Gartnavel, whose patients were not paid for their work, Woodilee patients received a salary for their employment and tended to spend it on tobacco.

As elsewhere, a patient's previous occupation often determined the work he or she did as an inmate. Workshops and tools, for example, were provided for artisans. Furthermore, since this asylum was built on farm land, the two surrounding fields were quickly put to use to provide patients with the therapeutic benefits of farm work and the institution with food. Indeed, two adjoining farms were purchased in 1902 when the asylum land was deemed insufficient to meet its requirements. In the early years, the farms produced beef, mutton, veal, pork, chicken, oatmeal, milk, butter, eggs, potatoes, soft fruit, rhubarb and vegetables. However, by the 1920s, the land was largely given over to grazing and crops of wheat, oats, turnips, cabbage, hay, grass and potatoes. Surplus produce was offered to other institutions.[70] Such agricultural work was used as a form of work therapy until the late 1960s.

Another important method of treatment was what might be termed 'industrial therapy'. This therapy developed from the Brabazon Employment Scheme which was first introduced to a Scottish asylum – Woodilee – in 1898.[71] The scheme, devised by Mary Jane Brabazon, Countess of Meath, in order to employ poorhouse inmates, was first practised at the Union Poorhouse in Tonbridge, England.[72] Inmates made craft goods – including embroidery, paintings, rugs and baskets – which were then sold and the proceeds put towards new materials. The fund thereby became self-perpetuating, with any surplus used to provide treats and incentives. Within Scotland, such employment was seen to be particularly appropriate and beneficial for those patients deemed 'physically unfit for strenuous work... whose mental condition must be stimulated and educated by a greater variety of light and interesting occupations'.[73] About fifty Woodilee patients were instructed one day per week by the volunteer ladies of the Brabazon Employment Society, although by the 1920s nurses were beginning to take over this work, with the produce still being sold in order to pay for outings.[74]

Day rooms, stocked with Bibles and books, were provided for patient relaxation. Outdoor recreation was also encouraged, with a bowling green laid out next to the asylum as soon as it was opened. The grounds were adapted so as to provide patients with a cricket ground, tennis courts, croquet lawns and curling rinks. The recreation hall was used for dances, concerts, plays and choral recitals. Staff joined patients for Monday evening dances in the hall. In addition, religious services were provided.

Appendix 2 lists those Physician-Superintendents who served Woodilee from its founding until the 1930s. The first Physician-Superintendent at Woodilee, James Rutherford, who served from 1874 to 1883, had previously been in charge of Argyll and Bute District Asylum, and subsequently took charge of the Crichton Royal Institution. He was to become a distinguished alienist, co-translating Wilhelm Griesinger's *Manual of Mental Diseases* in 1867 and acting as Honorary Secretary to the Scottish MPA.[75] However, the three significant figures for the period of this study were Robert Blair, Hamilton Marr, and Henry Carre. Robert Blair replaced Rutherford as second Physician-Superintendent of Woodilee from 1883 to 1902, having previously been an assistant physician at Gartnavel, but little other information is available on this physician.

More substantial information is available for Blair's successor, Hamilton Clelland Marr (1870–1936), arguably the most notable of Woodilee's staff. Marr graduated in medicine from the University of Glasgow and was attracted to the study of mental and nervous disorders from the outset of his career. He found employment as Woodilee's first assistant physician, and then as senior assistant medical officer to the Crichton Royal Asylum, Dumfries, before returning to Woodilee to the posts of Deputy Medical Superintendent and then, upon Blair's retirement, Superintendent between 1902 and 1910. He also became Mackintosh Lecturer in Psychological Medicine at St Mungo's Medical College, Glasgow, and extramural Lecturer in Mental Diseases at the University of Glasgow. Marr was subsequently appointed HM Medical Commissioner in Lunacy for Scotland in 1910, Senior Medical Commissioner for the General Board of Control, and President of the MPA.[76] Henry Carre was unanimously appointed to succeed Marr, having previously served as assistant medical officer at Woodilee since 1897. Before arriving at this institution, Carre had held junior posts in Scottish and English asylums.[77] He vacated the Woodilee Physician-Superintendent post upon retirement in 1936 and died in 1947.

However, while the employment of such senior physicians at these district asylums aided, or at least did not preclude, their ascent up the psychiatric ladder, many junior medical officers who started out at these institutions failed to achieve senior positions within psychiatry, or to specialise in psychiatry at all. Many opted, instead, for careers in general medicine, both in the general hospitals and infirmaries of the district, and as parochial medical officers, or else preferred the better remuneration offered by private practice.[78]

Figure 2.3, overleaf, sketches the number of total admissions and neurosyphilitic admissions to the asylum over the period from 1880 to 1920.[79] Over this forty-year period, there appears to have been a steady rise in admissions to the institution, although the years 1894 and 1915 witnessed a significantly larger influx of patients.[80] Between 1880 and 1920, Woodilee's total admissions fluctuated between 145 and 446 and neurosyphilitic admissions between 1 and 33, with neurosyphilitics constituting an annual average of six per cent of the total admissions.

Midlothian and Peebles District Asylum, Rosslynlee

As with Woodilee, Midlothian and Peebles District Asylum was established to receive the pauper insane of its district. The Midlothian and Peebles District Board of Lunacy appear to have experienced considerable difficulty in finding an affordable site that was suitable to the requirements of a county asylum. Of those placed at their disposal, they finally selected a piece of land on the Whitehill Estate with the combined advantages of a central situation

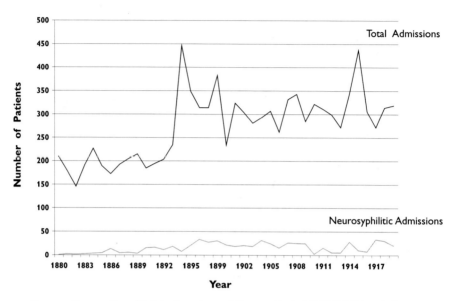

Figure 2.3

Admissions to Woodilee, 1880–1920

Source: *Barony Parochial Asylum Annual Report,* 1919, NHSGGCA30/2/20.

within the district, isolation from the village population, and proximity to the railway station of Rosslynlee (see Image 2.11). The grounds were of forty acres, acquired at a feu-duty of £4 per acre, with a further seventy acres leased shortly afterwards.[81]

Rosslynlee was opened for the reception of patients in 1874, in which year fifty-one patients were admitted, most of these transferred from the REA. The institution was equipped to provide accommodation in all for 230 patients, so as well as taking anyone whose circumstances brought them within the scope of the Poor Law Acts, the vacant beds were occupied by patients from other districts or by patients of a higher class who would pay a remunerative rate of board in return for the accommodation afforded to them. Indeed, by 1894, its Physician-Superintendent was ironically lamenting the relentlessly multiplying asylum pauper population and the fact that they would soon be driven to remove all private patients if this trend continued, which would inevitably lead to 'a considerable rise in the maintenance rate'.[82] Within two years, a number of private patients were indeed being transferred to other asylums, as well as incurable pauper patients being boarded out.

70

Image 2.11

*Midlothian and Peebles District Asylum, Rosslynlee, 1925.
Courtesy of Lothian Health Services Archive.*

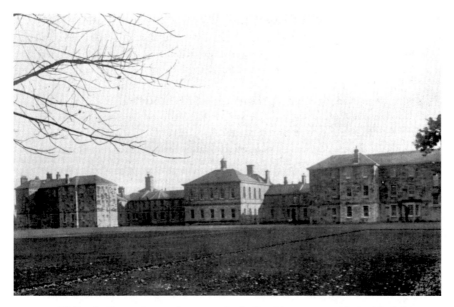

All Rosslynlee patients who were physically able were provided with daily employment. By 1902, it was estimated that about seventy per cent of all patients did some useful work. The more able-bodied men tended to engage themselves in outdoor labour, such as gardening, farming and laying out the asylum grounds, although the tradesmen employed themselves as tailors, shoemakers, masons, painters, smiths or carpenters. The female patients occupied their time chiefly with sewing, knitting, house and laundry work. Thus, as with the other three institutions, work was segregated very much along gender lines, as it was in the outside world. Taking its lead from Woodilee, the staff of Rosslynlee implemented the Brabazon Scheme into their programme of activities from 1905. Approximately thirty patients attended these classes on a weekly basis.

In its early years, quoits appears to have been the only outdoor game offered to Rosslynlee patients. Annual picnics to the Pentland or Moorfoot Hills were commenced in the summer of 1889 and continued until the war years. There was also a weekly dance and occasional concerts or dramatic entertainments. By 1902, the institution was playing host to formal cricket and curling matches, concerts and variety entertainments, dances, athletic games and an annual picnic.[83] By the 1920s, the institution was offering patients an array of sports, including golf, tennis, bowls, curling, football and hockey. Board games, periodicals and daily newspapers were also provided. Religious service was held every Sunday morning, attracting up to a hundred patients.

In terms of staffing, by the 1880s the staff of the asylum included a Physician-Superintendent, Chaplain, Steward, five farm or garden servants, five artisans, four women engaged in the kitchen or laundry, and fourteen attendants.[84] Physician-Superintendent Robert Cameron commented with pride on the asylum's low turnover of staff, particularly the attendants, whose duties were said to be 'among the most trying to which human patience can be subjected'.[85] By 1908, the ratio of attendants to patients was one to ten for day duty and one to fifty for night duty. In 1921, the post of Assistant Medical Superintendent was created. John Sibbald, Commissioner in Lunacy, noted this to be an important step for the asylum, given the fact that its administration with only one Medical Officer was 'always conducted under some difficulty'.[86]

Appendix 2 provides an overview of all Physician-Superintendents employed in Rosslynlee from its founding to the mid-twentieth century. Thomas Anderson, who had formerly been an assistant at the Southern Counties Asylum, Dumfries, was the first Physician-Superintendent of Rosslynlee between 1874 and 1880. He was replaced, due to illness, by Robert Cameron, who was first appointed Interim Superintendent and then promoted to a permanent post when Anderson was forced to retire due to his poor health. However, as the 1888 annual report of Rosslynlee intriguingly states, 'subsequent investigation of the affairs of the Asylum and its management necessitated some important changes in the staff'.[87] As a result, Cameron resigned the office of Physician-Superintendent after eight years in the post.

Richard Blackwell Mitchell (Image 2.12) was appointed as Cameron's successor, and filled the post for twenty-eight years, not retiring until 1916. Mitchell appears to have been the most significant of the Rosslynlee physicians. A native of Orkney, he received his medical education at the University of Edinburgh. At an early stage in his career, he devoted himself to the study of insanity, becoming assistant medical officer in the Fife and Kinross District Asylum and, later, senior assistant physician under Clouston at the REA. In 1909, Mitchell's assistant physician, James Sturrock, left upon being appointed Medical Officer to Perth Prison. James Henry Cubitt Orr was appointed to the vacated post, and promoted to Physician-Superintendent in 1916, a post he filled until his death in 1942.

Image 2.12

Richard Mitchell, Rosslynlee Physician-Superintendent, 1888–1916.
Courtesy of Lothian Health Services Archive.

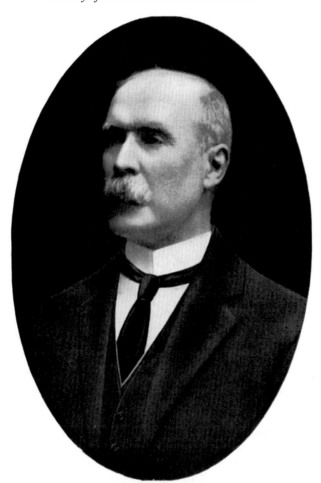

Finally, overleaf, Figure 2.4 plots the total number of admissions to the asylum and also the number of specifically neurosyphilitic admissions over the period from 1880 to 1930.[88] Admissions remained relatively steady throughout this period, except in 1902, which saw a sharp rise in the total number of admissions to the asylum, and the war years, during which admissions tended to be marginally higher than normal.[89] The years from 1880 to 1930 witnessed a fluctuation in total admissions to Rosslynlee of

Figure 2.4

Admissions to Rosslynlee, 1880–1930

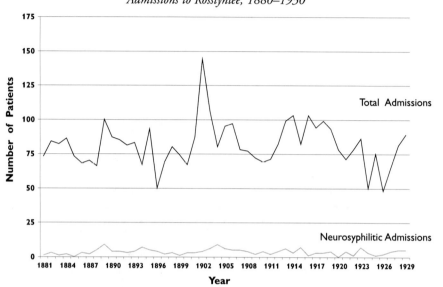

Source: *Midlothian and Peebles District Asylum Annual Reports,* 1880–1930, LHB33/2/1–3.

between 48 and 144, while neurosyphilitic admissions ranged between zero and 9, with neurosyphilitics constituting an annual average of five per cent of the total admissions over the period as a whole, the smallest proportion for the four Scottish asylums that form the basis of this study.

Comparisons

Two major contrasts can be discerned from the historiography of Scottish psychiatry which relate to the asylums selected for this study: the geographical contrast between 'east' and 'west' and the social contrast between 'royal' and 'parochial' asylum. In fact, a detailed exploration of each of these four asylums during the *fin-de-siècle* period suggests that such portrayed contrasts are stereotypical to an extent and in need of modification.

In terms of geography, Jonathan Andrews has argued convincingly that the level of coherence and significance found in psychiatry in the east of Scotland by the late nineteenth century constituted an outstanding 'Edinburgh School of Psychiatry'. In contrast, psychiatry in the west failed to achieve the same level of distinctive prominence and coherent identity.[90] However, this study would stress that early twentieth-century developments in Glaswegian psychiatry did raise its status substantially. Glasgow was the first Scottish university to have both an endowed lectureship in mental diseases and an endowed scholarship in aetiological research into insanity; while the success of Oswald's psychiatric out-patient clinic stood in marked contrast to Edinburgh's shortcomings in this field. Thus, it could be argued that by the 1920s, David Henderson, with his innovations based on clinical experience gleaned in Britain, Germany and the United States, was heading a psychiatric community which was on a par with its Edinburgh counterpart. Nonetheless, any talk of a distinct Edinburgh or Glasgow 'school' must also acknowledge the extent to which that east–west barrier was an artificial one, particularly when we take into account the constant interchange of staff and patients and the collective contributions to the joint pathological laboratories, which will be explored in Chapter 4.

With respect to social contrasts, it might seem an obvious conclusion that the Scottish 'royal' asylums would enjoy a higher status, attract better and more faithful staff, and reflect newer trends in psychiatric care. Certainly, the demands of administration, financial constraints and overcrowding did not entirely compromise the commitment of the chartered asylums to innovative clinical and pathological research. In particular, the REA and Gartnavel pioneered such advances in Scottish psychiatry as the provision of out-patient psychiatric care and laboratories to advance knowledge of the pathology of insanity. Furthermore, both asylums attracted or fostered figures of international renown to fill their posts and to further bolster their reputation as centres of excellence for psychiatric practice and research in the later-nineteenth and early twentieth centuries.

Clearly the district asylums began as the poor cousins of the Royals, with their lower profile, more transitory staffing, and obligation to focus upon the pauper insane. Nonetheless, some of these institutions quickly attracted figures who were subsequently to gain real prominence within Scottish psychiatry – as the careers of Rutherford and Marr at Woodilee demonstrate – and, as a result, it is arguable that medical posts within these institutions proved more secure and prestigious by the turn of the century. Indeed, it has been argued that the very creation of these asylums arguably allowed the expansion of psychiatry as a profession and the emergence of rather more prominent medical figures at their heads.[91] Furthermore, these parochial institutions were pre-eminent in employing new forms of work therapy for their patients. In particular, Woodilee was innovatively designed as a farm asylum and was the first Scottish asylum to utilise the Brabazon Employment Scheme. Thus, in a number of respects, Woodilee can be claimed to have made a significant contribution to psychiatry in the west of Scotland.

It is also important to acknowledge that there were connections and similarities between the royal and parochial asylums as well as divisions and differences. The staff of all four institutions selected for this study reveal a clear degree of commonality in terms of their social origins, attitudes, training and career patterns. Many of these alienists were trained at the Universities of Edinburgh and Glasgow under the same influential teachers, such as Laycock and Skae. Neither is there a clear division of patients. While the parochial institutions were intended exclusively to treat pauper patients, Rosslynlee was to branch out into providing care for private as well as pauper patients, and to resent its intended pauper focus. The royals similarly catered for a fairly mixed clientele. Moreover, there was a regular exchange of patients between these institutions, particularly the transfer of paupers from the royals once the parochial asylums began to open, as well as the transfer of patients to all four asylums from other institutions such as hospitals and prisons. While more work requires to be done on the parochial asylums, which will no doubt provide a more nuanced interpretation of these institutions and their place within Scottish psychiatry, this chapter suggests at least that those geographical and social contrasts commonly portrayed within the historiography of Scottish psychiatry are in need of revision.

Notes

1. For a more comprehensive overview, see F. Rice, 'Madness and Industrial Society: A Study of the Origins and Early Growth of the Organisation of Insanity in Nineteenth-Century Scotland, *c.*1830–1870', PhD thesis, 2 vols, University of Strathclyde (1981); R. Houston, 'Institutional Care for the Insane and Idiots in Scotland before 1820', parts 1 and 2, *History of Psychiatry*, 12 (2001), 3–31 and 177–97.

2. For a stimulating discussion of the 'mixed economy' of care for lunatics within the British and colonial contexts, see J. Melling and B. Forsythe (eds), *Insanity, Institutions and Society 1800–1914* (London: Routledge, 1999).

3. A charity had to be seen to be accountable and successful in 'value for money' terms and thus the charitable asylum followed a rather broader agenda than that of a purely medical or custodial facility by incorporating such elements as patient employment into its regular regime. See L. Walsh, 'The Property of the Whole Community: Charity and Insanity in Urban Scotland: The Dundee Royal Lunatic Asylum, 1805–1850', in Melling and Forsythe, *op. cit.* (note 2), 183–6.

4. R. Houston, *Madness and Society in Eighteenth-Century Scotland* (Oxford: Clarendon Press, 2000), 391.

5. A. Beveridge, 'Madness in Victorian Edinburgh: A Study of Patients Admitted to the Royal Edinburgh Asylum under Thomas Clouston, 1873–1908', Part 1, *History of Psychiatry*, 6 (1995), 21–54: 24.

6. For a detailed history, see J. Andrews, *'They're in the Trade... of Lunacy, They "Cannot Interfere" – They Say': The Scottish Lunacy Commissioners and Lunacy Reform in Nineteenth-Century Scotland* (London: Wellcome Institute for the History of Medicine, 1998).

7. Lunacy (Scotland) Act, clause XVII.

8. This contrasted favourably with the English Board of Lunacy, where six officials were responsible for overseeing the condition of 82,600 patients. See H. Sturdy, 'Boarding-Out the Insane, 1857–1913: A Study of the Scottish System', PhD thesis, University of Glasgow (1996), 266.

9. This was replaced by the Mental Welfare Commission in 1960.

10. Rice, *op. cit.* (note 1), 363.

11. J. Andrews, 'Raising the Tone of Asylumdom: Maintaining and Expelling Pauper Lunatics at the Glasgow Royal Asylum in the Nineteenth Century', in Melling and Forsythe, *op. cit.* (note 2), 202.

12. Harriet Sturdy's PhD thesis 'Boarding-Out' addresses this deficiency in the historiography, within the Scottish context. See Sturdy, *op. cit.* (note 8).

13. That is, 12 from Gartnavel and 14 from the REA.

14. *111th Glasgow Royal Asylum Annual Report*, 1923, NHS Greater Glasgow and Clyde Archives, NHSGGCA13B/2/224, 19.

15. J. Andrews and I. Smith (eds), *'Let There be Light Again': A History of Gartnavel Royal Hospital from its Beginnings to the Present Day* (Glasgow: Gartnavel, 1993), 104.

16. Ferguson's medical attendant, Dr Andrew Duncan, was said to be so moved by the poet's plight that he resolved to found a hospital in Edinburgh specifically for the mentally afflicted. However, it was not until 1792, many years after Ferguson's death, that a circular was issued by the Lord Provost of Edinburgh inviting subscriptions to this venture. See A. Mitchell, 'Memorandum on the Position of the Royal Edinburgh Asylum for the Insane', 1883, Lothian Health Services Archive (LHSA), LHB7/19/18, 9.

17. M. Thompson, 'The Mad, the Bad and the Sad: Psychiatric Care in the Royal Edinburgh Asylum (Morningside), 1813–1894', PhD thesis, Boston University Graduate School (1984), 93.

18. This latter request was not realised until 1906, with the opening of a new pauper asylum at Bangour.

19. The private patients' rates of board were on a sliding scale according to income. Some of these patients received financial assistance from the asylum charity fund, started in the 1850s to help impoverished middle-class, genteel individuals avoid the stigma of pauperism.

20. *24th Royal Edinburgh Asylum Annual Report*, 1836, LHSA LHB7/7/4, 6.

21. Thompson, *op. cit.* (note 17), 243.

22. The high proportion of Orcadian patients resident in West House arose from an agreement made in 1842 with Mr Balfour of Trinsby, Orkney, whereby in return for his own donation of £200 and two others of £150 and £50, the asylum would receive 'all the insane poor of Orkney for ever, to be maintained at the lowest rate of Board'. See E. Catford, 'Draft History of the Royal Edinburgh Hospital, 1774 to 1856', LHSA GD12/1, 63. This agreement remained operative for many years longer than it would otherwise have done because no district asylum was available to the parish authorities of Orkney. The link was further strengthened in 1873 when Clouston became Physician-Superintendent. Clouston was born on Orkney in 1840, into a family whose heritage stretched back twenty-four generations.

23. *73rd Royal Edinburgh Asylum Annual Report,* 1885, LHSA LHB7/7/9, 18.

24. See, for example, D. Bennett, 'Work and Occupation for the Mentally Ill', in H. Freeman and G. Berrios (eds), *150 Years of British Psychiatry, Volume II: The Aftermath* (London: Athlone, 1996), 193.

25. Cited in L. Ray, 'Models of Madness in Victorian Asylum Practice', *European Journal of Sociology,* 22 (1981), 229–64: 256–7.

26. *69th Royal Edinburgh Asylum Annual Report,* 1881, LHSA LHB7/7/8, 53.

27. Thompson, *op. cit.* (note 17), 123.

28. See A. Beveridge, 'Life in the Asylum: Patients' Letters from Morningside, 1873–1908', *History of Psychiatry,* 9 (1998), 431–69: 432.

29. M. Thompson, 'The Wages of Sin: The Problem of Alcoholism and General Paralysis in Nineteenth-Century Edinburgh', in W. Bynum, R. Porter and M. Shepherd (eds), *The Anatomy of Madness: The Asylum and Psychiatry,* Vol. III (London: Routledge, 1988), 123.

30. M. Barfoot, 'Love's Labours Lost: The Work, Exercise and Health of Pauper Inmates of Nineteenth Century Scottish Asylums', Scottish Labour History Society, Edinburgh, 1997, unpublished conference paper, 12.

31. Andrews and Smith, *op. cit.* (note 15), 18. See, also, A. Digby, 'Moral Treatment at the Retreat, 1796–1846', in W. Bynum, R. Porter and M. Shepherd (eds), *The Anatomy of Madness: Institutions and Society,* Vol. II (London: Routledge, 1985), 52–72; R. Porter, *Mind-Forg'd Manacles: A History of Madness in England from the Restoration to the Regency* (London: Athlone Press, 1987), 222–8.

32. Crichton Royal was the exception here.

33. Rice, *op. cit.* (note 1), 486.

34. In 1823, Sir Alexander Morison had approached Edinburgh University to create a chair in mental diseases, with himself as the occupant. The request was rejected and similar approaches by Morison to the REA, the Royal College of Physicians and the Town Council also failed. Undeterred, Morison went ahead anyway with a lecture course and has since been given

credit for instituting the first course of formal lectures in mental diseases in
Britain.

35. The MPA was created to represent the professional interests of alienists and
to improve the plight of the mentally ill. It founded the *Journal of Mental
Science* to facilitate communication between British alienists. However, very
few Scottish alienists became members, so it was decided to establish a
specifically Scottish branch in order to improve recruitment, of which W.A.F.
Browne became the first Secretary.

36. See G. Robertson, 'The Hospitalisation of the Scottish Asylum System',
1922, LHSA LHB7/14/10.

37. 'Obituary of George Matthew Robertson', *Lancet*, 1 (1932), 805–8: 805.
From its opening, Jordanburn was run in conjunction with the Mental Out-
Patient Clinic at the Royal Edinburgh Infirmary, a clinic which opened in
1923 upon Robertson's appointment as first occupant of the post of
Physician-Consultant in Psychiatry to the Infirmary. See, also, 'Obituary of
George Robertson', *Edinburgh Medical Journal*, 39:6 (1932), 397–404: 401.

38. See, for example, J. Andrews, 'A Failure to Flourish? David Yellowlees and
the Glasgow School of Psychiatry', parts 1 and 2, *History of Psychiatry*, 8
(1997), 177–212; A. Beveridge, 'Thomas Clouston and the Edinburgh
School of Psychiatry', in G. Berrios and H. Freeman (eds), *150 Years of
British Psychiatry, 1841–1991* (London: Gaskell, 1991), 359–88; F. Fish,
'David Skae, MD, FRCS, Founder of the Edinburgh School of Psychiatry',
Medical History, 9 (1965), 36–53.

39. These figures are given in the annual reports, of which there is a complete
run for this period.

40. The 1907 drop was due largely to the transfer of a large number of the rate-
paid patients to the district asylum at Bangour. The 1915 rise in admissions
was a war-time measure which temporarily reclaimed Bangour patients while
that institution was taken over by the War Office as a military hospital. The
1923 drop in admissions was due to the ending of this arrangement.

41. William Stark came from Dunfermline, Scotland. He had, by 1814,
established a great reputation as an architect, although he had never before
designed a hospital or asylum. His reputation instead rested on such
buildings as the interior of Glasgow Cathedral, the old Hunterian Museum
and St George's Tron Church.

42. Stark's Asylum appears to have been the first example of the Panopticon
Model being employed within British asylum design. Placed at the
institution's centre was an octagon, covered with a circular attic. Four oblong
wings, three stories in height, were attached to the octagon and radiated
obliquely outwards in opposite directions like the spokes of a wheel.

43. Rice, *op. cit.* (note 1), 378.

44. For further details of Gartnavel's changing environment, see Andrews and Smith, *op. cit.* (note 15), 25–9.

45. Rice, *op. cit.* (note 1), 449.

46. These included the erection of new boundary walls and an entrance gate, a cottage for patients suffering from infectious diseases and the complete installation of electric lighting, as well as the creation of a Reserve Fund to meet emergencies and pensions.

47. Andrews and Smith, *op. cit.* (note 15), 6–9.

48. Andrews, *op. cit.* (note 11), 207–8.

49. *67th Glasgow Royal Asylum Annual Report*, 1880, NHSGGCA13B/2/221, 10.

50. *84th Glasgow Royal Asylum Annual Report*, 1897, NHSGGCA13B/2/221, 11.

51. However, as Andrews points out, the total exclusion of paupers from Gartnavel was merely a realisation of earlier admission policies. Long before the 1870s, the asylum had been choosy about pauper admissions. While private cases were rarely turned away, paupers who were destructive, pregnant, chronic, moribund or infectious were frequently refused entry or quickly discharged. See Andrews, *op. cit.* (note 11), 208–9.

52. However, they did not replace tradesmen in the asylum – by 1845, resident tradesmen with their own workshops included a weaver, tailor, shoemaker and carpenter. See Andrews and Smith, *op. cit.* (note 15), 36.

53. *Ibid.*, 56–7.

54. *69th Glasgow Royal Asylum Annual Report*, 1882, NHSGGCA13B/2/221, 11.

55. *68th Glasgow Royal Asylum Annual Report*, 1881, NHSGGCA13B/2/221, 12.

56. Andrews and Smith, *op. cit.* (note 15), 35.

57. Rice, *op. cit.* (note 1), 486.

58. Andrews and Smith, *op. cit.* (note 15), 52.

59. J. Andrews and I. Smith, 'The Evolution of Psychiatry in Glasgow During the Nineteenth and Early Twentieth Centuries', in Freeman and Berrios, *op. cit.* (note 24), 310.

60. D. Henderson, *The Evolution of Psychiatry in Scotland* (Edinburgh: E. and S. Livingstone, 1964), 65.

61. Indeed, the success of this venture stands in marked contrast to the corresponding situation in Edinburgh. Calls there for a psychiatric clinic dated back to the 1870s and culminated in a concerted effort in 1902 by the city's most prominent alienists which failed to convince the managers of the Edinburgh Royal Infirmary. Thus, while Edinburgh alienists had to rely on teaching at the REA and an extramural clinic thirty-five miles away in

Stirling, the asylums of Glasgow could call upon the services of a centrally based out-patient clinic.

62. During this time he had the opportunity not only of conducting innovative clinical and pathological work but also of studying at first hand the methods of the care and treatment of the insane and the general administration, particularly of the New York State Hospital system, which at that time was considered to be unrivalled. See 'Obituary of D.K. Henderson', *British Medical Journal*, 1 (1965), 1194.

63. Andrews and Smith, *op. cit.* (note 15), 84–5.

64. Andrews and Smith, *op. cit.* (note 59), 313.

65. These figures are given in the annual reports, of which there is a complete run over this period.

66. G. Hutton, *Woodilee Hospital, 125 Years* (Glasgow: Greater Glasgow Health Board, 1997), 61.

67. *Ibid.*, 14.

68. 'Glasgow District Asylum, Woodilee, Lenzie: General Management of the Asylum, and General Rules for the Guidance of Attendants', 1900, NHSGGCA30/8/3, 3.

69. *23rd Commissioners of Lunacy for Scotland Annual Report*, 1881, NHSGGCA13B/14/59, xxiii.

70. Hutton, *op. cit.* (note 66), 52.

71. For a more comprehensive discussion of this Scheme, see E. Halliday, 'Themes in Scottish Asylum Culture: The Hospitalisation of the Scottish Asylum, 1880–1914', PhD thesis, University of Stirling (2003), Ch. 5.

72. Hutton, *op. cit.* (note 66), 65.

73. *13th Board of Control for Scotland Annual Report*, 1926, NHSGGCA13B/14/71, xxxi.

74. Hutton, *op. cit.* (note 66), 65.

75. Andrews and Smith, *op. cit.* (note 59), 314.

76. 'Obituary of Hamilton Marr', *British Medical Journal*, 1 (1936), 1234–5.

77. 'Obituary: Late Dr Henry Carre', *Scotsman*, 17 June 1947.

78. Andrews and Smith, *op. cit.* (note 59), 315–6.

79. Annual reports for this institution are not available after 1920 and are not complete for the period from 1880 to 1920. However, the 1920 Report provides a retrospective overview of the asylum admission figures from 1875.

80. The 1894 influx was due in part to the expulsion of pauper lunatics from the neighbouring Gartnavel asylum. Furthermore, two new 'chronic' blocks were completed and opened that year in Woodilee which provided extended accommodation for 850 patients. The reasons for the 1915 influx are less clear, although the wartime movement of patients is a likely explanation.

81. *1st Annual Report of the Midlothian and Peebles District Board of Lunacy*, 1871, LHSA LHB33/2/1, 4.

82. *10th Annual Report of the Midlothian and Peebles District Board of Lunacy*, 1894, LHSA LHB33/2/1, 16.

83. *18th Annual Report of the Midlothian and Peebles District Board of Lunacy*, 1902, LHSA LHB33/2/1, 27.

84. *4th Annual Report of the Midlothian and Peebles District Board of Lunacy*, 1883–8, LHSA LHB33/2/1, 25.

85. *3rd Annual Report of the Midlothian and Peebles District Board of Lunacy*, 1880–3, LHSA LHB33/2/1, 20.

86. *11th Annual Report of the Midlothian and Peebles District Board of Lunacy*, 1895, LHSA LHB33/2/1, 24.

87. *4th Annual Report of the Midlothian and Peebles District Board of Lunacy*, 1883–8, LHSA LHB33/2/1, 6.

88. The 'total admission' figures are taken from the annual reports. However, neurosyphilitic admission figures are not recorded in these reports, so that reliance here has been placed on the case notes.

89. The sharp rise around 1902 was claimed to be due to a 'fair increase in the number of private patients' as the 'merits and excellent accommodation of the asylum bec[a]me known'. See *18th Annual Report of the Midlothian and Peebles District Board of Lunacy*, 1902, LHSA LHB33/2/1, 7. During the war years, Bangour Asylum and Larbert Asylum in the Stirling District were converted into a military and naval hospital respectively, and the staff of Rosslynlee were asked to take in all patients from certain parishes in the Stirling District.

90. Andrews, *op. cit.* (note 38).

91. Andrews and Smith, *op. cit.* (note 59), 314.

3

Clinical Diagnosis

The diagnosis of the neurosyphilitic disorders evolved during the late nineteenth and early twentieth centuries, and ultimately the most statistically significant category, namely general paralysis of the insane (GPI), was differentiated both from the other neurosyphilitic diseases and from diseases such as alcoholic insanity and mania. Chapter 4 will assess the impact of the laboratory upon diagnosis in the second and third decades of the twentieth century, whereas this chapter will focus particularly upon those patients who were admitted to the Scottish asylums in the three decades before 1910, that is, before the Wassermann test began to be employed in the diagnosis of GPI. A brief historical overview of GPI will first be provided. Its main symptoms will be outlined, and for clarity have been divided into three sections – mental, physical and physiognomonic. The concept of differential diagnosis will then be explored, given the many disorders that GPI's variety of symptoms could cause it to resemble. Finally, the clinical identity of GPI will be considered more generally for this period.

General paralysis of the insane

GPI first appears to have been reported in Paris during the Napoleonic Wars.[1] In 1816, the French alienist Jean-Étienne Esquirol (1772–1840) noted that the majority of a series of 230 patients who were suffering from dementia were also afflicted with paralysis. The frequent incidence of paralytic symptoms among the insane, as well as the dismal prognosis associated with a diagnosis of paralysis, were thus already well known when the French physician Antoine-Laurent-Jesse Bayle (1799–1858) first announced his views on paralysis in his medical thesis of 1822.[2] Under the name 'arachnitis chronique', he described cases of what, by the 1830s, was known as 'general paralysis of the insane'. He rejected Esquirol's view that paralysis was a complication of insanity and postulated instead that paralysis and mental disorder were related symptoms of a definite disease caused by inflammation of the meninges of the brain (chronic arachnitis).[3] Bayle was henceforth credited with establishing GPI as a definite pathological entity.

The identification of GPI as a distinct disease category was the achievement of a small group of French alienists. During these early decades of the nineteenth century, the mindset of most British physicians appears to have been characterised by a comparative lack of appreciation for the significance of this disease. Indeed, this national difference may help to explain the divergence between the recorded incidence of GPI in the asylums of Paris and its novelty and comparative infrequency in Britain until the mid-nineteenth century. Esquirol was convinced that once British alienists 'learned better to distinguish the symptoms of paralysis which complicate insanity', they would find as many insane paralytics as there were in Paris.[4] In fact, in what he claimed to be the first monograph written on this disease by a British author, Thomas Austin argued in 1859 that GPI had 'doubtless existed from the earliest period of insanity' and simply 'eluded observation'.[5] The majority of British alienists appear to have argued that they had to 'learn to see' GPI, and that this unfamiliar disease had probably been significantly under-recognised in their own country. John Conolly, for example, claimed that he had never noticed a case of it until he visited Charenton, at which point he began increasingly to observe the disease back in Britain.[6] Careless classification in public asylums was commonly blamed for this lack of recognition, as well as the common refusal of private asylum keepers to admit paralysed patients whom they regarded as incurable.[7]

This phenomenon was noted similarly by Scottish physicians. W.A.F. Browne, Commissioner in Lunacy, stated that he 'saw the disease' in Paris in 1832, 'but did not recognise it in [Scotland] till 1839'.[8] According to the clinician–historian and epidemiologist Edward Hare, GPI became fairly commonly diagnosed in Edinburgh and Glasgow soon after.[9] Indeed, the proportion of Scottish asylum deaths deemed due to GPI in the period from 1858 to 1895 was given as 19.2 per cent in males and 4.7 per cent in females.[10] Having said that, outside Edinburgh and Glasgow, the disease appears to have remained rare or unknown for many years. The Edinburgh alienist David Skae (1814–73) related that a former pupil of his, who had been well acquainted with the disease in Edinburgh, could not find a single case among the 300 patients of the Montrose Asylum; while during the years 1869 to 1872, Batty Tuke discovered only four cases amongst 200 admissions to the Fife and Kinross Asylum.[11] As late as 1879, the English alienist Henry Maudsley (1835–1918) remarked that GPI was 'hardly ever met with in the highlands of Scotland'; while the 1893 annual report for Inverness District Asylum claimed that GPI was still 'practically unknown'.[12] Chapter 6 will explore why this disease may have been confined largely to the urban centres of Scotland or, at least, more commonly diagnosed there.

Until at least the 1860s, alienists in Britain and France grappled with the question of how insanity was related to the physical symptoms of GPI, and continued actively to negotiate its exact mental and physical parameters.[13] Nonetheless, by the late 1860s, British alienists seem to have accepted it as a distinctive disease with an identifiable brain pathology, predictable clinical history and a definite correlation between these two elements. This was acknowledged by the Medico–Psychological Association in 1869, when they endorsed a decision made by the International Congress of Alienists that GPI was 'a distinct morbid entity, and not at all... a complication, a termination of insanity'.[14] This viewpoint was soon reflected in medical textbooks; Bucknill and Tuke, for example, listing GPI as a complication in 1862, but a separate disease in 1874.[15]

Scottish physicians appear to have been more divided over the kind of insanity implicated in GPI. David Skae, Physician-Superintendent of the REA from 1846 to 1873, preferred to view the disease as a form of paralysis complicated with insanity.[16] Alternatively, Thomas Clouston, his successor from 1873 to 1908, did not attach insanity necessarily to GPI. His Gartnavel equivalent, David Yellowlees, was not disposed to go quite so far as Clouston, but nevertheless agreed to an extent. He said of some general paralytics: 'Look out for that man's mind, I do think it will go', but in other cases, 'you knew the man was unwell, yet his condition was such that you could not say there was anything insane about him.'[17] However, as Skae and Clouston concluded, the question of whether GPI was 'paralysis complicated with insanity, or a form of insanity complicated with paralysis' was 'a mistake entirely'. Whilst it might begin as either, it was 'always both at the end' of the patient's life, assuming that the patient lived long enough for the disease to run its full course.[18]

As British alienists began to unify behind the theory that GPI exemplified the alliance of physical and mental symptoms, they increasingly held it up as the best scientific model of mental disease. At this time, alienists were employing the French symptomatological method of classification proposed by Pinel and Esquirol. However, through the 1860s and 1870s, they began to debate the possibility of employing alternative and more rigorous forms of psychiatric classification. David Skae embarked upon one of the most ambitious critiques of the Pinel–Esquirol 'citadel',[19] in attempting to found an alternative 'somato–aetiological' classification based upon the natural history and causation of mental diseases.[20] Skae argued that symptomatological classification was inappropriate because the same physical disorder could cause quite different mental symptoms in different patients. Instead, through his own classificatory scheme, he attempted to correlate mental disorder with any accompanying physical affection, based on the contemporary belief that insanity was determined by some degree of bodily impairment.[21] Indeed, he presented GPI as the best model for this new 'rational and practical method of classification' since 'its natural history, including its symptomatology, progress, terminations, and pathology' were 'perhaps more complete than that of any other form of insanity'.[22]

Although Skae claimed that his classificatory scheme constituted his major contribution to psychiatry, it was in fact quickly subjected to a barrage of criticism, and does not appear to have been seriously employed by any other asylum.[23] The most scathing opposition came from James Crichton Browne (1840–1938), the distinguished Edinburgh-born alienist and Medical Director of the West Riding Asylum at Wakefield, who deemed the system 'philosophically unsound, scientifically inaccurate and practically useless'.[24] This attack by a former pupil and friend of Skae's led Clouston to counter-attack in a defence of the scheme, though with little success. Clouston argued that its greatest merit was as an aid to the physician 'in his efforts to discover the causes of the insanity' and 'in his treatment and prognosis'; and that 'no other mode of assorting mental diseases does half as much for us in these respects as Skae's'.[25] Clouston noted that it was also 'eminently British in character, not being strictly logical and consistent, or altogether scientific, but yet most practical and helpful to the practitioner of medicine'.[26] He continued to defend it into the 1890s.

Clouston also supported Skae's characterisation of GPI as the key to the future of psychiatry. Indeed, he largely rebutted Crichton Browne's charges by employing GPI as a test case, asking:

> Does he deny that General Paralysis... is a true cerebro–mental disease, a distinct clinical, symptomatological, and pathological reality?... The most distinct, the most real, the most undisputed, the truest cerebro–mental disease... cannot be provided for in [Esquirol's symptomatic] classification that he defends.[27]

Clouston argued that GPI was therefore 'by far the best justification' for the adoption of Skae's scheme, which aimed to distinguish 'the true diseases affecting the cerebral convolutions' rather than 'merely ticketing groups of similar symptoms with a name'.[28] Furthermore, Clouston had great faith that other mental diseases would ultimately be revealed to be as unique as GPI:

> Did we know everything about general paralysis and epilepsy, we should find the path of research into most other diseases of the nervous system comparatively easy. They would be the key to all the rest.... It is quite certain that under the term insanity there are included many pathological species of brain disease, just as distinct as general paralysis, which we shall ultimately be able to segregate and distinguish.[29]

Although the belief that GPI might prove the organic insanity *par excellence* was mooted more widely at this time, alienists were vague in such discussions and tended, instead, to focus upon the natural history of the disease – the collection of features which provided its unique identity.

By the mid-nineteenth century, medical textbooks provided a consistent but very lengthy list of those physical and mental symptoms which were considered characteristic of GPI, as will be discussed more fully below.[30] In comparison with its manifold symptoms, the progression of the disease was considered to be straightforward. Bayle described it as a disease of three stages. While some medical writers quickly rejected his rather rigid delineation,[31] Clouston seems to have reflected the view of the majority of British practitioners in embracing this stadial approach. His *Unsoundness of Mind* detailed the three stages fairly thoroughly, based upon decades of asylum observation.[32] In the first stage, patients would exhibit slight defects of speech, unco-ordinated facial muscles, eye irregularities and mental exaltation, to the point where the insidiously advancing mental symptoms became so evident as to convince the patient's friends of his madness. Unless the patient died of exhaustion or convulsions, he passed into the second stage of GPI, which Clouston argued was characterised by increased muscular incoordination, paralysis and mental enfeeblement. By this stage, patients were generally incontinent and suffered from pronounced delusions of grandeur. The final stage was said to be one of fairly complete paralysis and 'mental extinction'. Death might occur during an epileptic or apoplectic seizure, from asphyxia in paralysis or from acute lung disease, although slow decay and final exhaustion was said to be the cause of death in the majority of cases. Thus, the course of GPI was seen to be one of steady and progressive mental and physical deterioration. However, Clouston also argued that the course of the disease and its prevalent symptoms were 'very much influenced by the cause'. Thus, cases caused by excessive drinking exhibited 'much more acute and delirious excitement, a higher temperature, and a slower course'.[33]

Mental symptoms

The most documented symptom of GPI was probably the delusions, particularly the classical grandiose type. Such delusions typically related to ideas of importance, benevolence, and wealth. Even the most austere Physician-Superintendent might find himself warming towards a patient who, as Skae described, 'offers a cheque for £75,000 for the purchase of the asylum and promises to endow it with unbounded munificence, and to convert it into a paradise of brilliancy and bliss'.[34] Grandiose delusions tended to indicate the patient's weakness of mind and lack of insight into his own condition. In fact, when this symptom was absent in a patient, the physician seems often to have felt it necessary to draw attention to this fact. For example, John R., a 45-year-old married ship's captain, admitted to the REA in August 1897, was 'a case of GP without the usual expansive delusions'.[35] Similarly, Alexander H., a 32-year-old single mason, admitted in April 1894, had 'some unmistakable [physical] signs of GP... but emotionally he is depressed and has no exaltation'.[36]

Much more typical were said to be those patients who exhibited delusions of grandeur. James S. of Gartnavel, a 40-year-old married beer merchant:

> [Had] been buying great quantities of childrens' toys and fruit and... trinkets for his own adornment and when he arrived here he had a telescope and some other useless articles and indeed his whole aspect, his well pleased, contented, happy manner, his unconcern and his expansive ideas suggested at once General Paresis.[37]

Similarly, Robert I. of Woodilee, a 48-year-old married farm labourer, had 'delusions such as that America belongs to him because he bought it'.[38] William M., a 44-year-old married patient, had 'married 500 women or "slept 80 hours" nearly every morning; he speaks all the languages; in fact he "made" them; then he mutters inarticulately and calls it Japanese'.[39] John N., a 35-year-old married miner, had the '[d]elusion that he is related to the Queen. Says he intends to steal the Kohinoor diamond sell it and drink the proceeds.'[40] Alexander W., a 30-year-old single physician, admitted to Gartnavel in May 1898, was:

> [F]ull of delusions of grandeur. Believes that he has a practice worth ten millions a year – that he can give people new brains, lungs and bodies. That he has abolished death from the works: that he is himself the almighty: that he rules the world as Emperor of all the countries. Every other statement he makes is equally exaggerated and ludicrously unfounded in fact.[41]

It is later noted in the case notes of this patient, and not without irony, that he claimed to be 'able to remove the brain if diseased and to substitute another'.

However, general paralytics might alternatively be admitted suffering from delusions and hallucinations of suspicion or persecution. Elizabeth I., a 40-year-old married domestic, admitted to Woodilee in September 1905, 'says people come through the wall at night – when she lights the lamp they disappear'.[42] James Y., a 40-year-old married cloth inspector, 'imagines that he has been poisoned, that his father, mother, wife and other friends have a plot against his life'.[43] Alexander G., a 45-year-old single labourer, admitted to the REA in June 1883, '[t]hinks the clinical thermometer is an instrument meant to kill him, is full of suspicion regarding everyone about him, and thinks they are going to injure him in some way.'[44] Finally, Robert D., a 45-year-old married waiter, admitted in July 1896, was 'suspicious of his wife but this may have a sound origin', according to the admitting physician of the asylum.[45] Patients less commonly felt that they had done harm to others, such as Robert N., a 50-year-old widower, admitted to Woodilee in December 1896, who 'imagines that he has killed many people, that they are looking at him through the wall'.[46]

The devil figured prominently in a number of these delusions of persecution. William S., a 46-year-old married fishing tackle maker, admitted to the REA in June 1889, '[c]omplains of being tormented by devils and supposes his wife to be in league with them.'[47] John S., a 33-year-old single commercial traveller, admitted in August 1881, '[s]ays that "devils" come and beat him; that he is made of diamonds; that he changes his flesh every few weeks, and that yesterday walked 60 miles.'[48] James E., a 35-year-old married miner, admitted in October 1897, '[s]aw the devil under the bed – "the man with cloven feet".'[49]

There were, in addition, the mental symptoms relating to the 'dementia' of 'dementia paralytica', particularly loss of short-term memory. While remote events might still be recounted with accuracy until the later stages of the disease, recent events would be quickly forgotten, such as the fact that the patient had just eaten his dinner. Susan N. of Gartnavel, a 43-year-old married housekeeper '[h]ad no memory for time and did not know the day of the week.'[50] William Y., a 34-year-old single watchmaker and scientific instrument maker, 'does not know the year he was born and says this is 1899 when told he was wrong says it is 1999'.[51] Although the patient might behave erratically, his personality usually remained intact for a considerable length of time, during which routine duties could be carried out.

Extreme restlessness was another common symptom. Such patients were very troublesome to nurse 'on account of their restless, aimless, and purposeless excursions about the room'.[52] Mary D., a 35-year-old married lady, admitted to Gartnavel in December 1882, was '[r]estless, excited and very incoherent, could not answer the simplest question and was altogether in a very helpless condition.'[53] Allied to this, patients could be destructive and dirty in their habits, tearing their clothes and breaking windows and furniture. John S., a 36-year-old married bookbinder, admitted to the REA in December 1880, was 'very restless, noisy and destructive at nights, tearing his blankets into fragments and scattering about the contents of his mattress…. Has been smashing windows lately.'[54] The emotional side of the general paralytic might also be exaggerated and restless. There was perceived to be a noticeable disposition to indulge in fits of crying at unexpected moments. Alexander N., a 51-year-old married former umbrella manufacturer, was '[v]ery emotional and cries because as he says God will not give him all he wants.'[55] Similarly, Jane L., a 42-year-old single domestic servant, admitted to Rosslynlee in September 1905, was '[m]orbidly emotional and has great fits of weeping'.[56]

Finally, a prominent mental symptom related to GPI was larceny and the hoarding of other peoples' belongings. In their enfeebled state, general paralytics might collect other people's goods, or simply rubbish such as old bread crusts, imagining them to be valuable items. Thus, James E., a 40-year-old married tailor, admitted to Rosslynlee in July 1908, '[a]dmits picking up rags and handkerchiefs off the street and bringing them home and using them.'[57] Such patients had a reputation for being foolish and unmalicious thieves who would make no attempt to conceal their crimes, and who tended to hand back stolen items with good humour if challenged. Nonetheless, prior to being admitted to the asylum or diagnosed a general paralytic, such patients might get into trouble over such actions. An article in the *Journal of Mental Science* for 1873 documents six cases in which 'general paralytics had committed theft after the onset of the disease, and had, consequently, suffered a greater or less term of imprisonment, the disease remaining unrecognised both before the trial and for some considerable time afterwards'.[58] J. Burman, Resident Medical Officer and Superintendent of the Wilts County Lunatic Asylum, had to demonstrate that this was merely an early symptom of their disease, given their previous good character and absence of any reasonable motive for the crime. Burman noted that it was not difficult to understand a paralytic's propensity to steal given the abnormal exaggeration of his ideas as to wealth and property, and 'the blunting of the reasoning faculties and inability to properly comprehend consequences'.[59]

Such a symptom might explain why the admission certificates of sixteen of the sample of Scottish patients refer explicitly to a police station or prison. Robert E., a 32-year-old single fireman, had been imprisoned in Barlinnie prison for theft before being certified insane and transferred to the asylum.[60] William E., a 36-year-old married tailor, was nearly arrested but then seen to be a general paralytic and admitted to Woodilee instead.[61] John D., a 30-year-old single sailor and labourer, was apprehended by the police for a different reason. His delusions caused him to throw a stone through the window of a house, under the impression that the owner had been tormenting him. The patient was transferred from the police station to the REA.[62] Similarly, Alexander Y., a 38-year-old married moulder, 'fell into the hands of the police through disorderly conduct', and was said to be 'somewhat excitable, noisy and resistive'.[63]

Physical symptoms

The most important physical diagnostic sign of GPI was generally acknowledged to be the fully developed Argyll–Robertson phenomenon, or complete loss of the light reaction in one or both eyes.[64] Although normal pupils were present in up to ten per cent of early cases, by the late stage of the illness almost all paralytics were expected to display pupillary abnormalities.[65] For example, James C., a 39-year-old single labourer, admitted to the REA in June 1890, had 'pupils... very variable and abnormal – often unequal and irregular in shape'.[66] With Elizabeth I., a 40-year-old married domestic, admitted to Woodilee in the same month, the 'pupillary phenomenon' were stated simply to be 'rather striking'.[67]

Another distinctive physical symptom of the disease was said to be impairment in articulation. The patient would often 'speak thick', slur or mumble certain words, as though intoxicated. One medical commentator claimed that this disorder of speech was so typical that a correct diagnosis could often be made as the patient talked, and this defect certainly seems to have been one of the main physical symptoms on which alienists depended in diagnosing GPI.[68] Although this symptom could often be recognised simply during a conversation with the patient, the physical examination of a patient upon admission to the asylum appears often to have included test phrases such as 'British Constitution', 'Methodist Episcopal Church', 'Electricity' and 'Hippopotamus', which alienists deliberately encouraged the patient to repeat in a bid to reveal the disturbance. If asked to say 'trigonometrical', for example, a patient would tend to say 'trigomometrical' or 'trigonometical' instead. As the disease progressed further, medical textbooks claimed that the patient would generally become unable to form sentences, with speech being completely unintelligible by the terminal stage.

This symptom was understood to be so characteristic of GPI that a common phrase found in the Scottish case notes is simply 'speech like a GPI'. In only a small proportion of the case notes were the articulation difficulties more fully described. The speech of Margaret S. of the REA, a 44-year-old married housewife, 'resembles that of GP, she can only use a few words eg. "fine" – in answer to "how are you?"'[69] Susan Y., a 43-year-old married housewife, had '[s]peech very markedly hesitating and slurring (GP) and characteristic whining tone, eg. himapomatomusis (hippopotamus): general palal-I-silus.'[70] Robert L., a 36-year-old single labourer, had '[a]rticulation very thick, slurred and hesitating, just like that of an advanced case of General Paralysis.'[71] Alexander E., a 38-year-old single theatrical manager, admitted to Gartnavel in October 1895, had an affection of his speech, 'phrases such as "The National Hospital for the Paralysed and Epileptic" being to him an utter impossibility.'[72] Finally, William L. of the REA, a 33-year-old married clerk, was '[v]ery reticent, but when he does speak the tremulous character of his articulation is very striking. When asked how he is says f-f-f-ine in a stuttery way very like a general paralytic.'[73]

This trembling was a more widespread tendency. The lips, for example, might quiver 'not unlike those of a person about to burst into passionate weeping'.[74] A fine or coarse rapid tremor, particularly of the extended fingers, tongue and facial muscles, was often present. When the tongue was protruded, it had a tendency to tremble or waver from side to side. James H., a 36-year-old single saddler, had: 'Lips very tremulous, so that the disease is probably general paralysis.'[75] Similarly, Robert R., a 26-year-old single brewer's labourer, had the statement recorded in his case notes: 'His pupils and lips present no symptoms of paresis or incoordination but his tongue is tremulous. The tremors suggest GP.'[76] William D., a 40-year-old married retired wine and spirit merchant had 'marked tremor of the arms, legs and tongue indicative of General Paralysis'.[77] Finally, John E., a 49-year-old widowed retired sea captain, admitted in June 1892, had 'a marked tremor of the hands and fingers. There is no actual paralysis but a condition of general weakness. The tongue is large and flabby and very unsteady, and a finer tremor is also present in the muscle of the organ. The lips are tremulous'.[78]

Related to this, the patient's handwriting would be commonly affected, in an analogous manner to the speech. Writing was said to be unsteady, disorderly looking and lacking firmness in the lines, while the ends of the words, or whole words, were often omitted. Yet, very rarely would a patient recognise their mistakes. As the disease progressed, only an illegible scribble would be produced, as indicated by those letters of patients that were retained in the case notes and were either nonsensical or entirely indecipherable. Thus, physicians employed case-note phrases like 'the typical general paralytic calligraphy'. The handwriting of Alexander R. of the REA, a 45-year-old married ship's captain, was 'peculiar in that he leaves out words and letters'.[79] Similarly, it was said of James N. of Rosslynlee, a 57-year-old married naval seaman, that: 'In writing his letters were shaky, incomplete, disturbed and almost illegible.'[80] However, this calligraphy test was not considered to be of much diagnostic value, given that the standard of handwriting varied greatly in healthy people. As a practical test within the asylum, it might also fail due to nerves or distress suffered by the patient upon admission.

A further noticeable physical disturbance was that of gait, which usually became obvious somewhat later in the disease. This disturbance resulted in an irregular swaying walk with legs far apart, so that the patient would move in an unsteady manner like a drunken man. It was noted of Robert N. of Woodilee, a 38-year-old married carter: 'His gait is so ataxic that he is unable to walk alone. When assisted he throws his legs forward in a jerky manner and plants his feet in a very characteristic manner.'[81] The case notes of William N. of the REA, a 42-year-old married ship-carpenter, record: 'His gait is a characteristic one – he struts along piper fashion with the shoulders square.'[82] Mary S., a 44-year-old married housewife, was said to have a '[v]ery tottering gait – slightest touch sends her over.'[83] Similarly, John D., a

50-year-old married ironmonger, had a gait which was 'staggering and uncertain, resulting in minor accidents daily'.[84] In more detail, the case notes of Alexander C. of Gartnavel, a 43-year-old married house factor, record that his '[g]ait raises the question of general paralysis. He walks on a broad base and lurches a good deal, both in progression and in turning. He can stand well with his eyes shut but cannot walk on a band about four inches broad.'[85]

However, the most severe motor disturbances were almost certainly the convulsions and apoplectic phenomena which might appear at any stage of the disease, and were recorded to be present in up to sixty-five per cent of cases.[86] Elizabeth S. of Woodilee, a 40-year-old married dealer: 'Was stated by Attendant to have had two "epileptic fits", after which her speech became thick and stupid, and her pupils were found to be unequal.... The "epileptic fits" were probably congestive attacks.'[87] Such characteristic seizures sometimes led physicians to spot the other physical symptoms of GPI and to make a post-mortem diagnosis of GPI.

Finally, the patient would become bedridden, with a complete loss of intellectual and physical functions. Loss of consciousness and a series of convulsions usually signalled the end. As a typical example of a patient in the final throes of GPI, James G., a 39-year-old single coal merchant, admitted to the REA in September 1885:

> [H]as been in the third stage of the disease, completely paralysed for the last ten weeks. Two days ago was seized with congestive attacks, characterised by convulsions, at first confined to the right side, involving chiefly the upper limbs and the head which was turned to the right side and the eyes inhibited all concomitant deviation to the right: the left upper limb was afterwards convulsed also. He gradually sank and died.[88]

In a slightly less drawn-out manner, Robert N. of Rosslynlee, a 49-year-old married paper factory worker, 'had an epileptiform attack, recovering consciousness then passing into another. He had four of these altogether. He died at 11.15pm.'[89]

Physiognomy

Physiognomy, the study of human characteristics and personality based on facial configuration, had been debated for centuries, but its concepts were really formalised in the mid-eighteenth century when Johann Caspar Lavater (1741–1801), a Swiss pastor, wrote a classic German text on the subject.[90] Rees's 1819 *Cyclopaedia* defined physiognomy as 'the art of knowing the humour, temperament or dispositions of a person, from observation of the lines of his face, and the character of its members or features.'[91] By the early nineteenth century, physiognomy was becoming increasingly popular with physicians, who were employing this art to diagnose their patients, or at least

93

as an aid in seeking additional clues as to the nature of a patient's illness. Indeed, Bucknill and Tuke went so far as to claim that no physician could 'practise his art satisfactorily and successfully unless he' was a good physiognomist.[92]

While physiognomy was being seen as an aid to the study of medicine in general, Lavater had in fact recommended any student of physiognomy to commence with the insane, since they afforded 'extreme and crucial instances' of this art.[93] By the mid-nineteenth century, GPI was claimed to be one such disorder where the face of the patient clearly divulged their illness, for, as one commentator noted: 'The facial expression of the paralytic is peculiar.'[94] George Robertson, Physician-Superintendent of the REA, later defined this expression as 'somewhat expressionless and heavy'.[95] In a 1918 'Clinique', he gave a fairly fulsome description of those aspects of the general paralytic's appearance that he considered characteristic of the disease:

> There is a stolid vacancy and a want of play of feature which, though not obtrusive symptoms, are, when attention has been called to them, very remarkable and easy of recognition. Though the patient is frequently agitated by the most stormy passions; though his delusions, whether of exaltation or depression, are peculiarly calculated to leave their impress on the face; yet it remains comparatively unmoved during moments or hours, while fury or maniacal joy, moroseness or depression, are only too evident from the actions, the gestures, or the language of the patient. The mouth, which contributed so much to the variety and colouring of expression, remains nearly fixed, and the whole muscular machinery of facial expression is quiescent, and apparently incapable of being again set in motion by the ideas. The paralytic's lower jaw may descend in the act of laughing, but the reverse of Sardinian laughter is the result; he laughs with his heart, but hardly with his face.[96]

While most GPI textbooks published in the nineteenth and early twentieth centuries contain a small section devoted to the facial attributes of general paralytics,[97] none appear to give so much diagnostic importance to GPI physiognomy as does an article by David Skae. He claimed that general paralytics always had a peculiar expression of the countenance:

> [S]o peculiar and so easy to recognise, when frequently seen, and so very characteristic of the disease, that any one who has had a few years' experience among the insane could pronounce upon the existence of general paralysis from the aspect of the face alone.[98]

Image 3.1 shows Alexander Morison's portrait of a 36-year-old male in the final stage of general paralysis.[99]

Image 3.1

Alexander Morison's Portrait of a Man in the Final Stage of General Paralysis,
c.1840. Courtesy of the Royal College of Physicians of Edinburgh.

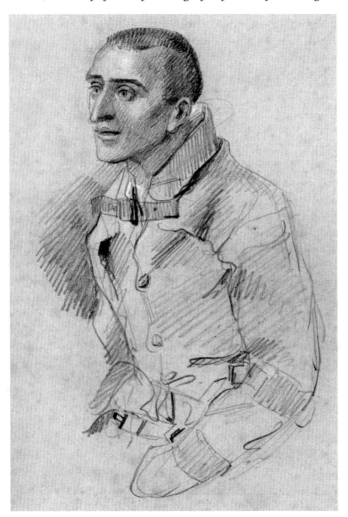

Although mental and physical symptoms clearly formed the central basis
of the diagnostic process within Scottish asylums during the late nineteenth
and early twentieth centuries, the diagnostic potential of the face was also
discussed to some degree. Under the 'State on Admission' section of each
asylum's case notes was the heading 'Appearance', which sometimes

contained comments on the general look or physiognomy of the patient, as might the admission certificates. The admission certificates of twenty-two GPI patients admitted to Woodilee (ten per cent) made reference to their appearance or expression, with descriptive phrases such as 'vacant', 'dull' and 'foolish'. In Rosslynlee, thirty-seven patients (twenty per cent) had their appearance or expression noted in the admission certificates, usually being described as 'wild', 'vacant', or 'dazed'. The 'physical state on admission' part of the case notes also contained numerous references to the 'wiped out' nature of the patient, held to be a typical GPI facet. For example, William P., a 48-year-old married labourer, admitted in August 1891, was 'dull, heavy, confused: partly "obliterated"'.[100] John M., a 32-year-old married soldier, had a 'dull "wiped out" expression', while Alexander L., a 45-year-old married millworker, had a 'somewhat washed out expression'.[101]

Ten of the patients admitted to Gartnavel (six per cent) with GPI had their general appearance noted on their admission certificates as a reason for admission. It was recorded in the case notes of James D., a 38-year-old married telegraphist in the General Post Office: 'There is no doubt that he is suffering from General Paralysis. In the first place he has the look of a general paralytic.'[102] When Robert N., a 33-year-old married marine engineer, was admitted in February 1908, his face was said to exhibit 'something of the mask like appearance'.[103] Finally, at the REA, as many as eighty-one neurosyphilitic patients (twenty-two per cent) were admitted with their expression or appearance noted as constituting a sign of insanity. This included the appearance of imbecility, melancholia, insanity or facility. However, more peculiar to GPI, John M., a 60-year-old single blacksmith, was 'expressionless' on admission.[104]

Clinical photography

Physiognomy had, therefore, the potential to be a useful diagnostic tool for physicians when completing the asylum admission certificates or providing the initial diagnosis upon a patient's admission to the asylum. However, it was difficult to incorporate this into the asylum documentation or published literature for future reference and possible re-diagnosis. This is where clinical photography came in.[105] The medical press enthusiastically advocated photography as 'the Art of Truth', as a means of allowing physicians to freeze or copy an instant of reality in a way that had previously been impossible due to the difficulties and subjective nature of hand-made pictures.[106] From the 1850s onwards, British and American medical journals regularly carried items on photography, reporting on both technical innovations and the diagnostic potential of the device.

Hugh Welch Diamond was probably the best known practitioner of psychiatric photography in nineteenth-century Britain. He used photographs as a diagnostic tool, to document the progress of treatment, and as an *aide mémoire* of individual patients.[107] As he stated in 1856:

> Photography gives permanence to these remarkable cases, which are types of classes, and make them observable not only now but for ever, and it presents also a perfect and faithful record, free altogether from the painful caricaturing which so disfigures almost all the published portraits of the Insane as to render them nearly valueless either for purposes of art or of Science.[108]

Additionally, Diamond argued that alienists should insert a portrait photograph of each patient in their case notes as part of a thorough administrative regime. This was said to be particularly important in relation to the criminally insane so that, if a lunatic escaped, he could be traced by sending his photograph to the police.

By the 1870s, photography was being employed within Scottish psychiatry. Aware that the naturalist Charles Darwin (1809–92) had advocated the scientific study of the physiognomy of the insane, whose emotions he believed to be intense and uncontrolled and thus ideal for scientific study, James Crichton Browne, the distinguished Edinburgh-born alienist and amateur photographer, sent Darwin the photographs of some paralytics he had requested in April 1871, with an apology:

> They are, I regret to say most unsuccessful and only indicate very imperfectly the labial tremor which I have described to you. The difficulty of photographing such shaky subjects is however immense and the artist a novice.... In all those whose photographs are now forwarded to you, the exalted extravagant profusive ideas have been well marked.[109]

Such difficulties, relating specifically to this disease, would be augmented by the usual problems that could accompany photographing the insane, including difficulties with concentration and sitting still, and delusions possibly making these subjects excessively nervous or suspicious of the camera. Image 3.2, overleaf, shows a female GPI patient who was photographed at the West Riding Lunatic Asylum, near Wakefield in Yorkshire, while Crichton Browne was Physician-Superintendent (1866–76).

Nonetheless, by the late nineteenth century, the camera was being employed in Scottish asylums in relation to general paralytics. Due to its purported capacity to copy reality, this device was by now considered a way to record and document the physiognomy of the insane, which was particularly useful in the case of general paralytics with their supposedly characteristic physiognomy. It was felt that photography could aid the study of GPI by illustrating a number of key features of the disease, such as the

Image 3.2

*Woman Suffering from GPI, Attributed to Sir James Crichton-Browne,
c.1869. Courtesy of the Wellcome Library, London.*

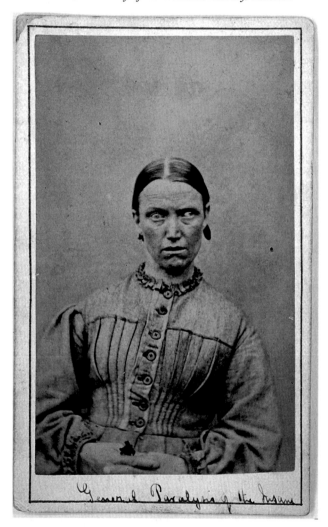

'washed out' facial appearance of the patient or the physical symptoms such
as tremors and the affected gait.

However, this use should not be exaggerated. Photography seems to have
had a very limited uptake within the four Scottish asylums, and for patients

other than the neurosyphilitics. Of the 181 Rosslynlee neurosyphilitics in my sample, only nine (five per cent) had their photograph taken and inserted into their case notes. Eight of these patients were admitted over the period from May 1893 to June 1900, with the final one admitted some time later in September 1915. Of the nine, only one was female, but this is unsurprising given that only thirty-three (eighteen per cent) in total were female. Unfortunately, no notes accompany these photographs and no mention was made of them within the annual reports or asylum minutes, so that we do not know the rationale underlying them. Two of these patients were admitted with mania, this diagnosis not being revised in the case notes until the post-mortem diagnosis. The remaining five were admitted with GPI.

In Gartnavel, an even smaller proportion of patients were photographed. A series of about nineteen photos were taken, all in 1890. This represented a broad cross-section of patients, in terms of their ages, genders and illnesses, and they were not all neurosyphilitics. The date of these photographs roughly coincides with a British Medical Association conference held in Glasgow, so they might have been taken for this specific purpose. At other times, photography had very limited use indeed in this asylum, for in no other year does it appear to feature in the case notes. This seems to tie in with the generally 'backward' nature of Gartnavel's case notes.[110]

Of the 361 REA neurosyphilitics in my sample, only twenty (six per cent) had their photograph taken and inserted into their case notes. The first of these was Margaret Y, a 43-year-old married housewife, admitted in August 1896 with GPI.[111] She had her photograph taken outdoors, probably in the hospital grounds, and was wearing fancy dress.[112] A further three general paralytics in the sample, admitted during the years 1896 and 1897, had photographs attached to their case notes. There then appears to be a gap until May 1905, when Susan A., a 44-year-old single woman, was admitted to the REA.[113] It might be noted that all five of these patients were female. A further fifteen neurosyphilitics in my sample had their photograph taken and inserted into their case notes between 1908 and 1919. These patients were of mixed gender and age. Although all twenty of these patients received a final diagnosis of GPI, their admission diagnosis was GPI in only fourteen of the cases. The remaining six patients were admitted with mania or manic-depressive insanity. Thus, there does not seem to have been one particular reason for photographing a specific patient. After all, if they were photographed because their faces revealed their GPI status, all twenty would presumably have received the diagnosis on admission, rather than having to wait until post mortem.[114]

Clearly these three asylums only made very limited use of the camera. However, the physicians of Woodilee were more exceptional in photographing almost half of their neurosyphilitics (104 of 210). The records of this institution suggest that almost all patients were routinely photographed upon admission, or at least all of those who could be made to sit still. These photographs also differ from those mentioned above, in that they are not simply portrait-style photographs. Instead, the patient is often posed beside a mirror, so that the photograph encapsulates both a front and side image of the patient. In fourteen cases, the patient's head leans against the mirror and wall, while in a further fourteen cases, the head of the patient is being held up by someone's hand, possibly a physician given that in one photograph you can see the sleeve of a white coat. These 104 patients were admitted between June 1906 and June 1928, unlike the other three institutions, whose use of photography was concentrated into two earlier decades – the 1890s and 1900s. The 104 patients were of mixed gender and age. Of these photographed neurosyphilitic patients, the vast majority were admitted with a diagnosis of GPI or juvenile GPI, except four who had to wait until post mortem for the GPI diagnosis.

Despite the systematic use of photography for Woodilee paralytics, no mention was made of it in the annual reports. As well as including photographs, the basic case-note pro forma for this institution also included a diagram of a head and ear, with notes regularly made on their shape and defining characteristics for each patient. Again, however, these diagrams were rarely incorporated into the admission and progress notes. As a result, on a practical level it is difficult to decipher exactly how much use was made of the diagrams and photographs within the asylum. There was a tendency in psychiatry to make the most of the available resources; to record what was seen and heard in an asylum, and to construct theories from such observations. These attitudes might go some way towards explaining the lasting influence of the science of physiognomy in psychiatry, or at least the continued noting of such information, even where it did not appear to be used.

Different types of GPI

The manic or expansive form of GPI was often called the 'classical' type of the disease because it was the first form to be recognised. This type was characterised by a maniacal attack involving intense feelings of joy and delusions of grandeur. The patient might believe that he was God or royalty; or that he possessed millions of pounds, many wives and businesses or properties. As the Edinburgh alienists David Skae and Thomas Clouston pointed out, such a patient would commonly be:

> [D]iverted from the highest enterprise or the most important duty by the
> simplest request; he forgets the conquest of Europe, or the immediate

commands of Her Majesty, for a walk round the airing-ground with an imbecile companion, to whom he talks condescendingly, promising him a dukedom or a bishopric.[115]

The exalted mood, absurd delusions of wealth and power, and cheerful frame of mind were said to make the diagnosis easy.[116] By 1880, this expansive form of the disease represented the usual textbook image of the general paralytic. Within the Scottish case notes, one need not look far to find examples of this form. Robert T., a 43-year-old single engineer, 'says he is God Almighty, and made me! "I made a damn'd good job of it too." He gallops round the world 4 or 5 times before dinner.'[117] William G., a 36-year-old married pedlar:

[S]tates that he is going to be one of the most outstanding stage performers in the world, which is a palpable delusion in his case. He has had a proposal of marriage from a beautiful woman, who has been so attracted by him that she offers him a dowry of £20,000 – another obvious delusion.[118]

Finally, Mary S., a 44-year-old married housewife, while not especially delusional:

[W]as very exhuberant and greeted the MO with great fervour, and straight away offered to embrace him. The offer was not accepted! She went off with the nurse to the ward, after bidding her husband an excessively affectionate adieu.[119]

General paralytics were made all the more pathetic by these grandiose notions in the face of their accompanying mental and bodily degeneration.

The depressed form of GPI, on the other hand, chiefly featured persistent depression, or at least mood fluctuations, in tandem with ideas and delusions of sin and persecution, impoverishment or hypochondriacal tendencies. A number of the Scottish general paralytics exhibited only such persecutory delusions. Some feared bodily harm to themselves, for example John Y., a 60-year-old widowed PO official, who suffered such auditory hallucinations as 'hearing by wireless that he is to be cut up'.[120] Similarly, John E., a 37-year-old single soldier, would 'not allow himself to be shaved, etc., for fear the attendants might cut his throat or drown him in his bath'.[121] Others feared for those around them, such as Robert T., a 36-year-old married soldier, who 'says that his brain has been removed and [speaks] about babies being killed'.[122] James Y., a 23-year-old single soldier, was profoundly depressed, 'weeping and moaning, and keeping clear of people in case he infects them'.[123] His capacity to 'infect' others almost certainly related to his syphilitic status, since a number of those patients who knew or at least believed themselves to be venereally diseased were said in their case notes to feel similarly dirty and infectious.

A number of the remaining Scottish paralytics exhibited a combination of expansive and depressive delusions. At Gartnavel, Alexander A., a 51-year-old married insurance agent, suffered both grandiose and persecutory delusions.[124] He believed himself to be a Lord of Balmoral and Dunblane, but also that the Gartnavel physicians wished to poison him with acid. James C., a 45-year-old single wine and spirit merchant, had an exaggerated idea of his own importance and abilities, stating 'that he has the best voice in the world, and is the world's best bridge player'.[125] However, after receiving malarial injections as a form of treatment, the delusions worsened so that he began to 'talk by wireless telephone with God, the Pope and the Chief of Dumfries Police'. It was also noted that he sat with his head hanging 'to allow the snakes and corpses in his brain to slip out through his eyes'.

While D.R. Brower and H.M. Bannister, representative of the majority of British clinicians, believed the expansive form consistently to be the typical type of GPI, L.P. Clarke and C.E. Atwood felt that the depressive form was, by the turn of the century, overtaking the grandiose form as the most popular type of the disease. They asked: 'Have the forms of GPI altered?'[126] By 1908, they claimed, only a tenth to a fifth of cases were grandiose, with the depressed type forming the majority of cases; while the German alienist Emil Kraepelin considered the depressed form to exist in more than a quarter of cases. Elsewhere, continental and Russian alienists complained that few modern writers were making a genuine attempt to differentiate types of GPI. However, it was proposed in various quarters that a considerable number of depressed and simple dementing types were being erroneously classed as melancholics and dements. This might explain why the expansive form of GPI had predominated for decades. Many depressed paralytics may have been erroneously diagnosed with another disorder simply because they did not conform to the 'classically' expansive form. In the specifically British context, Clarke and Atwood remarked that a number of writers had failed to diagnose GPI in the absence of euphoria, a view they believe to be due largely to William Julius Mickle's teaching two decades earlier.[127] Clouston himself saw the delusions of grandeur as the most striking symptom of GPI, although he noted that his predecessor, Skae, had found such a symptom in only half of the 108 Edinburgh cases he studied. Similarly, in reviewing 85 patients from a rural district outside Edinburgh, Clouston found that of the 68 men only 30, and 2 women out of 17, had exaggerated notions despite all being general paralytics.[128]

Thus, despite sharing a GPI diagnosis, it was perceived that some patients became depressed and others expansive and grandiose with approximately the same underlying organic brain damage. In fact, by the

1930s, a whole range of subtypes had begun to emerge, which were never fully defined and arguably muddied the identity of the disease. The five main subdivisions by this date were 'simple', 'demented', 'manic', 'melancholic' and 'agitated'.[129] The 'diagnosis' column of the REA admission register most clearly reflects this sub-division of GPI types in Scotland, containing, in fact, an even more complicated series of forms. Between 1909 and 1916, there were admissions of 'delusional dementia of GPI', 'general paralysis of the apathetic type', 'melancholic dementia of general paralysis', 'excited dementia of general paralysis', and 'dementia of organic brain disease (GPI)'.

Juvenile general paralysis

Until the 1870s, GPI was believed to be a disease exclusive to adults. However, in 1877, the first recorded case of 'juvenile general paralysis' was diagnosed when Thomas Clouston described the case of GPI in a boy aged sixteen, and pointed out that, both clinically and pathologically, his affliction differed in no significant way from the adult form of GPI, although the Edinburgh alienist added that this was an extremely rare occurrence in such a young patient.[130] Additional cases were subsequently reported in Germany, Austria, France, and further afield, with the disorder attracting attention from such eminent figures as Alois Alzheimer, Frederick Mott and Richard von Krafft-Ebing.[131]

Symptoms were typically seen to mimic those of adult paralytics, except perhaps that the dementia could be more severe and the course more prolonged, averaging about five years from the appearance of the initial symptoms to the fatal termination of the disease. Juvenile cases thus attracted the same bleak prognosis of progressive mental and physical deterioration. The symptoms might appear at any time after birth, although typically there were observed to be no noticeable symptoms until the child approached puberty. In terms of gender distribution, juvenile general paralysis was noted to occur with almost equal frequency in males and females, females dominating to only a slight extent, in marked contrast to the adult version of the disorder.

Juvenile GPI was estimated to constitute 1.6 to 1.8 per cent of all cases admitted to British asylums by the 1930s.[132] Within the four Scottish asylums, no cases of juvenile GPI were found in the REA sample or for the patient populations of Gartnavel and Rosslynlee. However, the Woodilee sample reveals that seven cases of juvenile GPI were admitted between 1916 and 1926, although the explanation for this comparatively high number remains unclear.[133]

Differential diagnosis

Due to the profusion of symptoms associated with GPI and the distinctive physical symptoms often being absent during the early stage of the disease, GPI could resemble a number of other disorders, making diagnosis problematic. Thus the method of 'differential diagnosis' was often employed in order to differentiate GPI from a number of related afflictions. The list of 'common differentials', that is, those disorders which GPI was deemed most likely to resemble, consisted of the other diseases in the neurosyphilis family – syphilitic insanity, cerebral syphilis and tabes dorsalis – as well as alcoholic insanity, mania, melancholia, epilepsy and senile dementia. Each will be considered below.

Syphilitic insanity

Both syphilitic insanity and cerebral syphilis attracted more attention on the continent than in Britain during the nineteenth century, although by the second half of the century some British medical interest had been awakened, particularly by the writings of Jonathan Hutchinson and John Hughlings Jackson, and by Thomas Clouston and David Henderson in Scotland.[134] Clouston classified syphilitic insanity into four chief forms: secondary, delusional, vascular, and syphilomatous insanity.[135] 'Secondary syphilitic insanity' was said to occur during the second stage of syphilis and was deemed both rare and curable. 'Delusional syphilitic insanity' was claimed to consist of monomania of suspicion and to lack motor symptoms, following at some distance of time an attack of syphilis in persons strongly predisposed to insanity. 'Vascular syphilitic insanity' apparently depended on the tendency of the poison to affect the blood vessels of the brain and cause slow arteritis, with diminished blood-carrying capacity and consequent slow starvation of the cerebral tissue. Finally, 'syphilomatous insanity' was said to depend on the tendency of the poison to affect the connective tissue, membranes, and bones, and to cause pressure, irritation and inflammation in the convolutions to any patient so afflicted.

The symptoms associated with syphilitic insanity were held by a number of medical commentators to make it one of the most difficult forms of insanity to distinguish from GPI. An Argyll-Robertson pupil seemed to be of little diagnostic value since it occurred in both diseases, but optic neuritis would likely point to syphilitic disease as it was uncommon in GPI. Tremors were believed to be seldom present in syphilitic insanity but common to general paralytics. Speech defects also favoured GPI, as aphasic states were the only form of speech disorders generally met with in cases of syphilitic insanity. However, the most important point the literature tended to stress was that, with anti-syphilitic treatment, the patient afflicted with syphilitic insanity often improved rapidly, whereas such treatment was deemed valueless in GPI.[136]

Within the four Scottish asylums, no cases of 'syphilitic insanity' were admitted in the period from 1880 to 1930 except to the REA, where a fairly significant forty-four cases within my patient sample received this diagnostic label. There are several possible reasons why only the REA employed this diagnosis. Since the physicians of this institution diagnosed far more of their admissions to be general paralytics than the other Scottish asylums, they may have felt more need to subdivide the 'catch-all' GPI category. There may also have been aetiological reasons behind the use of the label. Since, as Chapter 6 will discuss, Clouston was one of many physicians of this period who were slow to acknowledge a causative link between syphilis and GPI, 'syphilitic insanity' may have been perceived as a useful alternative label for those patients whose insanity appeared to be caused by syphilis. Moreover, Clouston's atypical adherence to Skae's classificatory system might also explain his interest in this more 'causative' diagnostic label.

Cerebral syphilis

One of the clearest descriptions of 'cerebral syphilis' – a manifestation of tertiary lesions in the brain or meninges – was provided in 1761 by the Italian anatomist Giovanni Battista Morgagni (1682–1771), who described gummata of the brain and pathological lesions in the smaller arteries.[137] David Henderson, Physician-Superintendent of Gartnavel, employed this diagnostic label in cases where syphilis affected the interstitial tissues of the central nervous system and was accompanied by mental symptoms.[138] Its symptomatology was considered very characteristic. Henderson detailed the most frequent physical symptoms to be headaches, dizziness, vomiting, sleeplessness, cranial nerve palsies, optic neuritis and hemiplegia. In addition to these physical symptoms, mental symptoms were frequently said to develop. As a general rule, such mental disturbance was noted to be acute in onset, and characterised by a dull, delirious, or confused state, with disorientation, poor power of retention and sometimes auditory and visual hallucinations.[139] These symptoms were said usually to appear within five years of the primary infection, and often within six months.

Such was Henderson's interest in this diagnosis that he presented a paper on it to the New York Academy of Medicine in March 1922.[140] He advised that, although this condition could be easily confused with GPI due principally to the common mental symptoms, more reliance could be placed on the physical signs. The presence of Argyll–Robertson pupils was comparatively rare in cases of cerebral syphilis, unlike in GPI. The speech defects of cerebral syphilis had not the distinctive character of the articulation in GPI, and were more often associated with ordinary aphasia.

Furthermore, the acute onset subsequent to syphilitic infection, and accompanied by headache and cranial nerve palsies, indicated cerebral syphilis affectation of the meninges rather than GPI.

This diagnostic label was little used within Scotland. There is no mention of cerebral syphilis in the Gartnavel annual reports and case notes, except in 1922 after Henderson had taken up the post of Physician-Superintendent. In that year, one patient was admitted to Gartnavel with this diagnosis. No other patient was admitted to any of the four Scottish asylum patient populations with this diagnosis in the period between 1880 and 1930.

Tabes dorsalis

'Tabes dorsalis' entered the clinical scene primarily as a result of work by the emerging German neurological school. The German neurologist Mauritz Romberg coined the term in 1840, and identified the important diagnostic sign that when a patient was made to stand and close his eyes, he lost his balance and fell. The French neurologist Guillaume Duchenne de Boulogne then elaborated Romberg's clinical description of tabes, but described it as 'locomotor ataxia' due to its most striking symptom, 'ataxie locomotrice progressive'. These two names for the condition, which were used interchangeably, reflect the equal importance which physicians generally afforded to the clinical and pathological features: 'tabes dorsalis' referred to the characteristic pathological lesion (wasting of the spine), and 'locomotor ataxia' to the corresponding clinical syndrome.[141]

Subsequent developments in the understanding of the disease proceeded independently in Germany, France and Britain. The majority of authors discussed this disorder as a syphilitic disease of the nervous system devoid of mental symptoms. Textbooks noted the classic symptoms of tabes dorsalis to include incoordination of the legs, which created a characteristic swaying and tottering gait in these patients – which physicians attempted to accentuate by asking the patient to close his eyes while he walked; excruciating 'lightning' pains throughout the body; sexual and urinary dysfunction; and multiple forms of joint disease elucidated by Jean-Martin Charcot during the 1870s.[142] The disease tended to run a chronic course, extending on average over a period of ten years.

However, within this diagnostic category there were two conditions believed to combine tabes with insanity: tabetic GPI and tabes with psychosis. Various authors noted that tabes could exhibit mental complications. Carl Westphal, a German alienist, was the first clinician to claim that he had observed the occurrence of GPI and tabes dorsalis in the same patient; and that this was a form of tabes which, many years after its onset, developed the general paralytic features of insanity.[143] Neurologists gradually came to recognise this close alliance between tabes dorsalis and GPI, and created 'tabo-paralysis' as a sub-group of GPI. Indeed, by 1903, an English discussion on the relationship between tabes and GPI found that most of the leading authorities, including Frederick Mott and Thomas Buzzard, were of the opinion that the two diseases were identical.[144]

In Scotland, the physician and neurologist Byrom Bramwell (1847–1931) claimed that 11.4 per cent of tabetics passed into GPI, and that one third of general paralytics presented signs of tabes. Thus George Robertson, Physician-Superintendent of the REA, warned that 'the appearance of mental troubles in a tabetic ought always to awaken the suspicion of general paralysis', particularly when accompanied by signs of mental weakness and loss of memory. Speech difficulties and 'a heavy, mask-like expression' were said to be the 'ominous physical signs'.[145] David Henderson, while Physician-Superintendent of Gartnavel, described how most of these 'combined' cases displayed the tabetic symptoms first; but that in some cases the two diseases seemed to develop coincidentally; while in a third, and much smaller group, the tabetic signs developed after the onset of the general paralysis.[146]

To complicate matters still further, a small number of physicians, such as the German alienist Emil Kraepelin, claimed to have observed cases of tabes with mental disorder whose onset, symptomatology and outcome differed absolutely from cases of GPI.[147] He argued that there must be a psychosis peculiar to tabes, which was of sudden onset and appeared at a later stage during its course than GPI. The disorder consisted principally of acute hallucinatory excitement. Memory and orientation appeared to remain intact, while speech and writing did not present the specific disturbances exhibited by general paralytics.

Within Scotland, 'tabes with psychosis' first appeared as a diagnostic category in the Gartnavel annual report of 1921, following Henderson's appointment. The Glasgow alienist's minority stance in this regard is most likely related to his psychiatric training in New York and Munich underneath the renowned Kraepelin and the Swiss alienist Adolf Meyer.[148] Henderson rejected the belief expressed by the majority of authors that tabes and GPI were essentially the same disease and that all mental disorders occurring in tabes were due to GPI or to a simple complication of it, instead concurring with Kraepelin that non-paralytic psychosis could occur in cases of tabes. Indeed, he published an article on the subject in 1911, which opened with the sentence:

> In tabes dorsalis, mental symptoms frequently develop; in the majority of
> such cases the mental symptoms are evidences of the onset of general

paralysis. In a certain number of cases, however, the autopsy has shown that the cortical changes of general paralysis are absent, and therefore the psychosis has arisen on a different basis.[149]

In order to differentiate between GPI and tabes, the test of closing the patient's eyes and watching its effect on balance and locomotion was commonly employed. A further differentiating factor was stated to be stuttering speech which, like the twitching of the lips and face, was scarcely simulated in tabes. Finally, memory retention and orientation seemed generally to remain intact in tabes cases, while speech and writing did not appear to present the specific disturbances normally noted in patients with GPI.

As with cerebral syphilis, tabes dorsalis and its variants were little used diagnostic labels within Scotland between 1880 and 1930. Only one patient was admitted to Gartnavel with tabes dorsalis during Henderson's period of Physician-Superintendency, and no other patients were admitted to the four Scottish asylums with this diagnosis. A small number of other patients were, however, admitted with combined GPI and locomotor ataxy between 1900 and 1919: one each to Rosslynlee and Woodilee, and six to Gartnavel.

Alcoholic Insanity

Moving outside of the neurosyphilitic family, a further series of mental diseases were said to require distinction from GPI. Thomas Clouston stated that, of all the list of common differentials, it was only alcoholism that gave the physician 'really great uncertainty in coming to a diagnosis' of GPI.[150] He noted M. Ball and E. Regis's finding that, while GPI differed essentially in its vital relations from all other varieties of insanity, it exhibited a very close parallelism with chronic alcoholic insanity. Alcoholic intoxication was seen as a common exciting cause of GPI, one possible reason why chronic and sub-acute alcoholism were often confused with general paralysis. More importantly, though, was their shared symptoms. Bonville Fox claimed that there was no method by which the exaltation of alcoholism could be distinguished with absolute certainty from that of GPI. Indeed, each separate physical symptom of GPI might exist in chronic alcoholism. In both there was said to be constant mental restlessness and confusion, marked tremors of the face and hands, and delusions of grandeur.

Potentially, one of the few ways to differentiate between the two disorders was said to be the fact that, in chronic alcoholism, there was typically a complete recovery of the patient, whereas the GPI prognosis was very poor. Furthermore, alcoholism saw only an incomplete affection of speech compared with GPI. In a fuller comparative discussion of both diseases, Reginald Farrar, assistant surgeon at Stamford and Rutland General Infirmary, held that:

> [W]hatever difference exists, clinically, between typical general paralysis and chronic alcoholism culminating in paralytic dementia, is due to the fact that, as Dr Clouston puts it, by a course of chronic soaking 'the finer points of moral character and feeling are rubbed off.' Whereas in the typical general paralytic, who is often at the commencement of his attack a vigorous and capable man of the world, rather above than below the average in intellectual capacity, the exaltation, grandiose delusions, and restless energy are but the insane exaggerations of his normal mental activities, thrown off the balance by some sudden disturbing agency, the tippler has been blunting and dulling his faculties by years of indulgence, till he has no intellect left to become deranged, and passes more gradually and insensibly into a condition of dementia. But the final result in both cases is the same, brain congestion, thickening of membranes, and erosion of the cortex giving rise to dementia, which ends in stupor, coma, and death.[151]

Two Scottish cases in my sample illustrate the confusion between these two conditions. Robert C., a 43-year-old married house factor, was diagnosed with GPI on his admission to Gartnavel in October 1885, but he was noted as displaying symptoms which 'may be due to the alcoholism and not GP'.[152] William U., a 45-year-old married clothier, admitted in September 1885, was described on admission as being:

> [E]xtremely stupid, unable to utter a syllable or seemingly to understand a request to do so simple an act as put out his tongue. He was irritable and inclined to use both his arms and feet in attacking those about him... his whole manner and aspect [suggest] very strongly General Paresis far advanced or else a marked case of alcoholism.[153]

One Woodilee paralytic was also diagnosed initially with alcoholic insanity.

Mania

Early in the course of GPI, the commonly exhibited acute maniacal excitement and delusions of grandeur were widely noted to cause the disease to be easily confused with mania. Both disorders could create a mixture of exalted and persecutory delusions, as well as some pupillary change in the patient. Tremors and twitching of the face and tongue, as well as affection of speech, could also be found in the monomaniac. Mania or monomania of grandeur, wealth, or pride, often occurred quite independently of GPI, but in doubtful cases of this sort, the French physician Esquirol diagnosed GPI by an occasional slowness in pronunciation, and by the fact that the patient could be 'calmed by a promise and induced to forego apparently cherished projects'.[154] The somatic signs, when well pronounced, also marked the case to be one of GPI. For example, the maniacal excitement which attended GPI was distinguished by the muscular tremors of the tongue and lips, and by the 'catch' of the voice. Furthermore, the type of excitement in each disorder differed:

> The excited state of general paralysis, which may be mistaken for acute mania, rarely lasts more than from ten to thirty days. After that time the excitement subsides, while the delusions and the muscular symptoms remain, and the nature of the disease becomes apparent.[155]

In the four Scottish asylums, the differential diagnosis of manic GPI from mania or the manic phases of manic-depressive insanity seems to have rested primarily on the demonstration of the physical symptoms. Jane C., a 50-year-old single lady's maid, who entered the REA in February 1893, was admitted as a case of acute mania and retained this diagnosis until about a third of the way into her progress notes, when her handwriting changed and she was then described as 'a marked case of GP'.[156] Other characteristic symptoms subsequently developed in this patient, including unequal and irregular pupils and slurred speech. Fifty-one REA patients in my sample (fourteen per cent) were diagnosed initially with mania, while the Gartnavel records include only four such re-diagnoses. Three Woodilee patients were initially diagnosed with mania due to their admission symptoms being incoherence in talk, violence, restlessness, excitement and delusions. For those GPI patients in the sample who were initially diagnosed with mania, it appears generally to have been because their physical symptoms had not yet developed.

Melancholia

W. Barker, a medical superintendent based both in England and Victoria, Australia, asserted: 'Melancholia is not commonly associated with general paralysis, although the emotional susceptibility and the easily excited tears would, perhaps, lead one to suppose the contrary.'[157] Yet, a fairly significant number of patients (forty-one) in my GPI sample were diagnosed initially with melancholia.[158] George Robertson, Physician-Superintendent of the REA, claimed to have regarded one patient as a case of melancholia for more than a year until he had an epileptic seizure, at which point Robertson decided the patient was in fact a general paralytic.[159] Given some of the symptoms of GPI, it seems hardly surprising that melancholia could be mistaken for general paralysis. Elizabeth N., a 49-year-old married housewife, was diagnosed with melancholia/GPI on admission to the REA in November 1894. Her progress notes record: 'Diagnosis of this case very doubtful on admission, thought to be melancholia (idiopathic)' due to the fact that she was '[e]xcited, incoherent, restless, talkative, talking rubbish, [and] delusional'.[160] In order to differentiate GPI from melancholia, Mickle advised that:

> Some of the somatic signs of GPI, the fact that the patients rarely maintain complete silence, that they show less of that rigid, fixed, contraction of the lineaments, and deep furrowing of the lines of expression, that is usually seen in the simple form of melancholia with stupor, are distinctive points.[161]

In addition, Maurice Craig, a physician and lecturer in psychological medicine at Guy's Hospital, London, pointed out that:

> The excitement of ordinary mania is not so unreasoning as that of general paralysis. The mental deterioration is greater in the latter disease. In mania and melancholia the memory is never really bad, as it may be in GPI. Speech defects, and failure of muscular power, altered handwriting, pupillary changes, and seizures all point to general paralysis.[162]

As with mania, the confusion between melancholia and GPI tended to occur at an early stage in the latter disease, before the physical symptoms had yet developed.

Epilepsy

Although stated to be far less likely to be confused with GPI, epilepsy did share several characteristic symptoms. Besides the convulsive seizures, there could be a shaky, thick speech and a jerky tremulousness of the lips and face, although, according to Mickle, 'as far as I have seen this only occurs to any marked degree in some chronic patients, subject to frequent, severe and general convulsions'.[163] However, upon closer examination, there were a number of differences between these two disorders. In epilepsy, the convulsive attacks often differed from those displayed by general paralytics, the physiognomy differed, and the 'irritable, suspicious, surly, impulsively violent state of the epileptic' contrasted with 'that more usual to the general paralytic'. Furthermore, it was seen as very rare for true epilepsy to begin after the age of thirty years, while general paralytics were typically aged between thirty and fifty. Only one REA patient in the sample received an initial diagnosis of epileptic insanity, which was altered to GPI at post mortem.

Senile dementia

When GPI appeared late in life, it was on occasion necessary to differentiate it from senile dementia. Clearly, the dementia from which GPI received its pseudonym, 'dementia paralytica', linked the two disorders. Such dementia-related symptoms as memory loss, disorientation, altered character and incontinence, were found in most general paralytics at some stage of their disease. The London-based lecturer George Fielding Blandford outlined the similarities between the two conditions – 'senile dementia... may be characterised by loss of memory, extravagant and indecent conduct, and delusions', all common symptoms of paralytics – and also listed the main differentials:

> There will, however, be an absence of the specific delusions and the maniacal condition; neither shall we find the inequality of pupils, the stutter, nor stumbling gait. In fact the failing mind in senile dementia is manifested usually long before any symptoms of bodily paralysis.[164]

As Maurice Craig, the English physician and lecturer, explained:

> [T]he diagnosis of dementia paralytic is often overlooked in the early stages of the disease, because physicians do not examine the patient carefully enough for physical signs and too frequently make their diagnosis from the mental symptoms alone.[165]

Margaret I., an 88-year-old single servant, was admitted to Rosslynlee in March 1910 with 'all the symptoms of a case of senile insanity being restless, irritable, confused and needing to be under constant supervision'.[166] Yet her diagnosis was recorded as GPI. A handful of Woodilee cases had to wait until post mortem for their GPI diagnosis. Eight of these patients received an initial diagnosis of dementia. Their symptoms upon admission were noted to be organic brain disease, not answering when questioned or taking any notice of their surroundings generally, and being restless, confused, noisy, excited, incoherent and delusional. Of those patients who did not receive an initial diagnosis of GPI, but whose diagnosis was altered to GPI at post mortem, no physical symptoms were recorded. Two Gartnavel paralytics were also diagnosed with dementia on admission.

The clinical identity of GPI

Given this whole spectrum of differential diagnoses, it is not surprising that a number of contemporaries commented on how difficult it was to diagnose GPI. They claimed that the onset of the disease could be so insidious that there was great difficulty in diagnosing in the earlier stages. The 'chief somatic signs' could 'for a time be absent, or ambigious, or slight', leaving the alienist initially with merely the mental symptoms.[167] The mental symptoms were, of course, those most likely to be confused with other disorders, such as mania and dementia. Thus Mickle advised that, 'in all such examples of insanity', particularly those which occurred as a first mental attack and in males aged between thirty and fifty, the medical attendant would be wise to 'keep in mind the possibility of general paralysis', and to 'systematically watch for any unequivocal indications thereof'.[168]

In fact, in some cases the diagnosis of GPI proved so problematic that it would not be given formally until death, once a post mortem had uncovered the distinct pathological changes in the brain. Even where a patient seemed to have all the characteristic symptoms of GPI in life, the fatal prognosis of GPI made some physicians wary to label the patient a general paralytic until death had intervened. As Clouston wrote:

> It may be said that as he has not died it is impossible to say that this is a case of true general paralysis. If he is not, he has had every symptom of the disease except its termination in death, and neither Dr Skae nor I, nor one of the score of assistant physicians here who have had charge of him, have had any doubt on the subject.[169]

There were occasional published reports of patients considered to be classic cases of GPI who had gone on to recover to some degree, hence throwing their diagnosis into considerable doubt. In 1903, Landel Oswald, Physician-Superintendent of Gartnavel, discussed in his annual report the fact that two GPI cases had been discharged 'improved' from the asylum 'nearly a year ago' and 'remained well'.[170] While they had both been considered to constitute 'typical cases' whilst residing in the asylum, since 'in both the classical symptoms of the disease were present', Oswald cautioned that 'true General Paralysis [was] believed never to be recovered from'. Similarly, the case notes of one REA paralytic state that he 'was examined some time ago by Dr John MacPherson who definitely diagnosed GPI, but the diagnosis is now doubtful owing to the marked improvement which has taken place under anti-syphilitic treatment.'[171] The fact of the patient's recovery was grounds for questioning the GPI diagnosis. While many of the Scottish patients in my sample were said to exhibit the core mental and physical symptoms that characterised GPI, only death, it seems, could truly clinch the diagnosis. This is one possible explanation for the fact that the Scottish asylum records contain a fairly significant number of patients who were given the GPI diagnosis only at post mortem.

A review of the Scottish case notes reveals the scale of what one might term 'initially erroneous diagnoses', that is, cases that were only re-diagnosed as GPI at death. There was, in fact, marked variation between the different asylums in this respect. At Woodilee, 20 of the sample of 103 patients admitted in the period between 1880 and 1910 (19 per cent) were re-diagnosed with GPI at post mortem, having been diagnosed upon admission with other disorders such as mania or melancholia. The figure was lower at Gartnavel and the REA, with the vast majority of these patients receiving their GPI diagnosis upon admission to the asylum. Whereas the case notes of both royal asylums reveal a low incidence of 'errors', at Rosslynlee, a surprisingly large 53 of the 115 patients (46 per cent) only received a GPI diagnosis shortly before or at post mortem. For this reason, REA physicians advised that the prevalence of GPI was much more accurately judged by the death-rate than by the admission-rate.[172]

Despite the difficulties in diagnosis and the inevitable errors, there appears to have been a fundamental stability in the symptoms associated with the disease for the period from 1880 to 1910. There was a general textbook consensus as to the core features of GPI, which included delusions, restlessness, a defective memory, speech and writing defects. This consensus is found, equally, in the admission certificates of those patients ultimately diagnosed with GPI in the four Scottish asylums, as Table 3.1 reveals. However, the central feature which emerges from this table is the mental and behavioural nature of all but one of these symptoms. On admission, 62 per cent (361) of all patients in the sample were recorded as having delusions, and a further 28 per cent (165) having symptoms of excitement.[173] Only a slightly smaller number of these patients exhibited signs of restlessness and memory defect upon admission.

At admission, the patient was often in a relatively early stage of the disease, and therefore the main symptoms presented for diagnosis were almost entirely mental. This would appear to be the central explanation for the substantial number of incorrect diagnoses during this period. This is in contrast to the later stages of the disease, where cases conformed far more to the textbook cases in displaying both the characteristic physical and mental symptoms. An initially erroneous diagnosis seems generally to have been made on the basis of these purely mental symptoms, which could be easily confused with other mental disorders.[174] As George Robertson frequently cautioned:

> [N]o one is justified in diagnosing a case of general paralysis from the mental symptoms alone. It is practically impossible to do so; you may suspect it, but you cannot diagnose it with any certainty. Any one who attempts to do so will, sooner or later, come a cropper.[175]

However, it was not just that other mental disorders had to be differentiated from dementia and GPI. Some eminent physicians believed that disorders such as mania and melancholia, by their nature, evolved into dementia. In their authoritative textbook, Bucknill and Tuke referred to 'the constant tendency of mania, and other forms of mental derangement, to pass into dementia'.[176] This observation chimes with the nineteenth-century concept of mania as a condition commonly leading to mental deterioration. Clouston, in discussing the prognosis of mania, claimed that there was complete recovery in about half the cases; death in 5 per cent; partial

Table 3.1

The Main Symptoms of GPI on Admission to the Four Scottish Asylums, 1880–1910

Symptom	No. of Patients
Delusional	361
Excited	165
Restless	152
Memory Defect	145
Confused	117
Incoherent	86
Unfit to be at Home	81
Incoherent in Talk	80
Violent	75
Speech Defect	71

Source: *Four Asylum Admissions Registers,* NHSGGCA13/6/78–9 and NHSGGCA30/10/1–3; LHSA LHB7/35/5–11 and LHB33/5/1.

---

recovery in 15 per cent; and in the remaining 30 per cent, dementia, adding that 'the bulk of chronic patients in asylums are of this class'.[177] It was widely believed that GPI could often be preceded by an attack of acute mania presenting the usual features but leaving the patient more or less demented when the maniacal symptoms passed off, and suffering the impaired speech and unsteady gait of the general paralytic.

This might explain why seventeen patients in the REA sub-sample initially had 'mania' written as their case-note diagnosis in the period between 1880 and 1910, which was then scored out and replaced with 'GPI' at some point during their stay. Five cases of 'melancholia' were similarly scored out and replaced with 'GPI' in the same period. Interestingly, this scoring out and altering to GPI is not seen for any other diagnosis except mania and melancholia. Perhaps this is simply accounted for by the fact that the physicians of the REA believed it natural for mania and melancholia to pass into dementia, and that a diagnosis of 'mania' later scored out and replaced with 'GPI' did not at any point constitute an 'inaccurate' diagnosis.

Several explanations have been advanced to account for the significant number of patients whose seemingly incorrect diagnosis upon admission to these four asylums was altered to GPI either during their stay or at post mortem. It is evident that the process of diagnosis was extremely complicated, due in part to the multitude of associated symptoms.

Moreover, the 'stadial' model of the disease and, in particular, the predominantly mental nature of the symptoms until a fairly late stage of the disease seems to have caused much of the initial diagnostic confusion. If we focus upon the case-note symptoms of those patients who received an ultimate diagnosis of GPI, the majority appear to have exhibited a fairly specific and tangible cluster of symptoms, but it would be difficult to make a case for the conceptual stability of GPI as a diagnostic category during this period. It remains to be seen what impact the laboratory made upon GPI's conceptual stability during the 1910s and 1920s.

Notes

1. For a fuller overview, see E. Brown, 'French Psychiatry's Initial Reception of Bayle's Discovery of General Paresis of the Insane', *Bulletin of the History of Medicine*, 68:2 (1994), 235–53.

2. Bayle presented this thesis, entitled 'Recherches sur les Maladies Mentales', for the Doctorate of Medicine to the Faculty of Paris, in which he detailed the results of his research at the Royal Asylum for the Insane at Charenton.

3. See, also, his pamphlet: A. Bayle, *Récherches sur L'Arachnite Chronique, la Gastrite et la Gastro-Enterite Chroniques, et la Goutte, Considérée Comme Causes de L'Aliénation Mentale* (Paris: Didot le Jeune, 1822), translated in M. Moore and H. Solomon, 'Contributions of Haslam, Bayle, and Esmarch and Jessen to the History of Neurosyphilis', *Archives of Neurology and Psychiatry*, 82 (1934), 807–29.

4. J. Esquirol, *Des Maladies Mentales Considérées sous les Rapports Médical, Hygiènique et Médico-Légal* (Paris: J. Baillière, 1838), translated by E. Hunt as *Mental Maladies: A Treatise on Insanity* (Philadelphia: Lea and Blanchard, 1845), 439.

5. Cited in E. Hare, 'The Origin and Spread of Dementia Paralytica', *Journal of Mental Science*, 105 (1959), 594–626: 596. See T. Austin, *A Practical Account of General Paralysis, its Mental and Physical Symptoms, Statistics, Causes, Seat and Treatment* (London: John Churchill, 1859).

6. J. Conolly, 'Clinical Lectures on the Principal Forms of Insanity: Lecture XI', *Lancet*, 1 (1846), 233–7: 233.

7. For example, the English physician, James Cowles Prichard (1786–1848), complained: 'Patients are dismissed from Bethlem when they manifest any indication of paralysis, and the events of such cases cannot... be correctly noted'. See J. Prichard, *A Treatise on Insanity* (London: Sherwood, Gilbert and Piper, 1835), 109.

8. Cited in Hare, *op. cit.* (note 5), 608.

9. Unfortunately the REA does not provide a 'form of insanity' table in its annual reports until the 1850s, so that it is not possible easily to chart the

epidemiology of the disease until then. The Gartnavel annual reports give such a table a little earlier, but not until 1859 is GPI included within it.

10. *38th Commissioners of Lunacy for Scotland Annual Report*, 1896, NHS Greater Glasgow and Clyde Archives, NHSGGCA13B/14/64, lii.

11. Cited in Hare, *op. cit.* (note 5), 608.

12. *29th Inverness District Asylum Annual Report*, 1893, Northern Health Services Archives (NHSA), HHB3/8/10, 16.

13. For a discussion of GPI's problematic identity in these early years, see J. Hurn, 'The History of General Paralysis of the Insane in Britain, 1830 to 1950', PhD thesis, University of London (1998), 40.

14. 'Report of a Quarterly Meeting of the MPA', *Journal of Mental Science*, 15 (1870), 635: 635.

15. J. Bucknill and D. Tuke, *A Manual of Psychological Medicine* (London: J. and A. Churchill, 1862 and 1874).

16. D. Skae, 'Contributions to the Natural History of General Paralysis', *Edinburgh Medical Journal*, 5 (1859-60), 885–905: 886.

17. Discussion, 'Quarterly Meeting of the Medico-Psychological Association, held at Glasgow', *Journal of Mental Science*, 22 (1876), 334–5.

18. D. Skae and T. Clouston, 'The Morisonian Lectures on Insanity for 1873', *Journal of Mental Science*, 21 (1875), 188–204: 192.

19. Other prominent attacks came from Luther Bell in America, Schroeder van der Kolk in Holland, and Bénédict-Augustin Morel in France. See D.H. Tuke, *Chapters in the History of the Insane in the British Isles* (London: Kegan Paul, 1882), 467.

20. See D. Skae, 'A Rational and Practical Classification of Insanity', *Journal of Mental Science*, 9 (1863), 309–19.

21. David Henderson argued that the 'rapid influx' of patients admitted to the REA during Skae's period of Physician-Superintendency encouraged his interest in classification. See D. Henderson, *The Evolution of Psychiatry in Scotland* (Edinburgh: E. and S. Livingstone, 1964), 53–4.

22. Skae, *op. cit.* (note 20), 318.

23. Indeed, Skae's most sympathetic biographer summed up the scheme as 'best forgotten'. See Frank Fish, 'David Skae, MD, FRCS, Founder of the Edinburgh School of Psychiatry', *Medical History*, 9 (1965), 36–53: 36.

24. J. Crichton Browne, 'Skae's Classification of Mental Diseases: A Critique', *Journal of Mental Science*, 19 (1875), 339–65: 341.

25. T. Clouston, 'Modern Medico–Psychology and Psychiatry', *The Hospital*, 11 May 1895, 91: 91.

26. Clouston's continued allegiance to Skae's system long after its rejection by most British authorities is perhaps partly explained by Skae and Clouston's close working relationship.

27. T.S. Clouston, 'Skae's Classification of Mental Diseases', *Journal of Mental Science*, 21 (1875), 532–50: 536.

28. Skae and Clouston, *op. cit.* (note 18), 2.

29. *Ibid.*

30. See, for example, the textbooks of Austin, Bucknill and Tuke, and Mickle, for a full description of all related symptoms.

31. For further details, see Brown, *op. cit.* (note 1), 244.

32. T. Clouston, *Unsoundness of Mind* (London: Methuen, 1911), 243–5.

33. Skae and Clouston, *op. cit.* (note 18), 12–13.

34. Skae, *op. cit.* (note 16), 894.

35. *Royal Edinburgh Asylum Case Book*, Lothian Health Services Archive (LHSA), LHB7/51/70/133.

36. *Ibid.*, LHB7/51/61/559.

37. *Glasgow Royal Asylum Case Book*, NHSGGCA13/5/124/133.

38. *Barony Parochial Asylum Case Book*, NHSGGCA30/4/3/453.

39. *Royal Edinburgh Asylum Case Book*, LHSA LHB7/51/57/317.

40. *Ibid.*, LHSA LHB7/51/69/277.

41. *Glasgow Royal Asylum Case Book*, NHSGGCA13/5/132/85.

42. *Barony Parochial Asylum Case Book*, NHSGGCA30/5/12/36.

43. *Ibid.*, NHSGGCA30/4/2/272.

44. *Royal Edinburgh Asylum Case Book*, LHSA LHB7/51/40/470.

45. *Ibid.*, LHSA LHB7/51/67/529.

46. *Barony Parochial Asylum Case Book*, NHSGGCA30/4/4/113.

47. *Royal Edinburgh Asylum Case Book*, LHSA LHB7/51/52/159.

48. *Ibid.*, LHSA LHB7/51/38/261.

49. *Ibid.*, LHSA LHB7/51/69/685.

50. *Glasgow Royal Asylum Case Book*, NHSGGCA13/5/102/399.

51. *Ibid.*, NHSGGCA13/5/146/241.

52. J. MacLachlan, 'General Paralysis of the Insane', *Glasgow Medical Journal*, 1 (1897), 423–30: 424.

53. *Glasgow Royal Asylum Case Book*, NHSGGCA13/5/102/381.

54. *Royal Edinburgh Asylum Case Book*, LHSA LHB7/51/34/751.

55. *Glasgow Royal Asylum Case Book*, NHSGGCA13/5/129/182.

56. *Midlothian and Peebles District Asylum Case Book*, LHSA LHB33/12/20/365.

57. *Ibid.*, LHSA LHB33/12/30/145.

58. J. Wilkie, 'Some Further Cases of General Paralytics Committed to Prison for Larceny, with Remarks', *Journal of Mental Science*, 20 (1874–5), 246–54: 246.

59. Cited in *ibid.*, 251.

60. *Barony Parochial Asylum Case Book*, NHSGGCA30/4/55/46.

61. *Ibid.*, NHSGGCA30/4/3/287.

62. *Royal Edinburgh Asylum Case Book*, LHSA LHB7/51/71/481.

63. *Barony Parochial Asylum Case Book*, NHSGGCA30/4/28/11.
64. This condition was named after the distinguished Scottish eye surgeon, Douglas Argyll Robertson (1837–1909). The phenomenon referred to pupillary changes consisting of irregularity of outline, inequality of size, and impairment (diminution or absence) of the light and convergence reflexes.
65. W. Bruetsch, 'Neurosyphilitic Conditions: General Paralysis, General Paresis, Dementia Paralytica', in S. Arieti (ed.), *American Handbook of Psychiatry* (New York: Basic Books, 1974), 140.
66. *Royal Edinburgh Asylum Case Book*, LHSA LHB7/51/52/723.
67. *Barony Parochial Asylum Case Book*, NHSGGCA30/4/12/36.
68. Bruetsch, *op. cit.* (note 65), 140.
69. *Royal Edinburgh Asylum Case Book*, LHSA LHB7/51/72/853.
70. *Ibid.*, LHSA LHB7/51/66/881.
71. *Ibid.*, LHSA LHB7/51/40/410.
72. *Glasgow Royal Asylum Case Book*, NHSGGCA13/5/130/88.
73. *Royal Edinburgh Asylum Case Book*, LHSA LHB7/51/45/535.
74. J. Bucknill and D. Tuke, *A Manual of Psychological Medicine* (London: John Churchill, 1858), 332.
75. *Royal Edinburgh Asylum Case Book*, LHSA LHB7/51/34/439.
76. *Ibid.*, LHSA LHB7/51/63/257.
77. *Glasgow Royal Asylum Case Book*, NHSGGCA13/5/135/15.
78. *Ibid.*, NHSGGCA13/5/127/298.
79. *Royal Edinburgh Asylum Case Book*, LHSA LHB7/51/70/133.
80. *Midlothian and Peebles District Asylum Case Book*, LHSA LHB33/12/27/11.
81. *Barony Parochial Asylum Case Book*, NHSGGCA30/4/4/298.
82. *Royal Edinburgh Asylum Case Book*, LHSA LHB7/51/75/533.
83. *Ibid.*, LHSA LHB7/51/72/853.
84. *Midlothian and Peebles District Asylum Case Book*, LHSA LHB33/12/30/150.
85. *Glasgow Royal Asylum Case Book*, NHSGGCA13/5/124/197.
86. Bruetsch, *op. cit.* (note 65), 141.
87. *Barony Parochial Asylum Case Book*, NHSGGCA30/4/2/303.
88. *Royal Edinburgh Asylum Case Book*, LHSA LHB7/51/45/143.
89. *Midlothian and Peebles District Asylum Case Book*, LHSA LHB33/12/13/225.
90. See J. Lavater, *Essays on Physiognomy, Designed to Promote the Knowledge and Love of Mankind* (London: John Stockdale, 1810).
91. Cited in L. Jordanova, 'The Art and Science of Seeing in Medicine: Physiognomy 1780–1820', in W. Bynum and R. Porter (eds), *Medicine and the Five Senses* (Cambridge: Cambridge University Press, 1993), 124.
92. Bucknill and Tuke, *op. cit.* (note 74), 292.
93. Cited in *ibid.*, 286.
94. Austin, *op. cit.* (note 5), 28.

Gayle Davis

95. G. Robertson, 'Clinique on General Paralysis', 15 February 1918, LHSA GD16, 9.

96. *Ibid.*, 29.

97. See, especially, Austin, *op. cit.* (note 5).

98. Skae, *op. cit.* (note 16), 887.

99. For a fuller description of this patient, see A. Morison, *The Physiognomy of Mental Diseases* (London: Longman and Co., 1840), 73.

100. *Midlothian and Peebles District Asylum Case Book*, LHSA LHB33/12/11/84.

101. *Ibid.*, LHSA LHB33/12/11/196 and LHB33/12/15/317.

102. *Glasgow Royal Asylum Case Book*, NHSGGCA13/5/129/390.

103. *Ibid.*, NHSGGCA13/5/138/148.

104. *Royal Edinburgh Asylum Case Book*, LHSA LHB7/51/101/193.

105. For a history of photography in medicine, see D. Fox and C. Lawrence, *Photographing Medicine: Images and Power in Britain and America Since 1840* (New York: Greenwood, 1988); J. Green-Lewis, *Framing the Victorians: Photography and the Culture of Realism* (Ithaca: Cornell University Press, 1996); M. Barfoot and A. Morrison-Low, 'W.C. McIntosh and A.J. MacFarlan: Early Clinical Photography in Scotland', *History of Photography*, 23 (1999), 199–210. For a detailed consideration of the role of clinical photography in late nineteenth-century Glasgow, see P. Summerly, 'Visual Pathology: A Case Study in Late Nineteenth Century Clinical Photography in Glasgow', PhD thesis, University of Glasgow (2003).

106. Fox and Lawrence, *op. cit.* (note 105), 21.

107. S. Burns, *Early Medical Photography in America (1839–1883)* (New York: The Burns Archive, 1983), 272–3.

108. Cited in A. Burrows and I. Schumacher, *Portraits of the Insane: The Case of Dr Diamond* (London: Quartet Books, 1990), 156.

109. Cited in J. Browne, 'Darwin and the Face of Madness', in W. Bynum, R. Porter, and M. Shepherd (eds), *The Anatomy of Madness: Essays in the History of Psychiatry*, Vol. I (London: Tavistock, 1985), 159.

110. Relative to the REA and Woodilee, Gartnavel's case notes were slow to incorporate a pro forma, or to include a diagnosis.

111. *Royal Edinburgh Asylum Case Book*, LHSA LHB7/51/86/881.

112. It is possible in such cases that a photograph was handed in by relatives of the patient rather than being taken by the asylum staff.

113. *Royal Edinburgh Asylum Case Book*, LHSA LHB7/51/85/605.

114. We do not, of course, know exactly when the case-note photographs were taken. One simply assumes that these were taken upon the patient's admission since this is the part of the case notes into which the photograph is inserted.

115. Skae and Clouston, *op. cit.* (note 18), 193.

116. Bruetsch, *op. cit.* (note 65), 138.

117. *Glasgow Royal Asylum Case Book*, NHSGGCA13/5/146/543.
118. *Ibid.*, NHSGGCA13/5/183/366.
119. *Ibid.*, NHSGGCA13/5/183/354.
120. *Ibid.*, NHSGGCA13/5/145/169.
121. *Ibid.*, NHSGGCA13/5/145/505.
122. *Ibid.*, NHSGGCA13/5/145/419.
123. *Ibid.*, NHSGGCA13/5/190/551.
124. *Ibid.*, NHSGGCA13/5/134/411.
125. *Ibid.*, NHSGGCA13/5/192/949.
126. L. Clarke and C. Atwood, 'Have the Forms of General Paresis Altered?', *Journal of Mental Science*, 54 (1908), 761–2: 761.
127. *Ibid.*
128. Skae and Clouston, *op. cit.* (note 18), 197.
129. The last of these was a somewhat rare form, generally accompanied by confusion, failure to recognise familiar people or places, motor excitement without mania, hallucinations of hearing and vision, convulsive movements and gnashing of teeth.
130. T. Clouston, 'A Case of General Paralysis at the Age of Sixteen Years', *Journal of Mental Science*, 23 (1877), 419–20: 419.
131. In 1895, Alzheimer collected thirty-seven published cases, to which he added three of his own. See J. Moreira and A. Penafiel, 'A Contribution to the Study of Dementia Paralytica in Brazil', *Journal of Mental Science*, 53 (1907), 507–21: 513. Mott published notes of twenty-two cases of juvenile GPI that had been diagnosed in the London County Asylums during a three-year period. See F. Mott, 'Notes on Twenty-Two Cases of Juvenile General Paralysis, with Sixteen Post-Mortem Examinations', *Archives of Neurology*, 1 (1899), 250–327.
132. Bruetsch, *op. cit.* (note 65), 148.
133. In September 1900, a Children's Home was built in connection with the asylum, the first of its kind in Scotland. Perhaps Woodilee therefore took in more young patients than the other asylums in this period, although even this would not explain the concentration of juvenile GPI cases into one decade.
134. See, for example, T. Clouston, *Clinical Lectures on Mental Diseases* (London: J. and A. Churchill, 1883), 464.
135. *Ibid.*, 466–9.
136. M. Craig, *Psychological Medicine: A Manual on Mental Diseases for Practitioners and Students* (London: J. and A. Churchill, 1917), 242.
137. D. MacKenzie, 'The Evaluation and Differentiation of Mental Disorders associated with Syphilis of the Nervous System', MD thesis, University of Glasgow (1950), 1.

138. He differentiated three main types: meningitis, endarteritis and gumma. See D. Henderson and R. Gillespie, *A Textbook of Psychiatry for Students and Practitioners* (London: Oxford University Press, 1927), 314.

139. D. Henderson, 'The Diagnosis of Cerebral Syphilis', *Review of Neurology and Psychiatry,* 9 (1911), 241–51: 242.

140. Reprinted as *ibid.*

141. 'Locomotor ataxia' expressed a characteristic feature of tabes, but did not occur in the first stage of the disease, the so-called 'pre-ataxic' stage. In fact, some cases might die without ataxia, so that the term 'tabes dorsalis' was generally felt to be the more appropriate.

142. See M. Romberg's classic account, *A Manual of Nervous Diseases of Man,* 2 vols (London: Sydenham Society, 1853), Vol. II, 395–401.

143. C. Westphal, 'Cases of Tabes Dorsalis and Paralysis Universalis Progressiva', *Journal of Mental Science,* 10 (1864), 207–20.

144. F. Mott, 'Tabes in Asylum and Hospital Practice', *Archives of Neurology,* 2 (1903), 1–10.

145. G. Robertson, 'The Morison Lectures, 1913: General Paralysis of the Insane', *Journal of Mental Science,* 59 (1913), 185–221: 198.

146. D. Henderson, 'Tabes Dorsalis and Mental Disease', *Review of Neurology and Psychiatry,* 9 (1911), 527–45: 530.

147. *Ibid.,* 531.

148. Indeed, Henderson dedicated his book, *A Textbook of Psychiatry, op. cit.* (note 138), to Meyer.

149. *Ibid.,* 529.

150. Clouston, *op. cit.* (note 32), 246.

151. R. Farrar, 'On the Clinical and Pathological Relations of General Paralysis of the Insane', *Journal of Mental Science,* 41 (1895), 460–82: 470.

152. *Glasgow Royal Asylum Case Book,* NHSGGCA13/5/124/197.

153. *Ibid.,* NHSGGCA13/5/124/171.

154. Cited in W. Mickle, *General Paralysis of the Insane,* 2nd edn (London: H.K. Lewis, 1886), 228.

155. Bucknill and Tuke, *op. cit.* (note 74), 304.

156. *Royal Edinburgh Asylum Case Book,* LHSA LHB7/51/58/593.

157. W. Barker, *Mental Diseases: A Manual for Students* (London: Cassell and Co., 1902), 99.

158. This is composed of twenty patients from Rosslynlee and twenty-one from the REA.

159. G. Robertson, 'Clinique on General Paralysis', 15 February 1918, LHSA GD16, 9.

160. *Royal Edinburgh Asylum Case Book,* LHSA LHB7/51/62/349.

161. Mickle, *op. cit.* (note 154), 238.

162. Craig, *op. cit.* (note 136), 241.

163. Mickle, *op. cit.* (note 154), 237.

164. Cited in *ibid.*, 234.

165. Craig, *op. cit.* (note 136), 243.

166. *Midlothian and Peebles District Asylum Case Book*, LHSA LHB33/12/24/28.

167. Mickle, *op. cit.* (note 154), 217.

168. *Ibid.*

169. Clouston, *op. cit.* (note 134), 371.

170. *90th Gartnavel Annual Report*, 1903, NHSGGCA13B/2/223, 18.

171. *Royal Edinburgh Asylum Case Book*, LHSA LHB7/51/108/505.

172. *96th Royal Edinburgh Asylum Annual Report*, 1908, LHSA LHB7/7/12, 19.

173. It can be noted that eleventh on this list was 'signs of GPI', mentioned for sixty-six patients. Bearing in mind that it was often family doctors who filled in these admission certificates, it is interesting that the GPI diagnosis was felt to be so definite that such a significant number of certificates contained reference to this particular disease, rather than the symptoms merely being listed and the alienist expected to reach his own diagnosis.

174. This might explain those journal articles specifically focused on diagnosing the early stages of GPI. See, for instance, G. Fleming, 'The Early Diagnosis of General Paralysis', *The Practitioner*, 112 (1924), 287–95; P. Knapp, 'The Early Symptoms of General Paralysis', *Journal of Nervous and Mental Disease*, 38:9 (1911), 513–21.

175. G. Robertson, 'Clinique on General Paralysis', 25 February 1920, LHSA GD16, 2.

176. Bucknill and Tuke, *op. cit.* (note 74), 304.

177. T. Clouston, *Clinical Lectures on Mental Diseases* (London: J. and A. Churchill, 1898), 205.

4

The Impact of the Laboratory

The laboratory had a dramatic impact upon clinical psychiatry and GPI,[1] with special reference to the asylum laboratories that were established in 1897 and 1909 in Edinburgh and Glasgow respectively. The work of these laboratories, and their role in the diagnosis and treatment of GPI will be discussed and, in particular, their application of the Wassermann test to the diagnosis and treatment of GPI. Although a range of diagnostic tests for GPI were available in the early twentieth century,[2] the Wassermann test was the most dominant, and one which provides an excellent means of studying the laboratory–clinic relationship at both published and case-note level.

The establishment of asylum laboratories in Scotland

By the 1890s, there seemed to be a growing feeling within British psychiatry that a significant gap had developed between Britain and the rest of Europe, particularly Germany,[3] with regard to pathology and technical sophistication.[4] Whereas British alienists had become, to a great extent, administrators of large asylums, German physicians appeared to constitute part of a neuro–psychiatric tradition and had a place in the clinics of university hospitals. In response, the first British asylum laboratory was opened in 1895, when London County Council established a laboratory at Claybury Asylum in Essex, in order to bring together research in fields such as neurophysiology, genetics and endocrinology.[5] From its opening until 1926, the laboratory was under the direction of the neuropathologist, Frederick Mott.[6] The Claybury Laboratory was utilised to train medical officers and their laboratory assistants in scientific pathology and served all Metropolitan Asylum Board asylums. It rapidly established itself as an internationally renowned centre of neuropathological research and was able to attract pathologists from around the world to undertake research there.

The Scottish Asylums' Pathological Scheme

The Edinburgh psychiatric profession was said to be so impressed by the laboratory at Claybury that, a year later, Thomas Clouston, Physician-Superintendent of the REA, began to organise a similar enterprise for Scotland. He referred to his scheme as 'this truly American Scheme', since further inspiration had been drawn from a Scheme of Research and Study recently set up by the State of New York in connection with its State asylums, which aimed to bring science 'to bear on the study of diseased brain and mind'.[7] The fact that the REA had the highest proportion of general paralytics in any Scottish asylum in this period may also have made a laboratory a more pressing issue, one of the first duties of the laboratory being an investigation into the aetiology and pathology of GPI. Thus, to further what was described by Thomas Clouston as the 'splendid original work of enduring importance' being conducted in the Pathological Department of the REA by Dr W. Ford Robertson,[8] a scheme began to evolve in 1896 to associate most of the Scottish asylums in pathological work. Once the aims of the Scottish Asylums' Pathological Scheme (henceforth SAPS) had been clearly established, Ford Robertson seems to have become the obvious candidate for the post.[9] He was thus appointed the first Pathologist under the scheme in 1897, and resigned as Pathologist of the REA to take up his duties as Laboratory Superintendent.[10]

The principal aim of the SAPS was to encourage pathological research among asylum doctors and to provide slides for clinical demonstration. It was noted that the Pathologist's duties were to examine and report on morbid specimens sent from the various asylums, to give instruction to the officials of the various asylums on microscopic technique as applied to the nervous system, and to undertake original investigations on neurological subjects. Furthermore, this 'conjoint laboratory of the Scottish Asylums' aimed to stimulate, support and facilitate scientific research of a similar nature in the individual asylums connected with it, rather than to suppress individual efforts: 'The general idea of the laboratory in no sense antagonises or supplants scientific research of a similar nature in the individual asylums. On the contrary', as the Commissioners in Lunacy for Scotland stated, there was reason to believe that the opportunities for prosecuting such work had been 'facilitated', and that, 'where an inclination exists to engage in it, the help of a central laboratory has been found of the greatest service.'[11] The Laboratory, therefore, also aimed to train assistant medical officers from the associated asylums in pathological methods, to circulate 'demonstration sets' for comparison, instruction and teaching purposes, and to purchase a collection of books and magazines for reference and lending purposes; such objectives reflecting a new level of commitment to 'foster a scientific interest in pathological research throughout the Associated Asylums'.[12]

The SAPS was soon funded by eighteen royal and district asylums and almost entirely maintained by voluntary contributions from the governing bodies of the Scottish asylums. However, the bulk of this funding came from three of the royal institutions: the REA, Gartnavel and Crichton. Besides providing spacious and suitable accommodation, special fittings and apparatus for the laboratory, the REA was spending at least £600 per annum on salaries and working expenses. The Commissioners in Lunacy inspected the Laboratory during 1901 and commended its ongoing contribution 'towards elucidating the many difficult and obscure problems of Mental Disease' as 'the best proof that the money spent on it by those Asylum Boards [was] well spent in the interests of the mentally afflicted'. Their annual report for that year continued:

> The Pathological Laboratory of the Scottish Asylums... has been successfully conducted, and has been productive of much scientific work of a high standard of excellence.... [T]he Text-Book recently published... by Dr Ford Robertson, the Superintendent of the Laboratory – based, it is understood, chiefly on his practical researches – might alone be held to justify the expenditure of money, and the great amount of care and labour which have been bestowed upon the founding and maintenance of this Institute.[13]

Membership of, and financial contributions to, the SAPS continued to evolve over the next few decades. Table 4.1, overleaf, shows the list of contributing asylums and their relative financial contributions to the Laboratory by 1930, one of the few years for which comprehensive data is available.[14]

The Scottish Western Asylums' Research Institute

It may be noted that these contributing asylums had a distinct east-coast bias. In fact, as early as 1908, the Lunacy Board had expressed concern that some asylums, chiefly in the west of Scotland, had withdrawn from the Scottish Asylums' Pathological Scheme.[15] This withdrawal seems to have been largely occasioned by the belief that the asylums in this area, perceiving the benefits that had accrued from similar laboratories elsewhere, could maintain a laboratory of their own. Thus in October 1909, the Scottish Western Asylums' Research Institute (henceforth SWARI) was founded to represent initially a group of eight asylums, and was situated in the grounds of Gartnavel.[16]

It was agreed that the SWARI Laboratory should be managed by a Board consisting of one representative from each contributing institution for each £100 or portion of £100 contributed by such institution, as well as the principal Medical Officer of each and the Professors of Practice of Medicine and Pathology at the University of Glasgow. The Managers of Gartnavel agreed to provide a house within their grounds, free of rent, taxes, coal, water and light, and with a separate entrance from the public road that was suitable for the purposes of the Laboratory; and to give, in addition, an annual financial contribution to the enterprise. The first Director of the SWARI, Ivy MacKenzie,[17] entered on his duties at a salary of £300 per annum in November 1909. It appears that their financial priority was to obtain good

Table 4.1

Asylum Contributions to the SAPS in 1930

Contributor	Amount			Percentage
	£	s	d	
Aberdeen District	62	5	10	5
Banff District	10	0	0	1
Bangour Village	79	5	4	6
Dundee Royal	10	6	3	1
Dundee District	48	12	8	4
East Lothian District	22	0	7	2
Royal Edinburgh Hospital	102	4	2	8
Fife and Kinross District	75	14	6	6
Glengall Hospital	57	8	9	5
Inverness District	40	0	0	3
Lanarkshire District Hartwood	111	8	11	9
Lanarkshire District Kirklands	10	10	0	1
Midlothian & Peebles District	30	18	3	2
Montrose Royal	85	8	1	7
Morayshire District	15	9	9	1
Murray's Royal	30	17	11	2
Perth District	36	10	10	3
Roxburgh District	33	18	4	3
Royal Scottish National Institution	20	0	0	2
Stirling District	90	3	4	7
Isle of Man	10	0	0	1
Grant from Carnegie Trust	34	12	11	3
Grant from Edinburgh University	110	0	0	9
Grant from Medical Research Council	125	4	9	10
TOTAL	1253	1	2	101

Source: *34th Scottish Mental Hospitals' Pathological Scheme Annual Report,* 1930, NHSGGCA21/2/4, 7.

---

personnel rather than sophisticated equipment,[18] and the representatives of the contributing asylums were said to consider themselves fortunate in obtaining MacKenzie as the first Director. It was made clear by the SWARI officials that there was no intention that the laboratory should 'in any way conflict with the laboratory in Edinburgh'. According to Landel Oswald, Physician-Superintendent of Gartnavel at this time, it was established 'for the same purpose, ha[d] the same ends in view, and hope[d] to have a like measure of success'.[19] The SWARI's main objectives were 'to stimulate, organise and carry out research relating to all forms of nervous and mental disorder, including their pathology, prevention and treatment', as well as to teach medical officers and post-graduate students the methods of studying and treating nervous and mental disorders.[20]

While both Scottish asylum laboratories were supported by the voluntary contributions of their associated asylums, financial problems seemed to threaten the Glasgow Laboratory from the outset. Indeed, the SWARI was soon inhibited by a variety of constraints, most particularly issues of finance, staff, resources, and the dislocation of war. In April 1913, when the SWARI seemed to be well established, MacKenzie intimated that he had accepted an appointment as Physician to the Victoria Infirmary, Glasgow, and could no longer devote the necessary time to the work of the SWARI. Difficulty was then experienced in securing the services of a suitably qualified director, with the £300 salary apparently not sufficient to attract experienced pathologists. Not until August 1914 was a new Director appointed, when Dr William Tulloch entered upon his duties. Tulloch was a skilled bacteriologist and had been an assistant in the Department of Pathology at the University of Durham. However, in May 1915, just as he was becoming familiar with the post, he resigned office in order to embark upon war service. Thereafter, until December 1919, the SWARI was closed owing to war conditions, although the various associated bodies continued to subscribe to the venture, and Wassermann testing was still conducted for the affiliated asylums. After initial difficulties in attracting suitable applicants, Dr William Whitelaw was appointed in December 1919.[21]

In view of the fact that the first three Laboratory Directors had resigned for financial reasons, and since contributors were so intent on obtaining specific and immediate results, in 1928 the SWARI's Chairman questioned whether it was desirable to continue the venture at all, or whether it should amalgamate with its Edinburgh counterpart. It was noted to be the unanimous opinion of the Executive Committee that the SWARI constituted a most valuable adjunct to the work of the associated institutions and that it would be 'nothing short of a disaster' were the scheme to be abandoned. It was felt that the option of amalgamating with the SAPS would not fulfil their ideal that any laboratory should be situated so as to be readily accessible to all associated institutions, in order to permit close personal contact between pathologist, asylum staff and patient; and that the asylums in and around Glasgow were sufficiently numerous and their patient populations large enough to form their own research unit. In the Committee's view: 'So far as close contact was concerned the laboratory might as well be situated in Inverness or London as in Edinburgh.'[22] Thus the SWARI survived, albeit temporarily. Its finances remained in deficit, and the Institute did not survive the formation of the National Health Service.

Technicalities of the test: the 'serological touch'

In 1906, the German bacteriologist August von Wassermann (1866–1925) perfected and published his method of serum diagnosis. The introduction of this 'Wassermann test' to detect syphilis in the blood and cerebrospinal fluid (CSF) coincided with the first decade of the SAPS and the conception of the SWARI, and was to constitute a substantial proportion of both laboratories' work. It may not seem surprising that grand claims were very quickly made for the potential of both test and laboratory, given the depressed nature of early twentieth-century psychiatry in Britain and the particularly depressing area of GPI. Published textbooks hailed the Wassermann reaction as the 'most reliable... single blood test available to the worker in mental disease'.[23] David Henderson, Physician-Superintendent of Gartnavel, shared this enthusiasm, claiming that the Wassermann test was positive in blood in practically one hundred per cent of GPI cases, and positive in CSF in about ninety-five per cent.[24] In this, Henderson seems to have been in tune with the majority of Scottish alienists. Their overriding confidence in the test's reliability would seem to be demonstrated by the fact that, of the 185 Scottish asylum patients tested in the period from 1909 to 1930, 151 (82 per cent) were tested only once.

Yet it had quickly been realised outside Scotland that it was possible to obtain a positive Wassermann reaction from a non-syphilitic blood sample, and a negative result from a syphilitic sample, without any major technical errors.[25] Physicians were discovering that between two and fourteen per cent of all Wassermann tests produced false positives and should thus be frequently repeated.[26] As W.J. Tulloch, the St Andrews-based bacteriologist and former Director of the SWARI, observed: if the attitude of the laboratory worker was 'that it is his duty to protect the non-syphilitic from unnecessary treatment, rather than to diagnose every case of the disease, active and latent', he was on safe ground.[27] If, however, he set out to get a one hundred per cent positive result rate in all types and stages of the disease, he would obtain positive results in non-syphilitics. For this reason it was strongly urged that, if in doubt regarding a result, the medical attendant should have the test repeated once, twice, or even three times.

One important strand of the Wassermann debate was the intricate technicalities of the test. The Wassermann reaction was defined by S. Grossman, an assistant medical officer based in Cardiff, as 'a complicated biological reaction, [requiring] expert knowledge, theoretical and practical, before any deductions can be made as to whether a patient suffers from neuro-syphilis or not'.[28] As well as being complicated, the test seemed to be a matter of individual preference in technique and in the use of the different sensitised haemolytic systems and antigens. Various serologists attempted to simplify the test, but even the simplest was apparently very complicated and required special apparatus and much time. The multiplicity of tests for syphilis led many authorities to plead for the procedure to be standardised. In the 1918 report of the Medical Research Committee (MRC) on the standardisation of Wassermann test pathological methods, they reassured that there was 'no process of biochemical diagnosis' that gave 'more trustworthy information' or was 'liable to a smaller margin of error than the Wassermann test' when it was performed 'with completeness and with proper skill and care'.[29] However, they did acknowledge that obvious advantages were to be gained from the standardisation of approved methods, and urged that Wassermann testing be undertaken only by pathologists with 'adequate training and experience in the performance of the tests and the control observations which are necessary to it'.[30] The MRC made it clear that no-one should attempt to undertake Wassermann tests who was not capable of the highest technical accuracy or in possession of full knowledge of the theory of the reaction. Mere acquaintance with ordinary laboratory procedure was not regarded as a sufficient criterion.

As well as technical difficulties, the Polish immunologist Ludwig Fleck (1896–1961) observed that interpretation was more of a mysterious art than a science, requiring a delicate initiation to be passed from one laboratory worker to another. The field of laboratory syphilology was 'a little world of its own... the serological touch... more important than calculation.'[31] Every laboratory used its own procedure, based upon precise quantitative calculations, but the experienced eye or the 'serological touch' was most important. Thus, a common view among serologists was that, while the Wassermann reaction was an infallible indication of the presence or absence of syphilitic infection, it had to be interpreted with intelligence and a regard for its essential limitations. Here lay the paradox of the Wassermann test. Introduced as the objective indicator of that elusive disease, syphilis, it soon became clear that it could be interpreted only through the 'intuition' of the pathologist. Furthermore, as the historian Ilana Löwy points out, paradoxically, it was precisely the delicacy and technical complexity of the Wassermann that was used to maintain confidence in the accuracy of the test.[32]

Attempts to standardise the test moved to an international level during the early 1920s and culminated in a series of recommendations issued by the League of Nations.[33] At the International Conference on the Standardisation of Sera and Serological tests, it was stated that: 'The desire for a standard serum test for syphilis has been voiced in many quarters', a desire that was easy to understand given:

[T]hat five reagents [are] employed in the test... that there is no general agreement as to the amount of each which should be employed; and that there are wide differences of opinion as to the source and method of manufacture of the antigen, as well as on the conditions of incubation and the degree of complement fixation which may be regarded as positive for purposes of diagnosis. Further, each laboratory employs its own method of noting results, and it is not surprising that the clinician who receives a report from a laboratory with whose standards and methods of notation he is not familiar is at a loss for a correct interpretation.[34]

Guidelines were soon being issued for laboratories to follow:

The careful standardization of reagents may appear tedious and lengthy, but it must be strictly observed. Scrupulous cleanliness in the care of glassware is also essential.... It is not... advisable that Wassermann reactions should be performed in laboratories where the required tests are few in number; they will be dealt with more satisfactorily at a central laboratory where large numbers of tests are made and where the various technical points are under constant supervision.[35]

The Wassermann test as a diagnostic tool

Table 4.2 gives the numbers of the Wassermanns (both blood and CSF) carried out by the Edinburgh laboratory for the REA and Rosslynlee over the period from 1909 to 1930. It is clear that there is a slight declining trend over this period in relation to the number of Wassermann tests conducted at the SAPS. Wassermann testing was first carried out at the SWARI from 1910 onwards, although regular testing was hampered during the Great War. However, as Table 4.3 reveals, and in contrast to the SAPS, laboratory testing at the SWARI shows fluctuations around a rising trend over the period. This can be explained at least partly by the defection of some SAPS member institutions to the SWARI venture during this period.

Wassermann testing appears to have constituted a substantial proportion of the work of both Scottish asylum laboratories in the two decades before 1930. Although we unfortunately lack comparable statistics for the proportion of tests devoted to the Wassermann in the early years of the laboratory, annual reports are available and provide this information for both laboratories for the year 1929. In that year, of 192 tests on specimens carried out at the Edinburgh laboratory, 97 (51 per cent) were Wassermann reactions, and a further 84 (44 per cent) related to CSF (colloidal gold, cell count and globulin).[36] The bulk of the specimens sent to the laboratory were to determine syphilis, despite the fact that the annual reports speak of the laboratory's work as being equally concerned with all types of insanity.[37]

Table 4.2		Table 4.3	
Wassermann Testing at the REA and Rosslynlee, 1909–1930		*Wassermann Testing at Gartnavel and Woodilee, 1910–1930*	
Year	No. of Tests	Year	No. of Tests
1909	9		
1910	15	1910	2
1911	4	1911	3
1912	11	1912	1
1913	12	1913	4
1914	7	1914	7
1915	6	1915	5
1916	3	1916	2
1917	0	1917	1
1918	7	1918	10
1919	7	1919	13
1920	3	1920	8
1921	5	1921	12
1922	3	1922	18
1923	0	1923	20
1924	7	1924	12
1925	2	1925	7
1926	4	1926	20
1927	2	1927	10
1928	6	1928	6
1929	2	1929	6
1930	2	1930	25

Source: Table 4.2, *REA and Rosslynlee Case Notes,* LHSA LHB7/51/34–120 and LHB33/12/5–36; Table 4.3, *Gartnavel and Woodilee Case Notes,* NHSGGCA13/5/123–48, NHSGGCA13/5/149–77, NHSGGCA13/5/178–94, NHSGGCA30/4/1–63 and NHSGGCA30/5/1–61.

While far more specimens were examined at the SWARI than the SAPS, a smaller proportion related to Wassermann testing. In 1929, of 903 specimens examined, 295 (33 per cent) were blood Wassermann tests, and 374 (41 per cent) were CSF-related (Wassermann, Lange Cell Count and globulin), with the remaining tests involving faeces, urine, blood and pieces of brain (26 per cent).[38] It is unclear why the Glasgow-based laboratory appears to have processed far higher numbers of specimens at this time, but once again it might in some part relate to the defection of some SAPS members to the SWARI.

The case notes of a sample of REA patients admitted between 1909 and 1930 who were given a final diagnosis of GPI indicate that 75 per cent were Wassermann tested (70 out of 93 cases). For Gartnavel, a similar proportion – 70 per cent of general paralytics – received one or more Wassermanns in this period (71 of 101). In the parochial asylums, however, this proportion was far less. Woodilee case notes record 111 patients to have been diagnosed as general paralytic in the period from 1909 to 1930, with 43 (39 per cent) Wassermann tested during their asylum stay. In the case of Rosslynlee, only one patient out of 72 admitted with GPI in this period was Wassermann tested, although a number were tested just before admission, with the results recorded in the case notes.

The case notes of all four institutions reveal that in two-thirds of the tested patients, testing was conducted within a month of admission, suggesting that the main purpose of testing was diagnostic. Staff were testing both patients already diagnosed with GPI and those whose diagnosis was in doubt but suspected to be GPI. However, as Chapter 3 revealed, the published literature considered GPI to be a definite clinical entity long before serological tests were introduced, its identity having been well-established on clinical grounds by the mid-nineteenth century. There was therefore a cluster of symptoms already strongly associated with the clinical diagnosis of GPI long before the first decade of the twentieth century. This raises the question of just how useful the laboratory could be to general paralytic patients, given the stability of the diagnostic category and supposed ease of diagnosis.

Despite supposedly being sure of the GPI diagnosis on admission, physicians requested that a Wassermann test be conducted in a number of cases. In the REA, this was true of 52-year-old widowed housewife, Elizabeth Y., and 39-year-old married coal carter, John S., both tested a month after admission in May 1915 and November 1918 respectively, where the results were found to be positive and the diagnosis did not therefore alter.[39] With James T., a 52-year-old married joiner, admitted to Gartnavel in October 1928 and diagnosed with GPI, the case notes record: 'Lumbar puncture was performed about a month ago [November 1928] – conclusive of patient having general paralysis.'[40] William P., a 37-year-old married car driver, admitted in July 1918, 'has looked very like a general paralytic, and his blood clinches the diagnosis.'[41] Regarding Margaret B., a 26-year-old married ropeworker, admitted in March 1919, Physician-Superintendent Henderson wrote to her family general practitioner: 'The possibility seems to me to be that this is a case of general paralysis. I shall be able to speak much more definitely, however, once I hear the result of the Wassermann reaction.' However, after the Wassermann was found to be positive, Henderson added: 'With this additional factor, I have now no doubt that the case is one of general paralysis.'[42] As a final example, the case notes of Susan N., an 18-year-old single pawn clerk, admitted to Woodilee in July 1921, recorded that '[t]he possibility of juvenile general paralysis has been entertained, but there are not yet sufficient signs and symptoms to confirm this diagnosis.' Subsequent to testing, it was noted: 'In view of the Wassermann reaction with the blood she is now regarded as a case of juvenile general paralysis.'[43] In such cases, the Wassermann result seems to have been used unproblematically to reinforce the initial diagnosis.

In other cases, a positive Wassermann reaction could alter a patient's diagnosis from something else *to* GPI. Thus, Mary S., a 44-year-old married housewife, admitted to Gartnavel in May 1923, had her diagnosis changed from manic depression to GPI on the basis of three positive Wassermann tests.[44] James M., a 56-year-old married clerk, admitted in February 1924 and diagnosed provisionally with organic brain disease,[45] was the subject of a staff meeting shortly after his admission to weigh up the various signs of his disease. At first sight there were features that spoke against a diagnosis of GPI: 'his personality was very well retained, his memory was still wonderfully good, and his mental activity in general was also very good.'[46] Nonetheless, Henderson was of the opinion that the case was one of GPI, 'facts in favour of this being that the seizures which the patient had had rapidly passed off, leaving no residuals: the fact of his pupils,' and the decisive result of his cell count and Wassermann. A post-mortem diagnosis of GPI was recorded. Since GPI was 'the great imitator' of other illnesses – particularly mania, manic depression and melancholia – alienists like Henderson seem to have been utilising the Wassermann test to differentiate GPI from these other disorders.

In cases such as these, the relationship between positive Wassermann test and GPI diagnosis seems straightforward. However, more complicated relations are evident elsewhere in the patient sample. Some patients were not diagnosed with GPI despite a positive Wassermann reaction and some of the clinical symptoms of GPI.[47] William S., a 40-year-old married coal miner, admitted to Rosslynlee in April 1928, was diagnosed with mania on admission, despite the fact that '[w]hen at Bangour, the serological reactions were blood WR +++, CSF WR +++, Pandy's test +++, Cells 49 per c.mm. Colloidal gold 555,555,431,10 (strong paretic).'[48] In the case of Jane F., a 38-year-old single fishworker, admitted to the REA in July 1911, her initial diagnosis of 'subacute delirious insanity' was retained due to her clinical symptoms – she was said, in particular, to exhibit considerable disorientation and restlessness – despite the fact that her CSF was 'most suspicious of GPI'.[49] Meanwhile, Mary C., a 35-year-old married housewife, admitted in

February 1913, had her diagnosis altered from manic depressive insanity to congenital deficiency and mania despite a positive Wassermann.[50]

The situation could be similarly complicated for those patients testing negative. William L., a 37-year-old married patient, admitted to Gartnavel in August 1923: 'Seems very like early GPI. Against it is the cell count of the cerebro-spinal fluid.'[51] However, this did not dissuade them from diagnosing him a general paralytic. In the case of Margaret Y., a 44-year-old single female, admitted to the REA in May 1905, the diagnosis of GPI was retained despite a negative Wassermann, based on the fact that the patient was 'a demented emotionally depressed general paralytic with well marked motor symptoms'.[52]

Moreover, patients could have their diagnosis altered from another diagnostic label *to* GPI despite a negative Wassermann being recorded in their case notes. Thus, 33-year-old married maltman, John N., and 49-year-old single tailoress, Elizabeth D., admitted to the REA in May 1903 and January 1905 respectively, had their diagnoses changed from mania to GPI despite a negative Wassermann.[53] In both cases, some of the physical and mental symptoms of GPI began to develop after admission. Finally, patients could have their diagnosis altered to a neurosyphilitic disorder without any laboratory input whatsoever. Thus, admitted in July 1920, 70-year-old widower John Y.'s initial diagnosis of senile dementia upon admission to Gartnavel was revised to tabes with psychosis without the use of serological testing.[54]

Indeed, a detailed reading of the case notes for these institutions reveals a complicated relationship between serological testing, clinical data, and GPI diagnosis. Indeed, six different possible relations can be detected between the Wassermann test and GPI diagnosis in each of the four asylums (see Figure 4.1). A patient could be diagnosed or re-diagnosed as a general paralytic with or without the aid of the laboratory, including where the test result was negative. Such observations suggest that the test itself was not over-enthusiastically used to define the diagnosis of GPI, with laboratory findings ignored or contradicted in a significant number of cases.

Despite this problematic relationship which the case notes illustrate between the laboratory and diagnosis, the published comments of a number of Scottish alienists at this time would indicate that the laboratory was quickly and gratefully integrated into the process of psychiatric diagnosis. As early as 1904, before the introduction of Wassermann testing and with regard to an obscure case of GPI, Clouston claimed to be most impressed by the conclusion of Dr G. Douglas McRae, assistant physician of the REA: 'It must be general paralysis, for I have been over to the laboratory and have found the characteristic diptheroid bacillus.' Clouston added: 'Whether he was right or wrong as to his conclusion, this spirit and this mode of work is

Figure 4.1

*Relations between Wassermann Testing and GPI Diagnosis
in the Scottish Asylums*

GPI diagnosis without testing	GPI diagnosis with testing +ve	GPI diagnosis with testing −ve
GPI re-diagnosis without testing	GPI re-diagnosis with testing +ve	GPI re-diagnosis with testing −ve

that of modern science, a method not dreamed of in the diagnosis of mental disease ten years ago.'[55] For many who published in the early years of the test, the new 'Wassermann' definition of GPI seemed triumphant over the old clinical criteria. Thus, by 1912, George Robertson, Physician-Superintendent of the REA, could pronounce that:

> The accurate diagnosis of some of the organic diseases of the brain has now reached such a degree of complexity that it can only be arrived at after a chemical examination of the blood and other fluids has been made by an expert in the laboratory.[56]

This comment particularly related to GPI, a disease which the laboratory had apparently revolutionised:

> Till little more than three or four years ago there was no certainty in some cases that the diagnosis was a correct one. Early cases were not always diagnosed, and cases were not rarely found to have been wrongly diagnosed.... This uncertainty has sometimes proved intolerable when important issues were at stake, and a piece of the brain has actually been removed during life for microscopical examination to settle this question. We are now able to diagnose this disease with absolute certainty in the earliest stage by means of chemical and microscopical tests. If the Wassermann reaction be negative in the spinal fluid as well as in the blood-serum then general paralysis may now, with almost absolute certainty, be excluded in spite of clinical symptoms.[57]

Robertson's neat conclusion suggested that psychiatry was no longer reliant upon either observation of symptoms (mental and physical) or the patient's history as supplied by patient or patient's family. Laboratory tests would not just complement clinical evidence but in fact easily outweigh it.

However, such positive verdicts of serology's rightful place within clinical psychiatry were increasingly interspersed with more critical comments and articles. Another group of physicians voiced grave concerns about the tendency of the laboratory to usurp the place of clinical experience. David Henderson, Physician-Superintendent of Gartnavel, recognised the test's limitations. While 'usually an aid to diagnosis', he added that 'one must not forget that it is by no means a specific reaction, and it requires to be interpreted with caution and in the light of the whole clinical picture'.[58] By 1933, in response to such criticisms, SWARI officials were explicitly reaffirming one of their aims as being to maintain a critical attitude towards established methods for the serodiagnosis of syphilis, and more especially the Wassermann test upon which, it was felt, too complete reliance was being placed.[59]

Such reservations were gathering strength elsewhere in Britain. In 1911, the army surgeon H.C. French, for example, eloquently cautioned against the allure of the laboratory:

> I put the clinical aspect [of diagnosis] last, but in my opinion it is by no means the least valuable. It does not perhaps glitter like the gold of the spirochaete, nor sound like the brazen cymbal of a positive Wassermann reaction, but as regards induration in the chancre it has the intrinsic merit of home manufacture.... Whatever each individual may think about the relative significance of Wassermann reactions, the fact must be admitted that in many instances we are as dependant [*sic*] today upon a correct clinical interpretation of what we see as in the past when John Hunter wrote.[60]

A decade later, C.F. Marshall and E.G. Ffrench still felt the need to warn against the 'dangerous tendency at the present day to exalt the value of laboratory diagnosis' and to 'neglect that of clinical experience'. These commentators warned that a diagnosis based upon laboratory tests alone could 'lead to disastrous consequences both to the patient and the practitioner'.[61] This smacks of the ethos prevalent among *fin-de-siècle* London consultants as described by the historian Christopher Lawrence,[62] which emphasised the intuitive aspects of the clinician's art and denied that these could be superseded by the findings of laboratory science. It was felt by such groups that laboratory techniques were in danger of reducing the complexities of diagnosis to a routine procedure. GPI was a definite clinical entity long before laboratory tests were introduced to the asylum, and these tests might introduce a fallacy, which presumably the clinical judgement of the physician would not. It seems that, rather than accept science into the asylum as a way to further their status as *bona fide* men of medicine – psychiatry of course requiring its status within medicine to be bolstered more than most medical specialities – the clinical experience which alienists alone possessed was deemed far more reliable.

The situation thus appears to have been complex and divided between those clinicians who welcomed the Wassermann and those who resented or mistrusted it. Although the test was received by many as a triumphant tool of science, ambivalence towards the claims of the laboratory was as clear within psychiatry as in other areas of medicine. From the introduction of the Wassermann test, there were those who deplored the separation and mutual suspicion between clinical and laboratory experts. In a most fulsome outline of these opposing factions, the venereologist Colonel L.W. Harrison noted that:

> Often… I find clinicians and pathologists working in watertight compartments and not a little mutual suspicion between two classes of worker whose close co-operation is essential to progress. As an example, you know that not a little criticism has been levelled at the reliability of the serum tests of syphilis. I think that much of this criticism springs from a lack of knowledge….[63]

Clinicians, Harrison claimed, criticised the Wassermann test because they did not understand it, whereas pathologists worked in blinkered isolation and took no interest in the concerns of the clinician. He referred to 'the folly and danger of rivalry instead of co-operation' between the two.[64] Harrison argued that serologists would have to convince clinicians of the value and reliability of the Wassermann reaction, but in carrying out this task they appeared to be confronted with an insurmountable problem: if the outcome of the Wassermann reaction confirmed the clinicians' judgement, this would be fine, but it would not add anything new to what clinicians already claimed to know. The situation would be different if laboratory reaction and clinical judgement pointed in opposite directions, but in that case the serologist would be hard-pressed to persuade the clinician of the accuracy of the result.

A clear reflection of the degree of concern felt over this issue was the efforts of the SAPS contributing asylums to unite clinic and laboratory worker. Meetings were held from 1936 onwards in an attempt to bridge the gap between both sides. Various suggestions were made for better contact between pathologist and asylum staff, including the proposal that members of staff from each contributing asylum might come to the SAPS where the Chief Pathologist would meet with them and discuss individual cases. The first of these meetings was held on 27 May 1936 when Henry Biggart, Laboratory Pathologist, met eleven members of staff from various related asylums. Some hours were noted to have been spent in demonstrating and discussing several of the more interesting recent cases sent from their asylums. Scottish pathologists were also visiting several of the more accessible asylums to discuss clinical and administrative problems, although such visits were of necessity infrequent and did little towards advancing 'the laboratory side of the picture' according to the 1936 annual report.[65]

These discussions resonated with wider negotiations going on within the United Kingdom. Thus, in January 1929, the General Paralysis Sub-Committee of the Medico-Psychological Association (MPA) attempted to resolve the contentious issue of how far clinicians could rely on the Wassermann test to aid diagnosis. They questioned whether the diagnosis of GPI was justified on laboratory findings alone, or should always be supported by mental and/or physical signs.[66] John Brander, Deputy Medical Superintendent of Bexley Mental Hospital, claimed that, while previously they had been able clearly to diagnose GPI, the introduction of serological methods caused many other conditions now to be classified as GPI. In the ensuing discussion, the preponderance of opinion favoured the view that no single test or combination of tests was sufficient to establish the diagnosis of GPI, and that diagnosis must be a combination of mental symptoms, physical signs and laboratory findings.

The changing identity of GPI?

In 1914, a contributor to the *British Medical Journal* claimed that the discovery of the spirochaete and the Wassermann test had 'thrown the whole subject of syphilis into the melting-pot, from which new conceptions of the disease [were] emerging'. It was argued that these reconceptions were 'still malleable' and that 'fresh investigations [were] daily entailing their remodelling'.[67] As a result of the extent to which positive Wassermann reactions were being found in patients displaying symptoms not previously understood to lie within the pathogenesis of syphilis and negative reactions in patients displaying the clinical symptoms, it seems that clinicians and pathologists were amending and building upon previous understandings of the aetiology and diagnosis of both syphilis and, by extension, GPI. The Wassermann test, it appears, was redefining these diseases.

Thus, in the first decade or two after the Wassermann entered psychiatry, a number of retrospective studies attempted to correct past diagnostic errors with the aid of the laboratory. One such study, conducted in Danvers State Hospital, Massachusetts, analysed the blood serum of those patients who had been admitted prior to 1912 – the year when Wassermann testing became a routine part of the admissions procedure at that institution – and given a diagnosis of GPI. Fifty-eight such patients remained in 1914. It was found that, had the Wassermann and spinal fluid tests been available at the time these fifty-eight patients presented for diagnosis, GPI would have been immediately excluded in some instances. As the study concluded, while 'clinical observation over a sufficient length of time will correct the diagnosis in the majority of cases', this method had 'very obvious disadvantages'.[68] Such accounts suggest that the Wassermann test allowed the diagnosis of GPI to be made much more accurately than had previously been possible.

However, the 1929 discussion of the MPA provided an interesting contrast to such earlier claims that the test had tightened the diagnosis of the disease.[69] The diagnostic developments of the early twentieth century were, they suggested, giving rise to an increasingly fragmented and unstable developing identity where GPI was concerned. Alienists agreed that the clinical features of GPI appeared to have become increasingly diverse, particularly in the years which followed the Great War. John Brander, the Bexley-based physician, was a fervent exponent of the view that the identity of GPI, confidently established by the clinical methods of an older generation of alienists, was being broadened and muddied by an over-zealous faith in the laboratory. 'Let it be remembered', he pointed out, 'that the diagnostic criteria of this disease and its fatal progression were developed many years before the days of the...Wassermann test.'[70] Brander concluded that there was 'far too great a tendency to attribute to syphilis any mental disorder which happens to be associated with a positive Wassermann Reaction.'[71] His objections demonstrate that, to some at least, the question of how GPI should be defined had not been improved by the widespread application of laboratory criteria.

The General Paralysis Sub-Committee of the MPA took up Brander's charges, but did not uphold them. The mistakes that Brander referred to, the meeting decided, had occurred back in the period from 1910 to 1912 when the test was new and 'some modern men had placed too much stress on laboratory findings'.[72] Since then things were said to have changed, and 'the present teaching was for the clinical findings to have the predominance every time'.[73] It was generally agreed that more varied clinical phenomena were now being treated as GPI, but whereas Brander maintained that this was due to changes in diagnosis resulting directly from over-reliance on Wassermann testing, the majority contended that the disease was in fact manifesting in new forms, many of which were treatable.

Although the Wassermann test seems quickly to have become a mainstay of asylum practice, we should be cautious in suggesting that it transformed GPI from a symptom-defined to a laboratory-defined disease.[74] We cannot assume, for example, that it really led to great changes in either the number of general paralytics diagnosed, or the way in which the diagnosis was made. Edward Hare, in his epidemiological study of the disorder, noted: 'I cannot find that, on the whole, there was any sudden fluctuation in the reported incidence or mortality of the disease after the introduction of objective methods of diagnosis.'[75] This is reinforced by the Scottish figures. As Table

4.4 reveals, at least three of these Scottish asylums exhibited marked fluctuations in their GPI admission figures, with the possible exception of Rosslynlee, whose numbers never reached more than nine admissions per annum. There cannot be said to be any significant long-term rise or fall in GPI admissions in the years around the introduction of laboratory testing. In the REA, Gartnavel and Woodilee,[76] while a noticeable rise can be discerned in the years around the beginning of the Great War, we see an equally abrupt decline in the diagnosis of the disease over the following decade, and this trend has also been charted south of the Border.[77]

Such a reduction is open to a number of interpretations. It is certainly possible that a proportion of the drop in GPI admissions was due to the Wassermann test reducing the number of patients in which the diagnosis was made, but it is unlikely that this was considerable. The War may also have been a factor in the reduction in cases. Certainly, such figures counter the claim that the test was used to over-diagnose GPI in asylums through an exaggerated faith in laboratory criteria. Even for those asylums where admissions continued to rise, the rise was very small indeed and in line with the pre-Wassermann period. George Robertson, a self-confessed devotee of the Wassermann reaction, estimated that the test had increased the diagnostic accuracy of GPI by six to fifteen per cent, primarily by differentiating it from two conditions that presented themselves very similarly – cerebral syphilis and alcoholic insanity.[78] For the REA, Robertson's statement is validated by the case notes, for the majority of 'erroneous' diagnoses – that is, those patients admitted with another disorder then re-classified as general paralytics later in their stay or at death – occurred in the pre-Wassermann period. This is also true of Woodilee, where few patients had their initial diagnosis changed to GPI after admission in the post-1910 period. The Rosslynlee case notes record erroneous initial diagnoses throughout this period, as one might expect given this institution's seeming reluctance to use laboratory methods. However, Gartnavel is quite different in this regard, where the majority of erroneous diagnoses changed to GPI were in fact recorded in the post-Wassermann period.

Despite the supposed impact of the laboratory on methods of diagnosis, it is significant that there appears to have been relatively little impact on the symptoms which alienists associated with GPI during this fifty-year period in Scotland. For all four asylums, the admission certificates of GPI patients retained the core cluster of symptoms found in the pre-laboratory period, recording in particular 'delusions', 'restlessness', 'excitement', 'incoherence', and 'memory impairment'. Only one or two of the core symptoms differed before and after the Wassermann test was introduced. Both Rosslynlee and the REA admitted fewer 'threatening', 'dangerous' and 'violent' patients in the Wassermann period than before. In the Gartnavel case notes, only

Table 4.4

GPI Admissions to the Four Scottish Asylums, 1880–1930

Years	REA	Gartnavel	Woodilee	Rosslynlee
1880-84	87	25	8	7
1885-89	94	39	29	23
1890-94	182	34	67	23
1895-99	162	20	131	13
1900-04	272	48	111	28
1905-09	205	32	92	20
1910-14	103	54	63	22
1915-19	201	67	90*	11
1920-24	105	29	0	16
1925-29	38	16	0	16**

* Until 1917 only

** Until 1928 only

Source: *Royal Edinburgh Asylum Annual Reports*, 1880–1930, LHSA LHB7/7/8–14; *Glasgow Royal Asylum Annual Reports*, 1814–1940, NHSGGCA13B/2/221–224; *Barony Parochial Asylum Annual Report*, 1919, NHSGGCA30/2/20; *Midlothian and Peebles District Asylum Annual Reports*, 1880–1930, LHB33/2/1–3.

'confusion' was noted much more frequently in the Wassermann-era admission certificates.[79] In contrast, in Woodilee, a number of symptoms became much more commonly noted in the Wassermann period. These principally included 'signs of organic brain disorder', 'problems with articulation', and patients being 'dirty in habits'. Woodilee also witnessed a marked increase in the number of delusions of persecution and suspicion after the Wassermann was introduced. Nonetheless, on the whole, the core cluster of GPI symptoms barely altered in the Wassermann period from that described in the previous chapter on pre-1910 admissions so that it is difficult to substantiate the claims of Brander and his supporters. Patterns of diagnosis for the Scottish asylums simply do not reveal a level of discontinuity that would indicate a major change in the number of patients diagnosed with GPI as a result of the Wassermann test, or a wholesale broadening of this diagnostic label.

Serological cure

This chapter has been concerned principally with the use of the Wassermann test in diagnosing GPI. However, the test was also used in conjunction with treatment regimens in order to determine whether the treatment had been successful and to what extent the patient had been cured. Indeed, the dermatologist Albert Neisser, instrumental in the development of the original test, had been primarily motivated by a therapeutic, and not a diagnostic, interest in the development of a serological test for syphilis.[80]

Although in the four Scottish asylums the majority of patients appear only to have been tested upon admission, and thus probably for diagnostic reasons, a small number were multiple-tested during their stay.[81] Of the post-1908 sampled admissions, only seven per cent of Woodilee patients and ten per cent of RAE patients were multiple-tested. Gartnavel physicians, however, had as many as twenty-five per cent of their patients multiple-tested. The purpose of this multiple testing appears to relate to the desire to measure efficacy of treatment. After all, as London Lock Hospital's surgeon Charles Gibbs and pathologist H. Wansey Bayly noted: 'Without the Wassermann reaction we have no means of judging, in the great majority of cases, as to when cure has taken place.'[82]

Thus, we can generally link multiple-testing patterns in patients to their treatment regimes. Such seems to have been the case for Alexander C., a 36-year-old married clerk, admitted to Gartnavel in February 1917, who had a Wassermann test, followed by:

> [A] course of salvarsan, five injections in all, the maximum dose on the last two occasions. In addition a very copious mercurial and iodine course was administered, but the blood gave a positive reaction after all. After the third injection there appeared to be a marked improvement, but the effect was only temporary.[83]

James O., a 28-year-old married patient, admitted in July 1930, had three tests over a period of four months in late 1930, whilst receiving a course of malarial and tryparsamide treatment.[84] Robert N., a 53-year-old married mechanic, admitted to Woodilee in July 1925, received three Wassermann tests, one before and two after malarial therapy.[85] 41-year-old widowed tracer, William U.'s six tests related to a course of fourteen injections of tryparsamide administered in March and April, 1924 and 1926.[86] The results of both of these patient's tests were consistently positive, and both were discharged 'relieved', although not 'recovered'. Finally, 44-year-old married housewife Elizabeth N., admitted to the REA in April 1928, received malarial therapy followed by tryparsamide and bismuth injections, with four Wassermann tests being taken just before and six months after the malarial treatment.[87] A large number of specimens sent to the SWARI by 1930 were blood and cerebro-spinal fluids from the general paralytics undergoing malarial treatment. As its annual report for 1929 stated: 'The results of treatment are carefully followed out, repeated examinations of the blood and CSF being made.'[88]

Once alienists began to use the test in this manner, it was quickly realised that many patients continued to test positive well beyond the point at which standard treatment was stopped. Thus, Alexander N., a 49-year-old single iron worker, admitted to Gartnavel in November 1911, was described in the progress notes as being 'physically much better than he has been for some time. He was advised, however, to go on with sulpharsenol treatment in London in view of the still positive Wassermann.'[89] It seems that it was no longer enough to remove external signs of the disease – a negative Wassermann became the definitive sign of cure. Thus, in 1914, George Robertson observed that:

> Our conception of the curability of syphilis has entirely changed since the Wassermann reaction has been employed to control its treatment. In the past many were unfortunately content to remove the external manifestations and call this a cure.... We know now that while the manifestations of tertiary syphilis respond wonderfully to salvarsan and mercury, it is not possible in some cases to remove the positive reaction from the blood.... Cure... is tested, not by the disappearance of all visible manifestations of the disease, but by a permanently negative Wassermann reaction, for anything else is futile.[90]

Treatment regimes and definitions of cure were thus developed simultaneously and in response to laboratory testing.

This was especially so given the greater treatment opportunities of the first decades of the twentieth century, as the following chapter will discuss. Testing on admission could in part relate to the perceived necessity of early treatment, on the grounds that the sooner a case was diagnosed, the sooner anti-syphilitic treatment could begin. This was at least partly a reflection of the faith being placed in new treatments like salvarsan in the early 1910s and malarial therapy in the early 1920s, provided that diagnosis was made early enough. The developing treatment armoury for GPI seems to have positively encouraged alienists to make the diagnosis, whether the laboratory verified that clinical judgement or not. This is well illustrated by the practice in Gartnavel, where on a number of occasions a course of anti-syphilitic treatment was administered before or without serological testing, further suggesting a precedence of clinical over pathological and a general 'better safe than sorry' attitude.

An advertisement, by the UK pharmacy Boots, for a brand of arsenical in 1925 took the new stamp of laboratory authority for granted: 'Approved by the Ministry of Health. Stabilarsan has a more permanent effect upon the Wassermann reaction... than any other arsenical.'[91] The Wassermann test was becoming central to a new definition of 'cure'. No longer did the disappearance of clinical symptoms constitute recovery. A convincing period of negative testing was also now required or, as an Edinburgh MD thesis of this period put it, 'a clinical and serological recovery'.[92] However, this change in the conception of GPI can only fully be understood within the context of the 'therapeutic revolution' which occurred in the treatment of GPI during the early twentieth century.

Notes

1. This chapter will focus exclusively upon those patients believed to have GPI because the other diseases within the neurosyphilis family were so rarely tested that no meaningful analysis could be made.

2. In 1912, the most specialised diagnostic test for GPI was introduced, Lange's colloidal gold. Lange discovered that an abnormal amount of protein substance in the CSF precipitated colloidal gold from solution, and that this precipitation occurred within certain dilution limits which were more or less specific to syphilitic conditions. However, the colloidal gold test does not appear to have been introduced to Scottish asylums until the early 1920s, and even then sparingly.

3. For a consideration of the development of laboratory science in German psychiatry, see E. Engstrom, *Clinical Psychiatry in Imperial Germany: A History of Psychiatric Practice* (Ithaca: Cornell University Press, 2003), Ch.4.

4. The main hurdle seemed to have been that alienists were too burdened by administrative duties. See A. Beveridge, 'Thomas Clouston and the Edinburgh School of Psychiatry', in G. Berrios and H. Freeman (eds), *150 Years of British Psychiatry, 1841–1991* (London: Gaskell, 1991), 380.

5. In 1915–16, the laboratory was moved to new premises at the Maudsley Hospital, Denmark Hill, London. See E. Jones, S. Rahman and R. Woolven, 'The Maudsley Hospital: Design and Strategic Direction, 1923–1939', *Medical History*, 51 (2007), 357–78.

6. Frederick Walker Mott (1853–1926) completed his medical studies at University College London, in 1881. After travelling and studying abroad, Mott was appointed Assistant Professor of Physiology in Liverpool in 1883, but returned to London the following year as Lecturer in Physiology at Charing Cross Hospital Medical School. After his 1895 appointment at Claybury, Mott's research began to focus upon the pathology of the nervous system and mental disease. For a fuller history, see A. Meyer, 'Frederick Mott, Founder of the Maudsley Laboratories', *British Journal of Psychiatry*, 122 (1973), 497–516; S. Mathews, 'Matter of Mind? The Contributions of Neuropathologist Sir Frederick Walker Mott (1853–1926) to British Psychiatry c.1895–1923', PhD thesis, University of Manchester (2006).

7. *86th Royal Edinburgh Asylum Annual Report*, 1898, Lothian Health Services Archive (LHSA), LHB7/7/10, 23.

8. *83rd Royal Edinburgh Asylum Annual Report*, 1895, LHSA LHB7/7/10, 18

9. William Ford Robertson (1867–1923) studied in Edinburgh from 1886 to 1891. Even during his undergraduate course, he was said to have shown a particular interest in pathology as taught by Professor William Russell, who was at that time Pathologist to the Edinburgh Royal Infirmary. After graduating, Ford Robertson held several Resident appointments, including house-physician at the Edinburgh Royal Infirmary. Despite the poor prospects at this time of pathology as a specialty, Ford Robertson devoted his professional life to it. In 1893, he became Pathologist to the REA, in succession to Dr James Middlemass, who had been appointed one of its assistant physicians. Robertson's contributions to the medical literature were many. He published on the histology of insanity, GPI and tabes, dementia praecox, and the parasitic origin of cancer – for further details on the last of these, see D. Gardner, *Surgeon, Scientist, Soldier: The Life and Times of Henry Wade, 1876–1955* (London: Royal Society of Medicine, 2005), 61–4 and 88–9. Robertson wrote one of the earliest Scottish psychiatric textbooks on pathology, *A Textbook of Pathology in Relation to Mental Diseases* (Edinburgh: William Clay, 1900), which remained the standard work of reference on the subject at the time of his death.

10. The first site of the SAPS laboratory was 12 Bristo Place, rented from the Royal College of Physicians of Edinburgh. This arrangement ended in 1900 when alternative premises were obtained, first in the Royal College of Surgeons of Edinburgh, and then in the grounds of the REA. In 1926, the Laboratory relocated once more, this time to the Department of Clinical Medicine at the University of Edinburgh, and by the 1930s, the Laboratory was housed at the Royal Infirmary of Edinburgh.

11. *Barony Parochial Asylum Annual Report*, 1905, NHS Greater Glasgow and Clyde Archives, NHSGGCA30/2/14, 80.

12. *89th Royal Edinburgh Asylum Annual Report*, 1901, LHSA LHB7/7/10, 18–19.

13. *Ibid.*, 17–18.

14. Annual reports for this Laboratory have only been traced for the years 1929, 1930, 1936, 1945 and 1947.

15. *55th Board of Control for Scotland Annual Report*, 1913, NHSGGCA13B/14/69, c.

16. When the Laboratory was inaugurated, the associated bodies were Gartnavel, Gartloch, Woodilee, Hawkhead, Kirklands, Smithston, Riccartsbar and Dykebar asylums.

17. Ivy MacKenzie (1877–1959) was to become one of Glasgow's most distinguished consultants. He graduated from the University of Glasgow MB, ChB in 1902, and MD with honours in 1912. He was employed as a consultant to the Victoria Infirmary, Glasgow, at the early age of thirty-six, and was concurrently Visiting Physician to the Eastern District Hospital,

where he had charge of the mental observation wards. In addition, he was Consulting Physician to the Glasgow District Board of Control, and a certifying physician in lunacy from 1914. Later, he became well known in medico–legal circles, recognised as an outstanding witness in both criminal and civil actions. His publications included contributions to anatomy, pathology, bacteriology, cardiology, neurology, and psychiatry.

18. *96th Glasgow Royal Asylum Annual Report*, 1909, NHSGGCA13B/2/223, 17 & 36.

19. *Ibid.*, 16.

20. *Scottish Western Asylums' Research Institute Minute Book*, NHSGGCA21/1/1, 1.

21. Whitelaw was recognised to be a skilled pathologist and bacteriologist. He had been for several years assistant pathologist at the Victoria Infirmary, Glasgow, and had served as pathologist and bacteriologist with the military forces at home and abroad.

22. *20th Scottish Western Asylums' Research Institute Annual Report*, 1929, NHSGGCA21/2/1, 10.

23. E. Southard and M. Jarrett, *The Kingdom of Evils* (London: Allen and Unwin, 1922), 458.

24. D. Henderson and R. Gillespie, *A Textbook of Psychiatry for Students and Practitioners* (London: Oxford University Press, 1927), 299.

25. This was most clearly demonstrated at the 1920s Wassermann Congresses held by the League of Nations where the best serologists from various countries examined the same blood samples simultaneously but independently.

26. A. Brandt, *No Magic Bullet: A Social History of Venereal Disease in the United States since 1880* (New York: Oxford University Press, 1985), 152.

27. W. Tulloch, 'Notes on the Wassermann Reaction', *Edinburgh Medical Journal*, 27 (1921), 34–55: 53.

28. S. Grossman, 'The Value of Simple Laboratory Tests in the Diagnosis of Neuro-Syphilis as Compared with the Wassermann Reaction', *Journal of Mental Science*, 71 (1925), 439–42: 439.

29. *Medical Research Committee and Medical Research Council: Reports of the Special Committee upon the Standardisation of Pathological Methods: The Wassermann Test*, 1918, The National Archives (TNA), Public Record Office (PRO), FD4/14, 21.

30. S. Mann and F. Partner, 'The Wassermann Reaction in Mental Hospital Practice', *Archives of Neurology*, 10 (1931), 1–14: 1.

31. L. Fleck, *Genesis and Development of a Scientific Fact* (Chicago: University of Chicago Press, 1979), 53. This work was first published in German in 1935. Fleck was among the first systematically to apply sociological principles to scientific knowledge, in relation to syphilis and the Wassermann reaction,

the field of science in which he was an active researcher.

32. Cited in H. van den Belt, 'Spirochaetes, Serology and Salvarsan: Ludwik Fleck and the Construction of Medical Knowledge about Syphilis', PhD thesis, Wageningen Agricultural University, The Netherlands (1997), 152.

33. The standardisation of sera and other biologicals was a major part of the programme of the League of Nations' Health Organization, from its foundation in 1921 to the outbreak of the Second World War. Many League projects were connected to national and military interests, including the effective control of syphilis since it affected the fertility of the population and the health and effectiveness of the armed forces. See P. Mazumdar, '"In the Silence of the Laboratory": The League of Nations Standardizes Syphilis Tests', *Social History of Medicine,* 16:3 (2003), 437–59.

34. 'International Conference on the Standardisation of Sera and Serological Tests', *Lancet,* 2 (1922), 1238–40: 1238.

35. Mann and Partner, *op. cit.* (note 30), 2.

36. *33rd Scottish Asylums' Pathological Scheme Annual Report,* 1929, NHSGGCA21/2/3, 7.

37. Asylum inmates could, of course, be infected with syphilis without this having progressed to GPI, and their mental symptoms might not be related to their venereal infection. However, evidence would suggest that the majority of these patients were being referred to the laboratory in relation to a possible GPI diagnosis.

38. *20th Scottish Western Asylums' Research Institute Annual Report,* 1929, NHSGGCA21/2/1, 14.

39. *Royal Edinburgh Asylum Case Books,* LHSA LHB7/51/97/701 and LHB7/51/103/885.

40. *Glasgow Royal Asylum Case Book,* NHSGGCA13/5/187/632.

41. *Ibid.,* NHSGGCA13/5/145/491.

42. *Ibid.,* NHSGGCA13/5/190/817.

43. *Barony Parochial Asylum Case Book,* NHSGGCA30/4/51/61.

44. *Glasgow Royal Asylum Case Book,* NHSGGCA13/5/183/354.

45. Of which GPI is a form.

46. *Glasgow Royal Asylum Case Book,* NHSGGCA13/5/181/285.

47. Again, such inmates could have syphilis without having a form of neurosyphilis, but they only appear in the samples used for this study because they received a final diagnosis within the neurosyphilitic disease group.

48. *Midlothian and Peebles District Asylum Case Book,* LHSA LHB33/12/35/69.

49. *Royal Edinburgh Asylum Case Book,* LHSA LHB7/51/94/301.

50. *Ibid.,* LHSA LHB7/51/94/789.

51. *Glasgow Royal Asylum Case Book,* NHSGGCA13/5/182/292.

52. *Royal Edinburgh Asylum Case Book,* LHSA LHB7/51/85/605.

53. *Ibid.*, LHSA LHB7/51/82/365 and LHB7/51/85/345.
54. *Glasgow Royal Asylum Case Book*, NHSGGCA13/5/147/205. Of course, as Chapter 1 indicated, the case notes may not have recorded comprehensively all those laboratory tests undertaken.
55. *92nd Royal Edinburgh Asylum Annual Report*, 1904, LHSA LHB7/7/11, 21.
56. *100th Royal Edinburgh Asylum Annual Report*, 1912, LHSA LHB7/7/12, 21.
57. G. Robertson, 'The Morison Lectures, 1913: General Paralysis of the Insane', *Journal of Mental Science*, 59 (1913), 185–221: 196.
58. D. Henderson, 'The Diagnosis of Cerebral Syphilis', *Review of Neurology and Psychiatry*, 9 (1911), 241–51: 244–5.
59. *Scottish Western Asylums' Research Institute Annual Report*, 1933, NHSGGCA21/2/2, 6.
60. Cited in J. Hurn, 'The History of General Paralysis of the Insane in Britain, 1830 to 1950', PhD thesis, University of London (1998), 154–5.
61. Correspondence, 'The Value of the Wassermann Reaction', *British Medical Journal*, 1 (1921), 686: 686.
62. C. Lawrence, 'Incommunicable Knowledge: Science, Technology, and the Clinical Art in Britain, 1850–1914', *Journal of Contemporary History*, 20 (1985), 503–20.
63. L. Harrison, 'The Role of the Pathologist in the Recognition and Treatment of Syphilis', *British Medical Journal*, 2 (1911), 686–7.
64. Correspondence, *op. cit.* (note 61), 686.
65. *39th Scottish Mental Hospitals' Pathological Scheme Annual Report*, 1936, NHSGGCA21/2/5, 7.
66. Discussion, 'General Paralysis', *Journal of Mental Science*, 75 (1929), 1–30: 1–2.
67. H. Armstrong, 'On Some Clinical Manifestations of Congenital Syphilis', *British Medical Journal*, 1 (1914), 958-61: 960.
68. *Ibid.*, 332.
69. Discussion, *op. cit.* (note 66).
70. J. Brander, 'The Diagnosis of GPI as a Clinical and Pathological Entity', *Journal of Mental Science*, 74 (1928), 673–86: 675.
71. *Ibid.*, 683.
72. Discussion, *op. cit.* (note 66), 290.
73. *Ibid.*, 280.
74. As, for example, Cunningham portrays the transformation of plague at the beginning of the twentieth century. See A. Cunningham, 'Transforming Plague', in A. Cunningham and P. Williams (eds), *The Laboratory Revolution in Medicine* (Cambridge: Cambridge University Press, 1992), 209–44.
75. E. Hare, 'The Origin and Spread of Dementia Paralytica', *Journal of Mental Science*, 105 (1959), 594–626: 613.

76. Figures for Woodilee are only available until 1920 due to the lack of subsequent annual reports.

77. In her study of GPI in England, Hurn has found a similar pattern of diminishing GPI admissions by this period. See Hurn, *op. cit.* (note 60), 171–2.

78. Robertson, *op. cit.* (note 57), 215. Such estimates were based upon studies in which diagnoses during life were compared with post-mortem diagnoses.

79. However, it should be mentioned that overall, Gartnavel physicians recorded a greater diversity of symptoms in their general paralytics than the other asylum physicians during this period.

80. Belt, *op. cit.* (note 32), 156.

81. I am taking 'multiple' to mean tested more than once.

82. C. Gibbs and H. Bayly, 'The Comparative Value of the Various Methods of Anti-Syphilitic Treatment', *Lancet*, 1 (1910), 1256–7: 1256.

83. *Glasgow Royal Asylum Case Book*, NHSGGCA13/5/144/396.

84. *Ibid.*, NHSGGCA13/5/189/814.

85. *Barony Parochial Asylum Case Book*, NHSGGCA30/4/57/12.

86. *Royal Edinburgh Asylum Case Book*, LHSA LHB7/51/112/201.

87. *Ibid.*, LHSA LHB7/51/117/937.

88. *Scottish Western Asylums' Research Institute Annual Report*, 1929, NHSGGCA21/2/1, 15.

89. *Glasgow Royal Asylum Case Book*, NHSGGCA13/5/140/574.

90. Robertson, *op. cit.* (note 57), 213.

91. Advertisement in *British Journal of Venereal Disease*, 1:1 (1925), front inside cover.

92. N. McLeod, 'General Paralysis of the Insane with Special Reference to its Treatment by Malaria', MD thesis, University of Edinburgh (1928), 45.

5

Treatment

Numerous therapies were employed in the Scottish asylums to treat the neurosyphilis disease group, particularly GPI, in the fifty years before 1930. This chapter shall give a comprehensive overview of such therapies, and explore the ways in which alienists in the four asylums utilised those remedies and with what level of success. The latter will involve the case notes being compared and contrasted with the published literature, as Chapter 4 did in relation to the Wassermann test. Efficacy will not be measured retrospectively, but in terms of both how contemporary physicians conceived it, and as judged from the recovery rates of the neurosyphilitics residing in the four Scottish asylums.

A hopeless disease

The published work of William Julius Mickle, Medical Superintendent of Grove Hall Asylum in London, and an authority on GPI, typifies late nineteenth-century writing on this disease. Four hundred and fifty pages of his *General Paralysis of the Insane* were devoted to descriptions of clinical and pathological findings, while a mere eight pages addressed therapy and hygiene.[1] This suggests that the diagnosis of GPI was something of a 'gateway to death', automatically constituting a prognosis of 'incurable'. Little had changed in this regard over the nineteenth century. As T. Austin, the Medical Officer of Bethnal House Asylum, lamented in 1859:

> The treatment of general paralysis is a subject which I approach reluctantly, and not without a feeling of despondence. The manifest hopelessness of the majority of cases, which have come under my notice, has induced me to regard the disease rather from a physiological than a therapeutic point of view; rather as a rich and unexplored mine of physico–psychical curiosities than as a curable malady.[2]

More bluntly, Thomas Clouston, Physician-Superintendent of the REA, called GPI the 'one absolutely hopeless disease' within the asylum, 'which, being once recognised, the patient's doom is held to be sealed, without a chance of respite'.[3]

However, by the second decade of the twentieth century, as Clouston's successor, George Robertson, noted: 'For a disease that is believed to be

153

incurable and fatal it is surprising how many remedies have been found'.[4]
Table 5.1 shows the various forms of therapy seen in the sampled
neurosyphilitic case notes of the four asylums in the fifty-year period up
until 1930.[5] Palliation was the mainstay of therapy throughout the period,
as well as a significant amount of sedation, in keeping with general asylum
regimens. Traditional syphilitic remedies were also utilised – mercury and
iodides – despite the dubious connection between GPI, tabes dorsalis and
syphilis until the early twentieth century. By the first decades of the
twentieth century, sera were being used experimentally on Scottish general
paralytics, although only in the REA. This period also witnessed the use of
the arsenical therapies, salvarsan and tryparsamide, in the four asylums,
though to only a very small extent in the case of the district asylums. Finally,
the 1920s saw the introduction of a new, and less orthodox, form of
treatment, malarial therapy, which was claimed to usher in a new era in
neurosyphilis therapy, and which was employed in all four Scottish asylums
during the later 1920s.

Remission

Before considering the efficacy of the therapeutic developments of this
period, it is important to mention that a characteristic of GPI was its
tendency to produce spontaneous remissions. William O., a 51-year-old
single law clerk, was admitted to the REA in January 1884. By the end of his
nine-month stay, his case notes mentioned: 'There is now a remission of the
mental symptoms of his disease, and Mr [O.] is at present rational in speech
and behaviour.'[6] Similarly, for John O., a 66-year-old married cashier,
admitted in May 1913, 'the paretic condition' was reported to be 'stationary
at present'.[7] Elizabeth E., a 46-year-old married housewife, admitted to
Gartnavel in July 1926, was 'seen to have improved her mentality during her
stay and remained stable for a fortnight', and was thus released on three
months probation.[8] Alexander N., a 55-year-old married labourer, was
discharged from Rosslynlee on a twenty-eight-day pass in July 1900,
'remaining on a remission of GPI.'[9] It is interesting that the degree of
remission in cases of GPI, though known to be only temporary, was
sufficient in a number of such cases to result in a discharge, even if only of
a probationary nature. These remissions were of three kinds:[10] firstly, there
was the simultaneous remission of the mental and motor symptoms;
secondly, there was remission solely or chiefly relating to the mental
symptoms, this being the most frequent type of remission; finally, on rare
occasions, there was a remission solely of the motor symptoms, without any
improvement in the mental condition of the patient.

Exactly what happened during these remissions was a matter of much
interest and debate, though an issue that was never satisfactorily resolved.

Treatment

Table 5.1

Neurosyphilitic Treatments in the Four Scottish Asylums, 1880–1930

Treatment	No. of Patients
Sedatives	167
Iodides	58
Malaria	24
Tryparsamide	14
Mercury	12
Serums	11
Salvarsan	8
Bismuth	2

Source: *Four Asylum Case Notes*, 1880–1930, LHSA LHB7/51/34–120, LHB33/12/5–36, NHSGGCA13/5/62–7 & 123–48, NHSGGCA13/5/ 98–122 & 149–94, NHSGGCA30/4/1–63, and NHSGGCA30/5/1–61.

The most popular explanation was that the activity of the spirochaetes was reduced 'either as a result of the lack of virility on the part of the spirochaetes or due to the proliferation of immunity bodies by the host'.[11] It was asserted by Jules Baillarger, the French neurologist, that remissions were most frequent when the disease began with a maniacal attack. When the remission ended and the disease resumed its course, it might be ushered in by an apoplectiform or epileptiform seizure. As Mickle dramatically explained, it was 'as if the disease had silently gathered force until "discharge" with explosive violence took place.'[12] The disease might otherwise commence with emotional and depressed ideas, maniacal restlessness and expansive symptoms, or with increasing dementia. Remissions did not seem to have a typical length, quite commonly lasting several weeks or several months. However, it was suggested by some that longer remissions were experienced by those patients receiving treatment of some sort. The American alienist H.C. Solomon stated that remissions of one to three years duration were very frequent in patients who had received treatment, occurring at least five times as often in the treated than in the untreated group, and lasting much longer.[13] However, spontaneous remissions and improvements also occurred without treatment of any sort.

Nineteenth-century therapies

Throughout the nineteenth century, neurosyphilitic treatments were practically confined to the alleviation of symptoms. After all, despite the prognosis, physicians could not be seen to do nothing except merely

155

'contemplate death... like men in a boat about to be swept over a fall, paralysed with despair'.[14] The patient was thus to be removed from employment at once and placed under the constant supervision of a relative or valet if treated at home or in a private house. If unsafe or certifiable, it was advised that the patient be placed at once under suitable hospital or asylum care. In fact, W. Barker, an alienist based both in England and Australia, felt that in any case of GPI, 'the first and only justifiable step [was] removal to an asylum'.[15] Complete rest was considered absolutely necessary, 'and a general paralytic ought never to be sent travelling on the Continent'.[16] The quieter the patient was kept, it was claimed, the more slowly would the disease develop, and the less likelihood of acute excitement supervening. On the other hand, gentle exercise, possibly out-of-doors, was recommended where the patient was able to cope with it. However, as Maurice Craig, a London-based physician and lecturer in psychological medicine, pointed out, moderate exercise was 'by no means easy to carry out, as the patient [was] usually restless and full of energy and [would] not be satisfied with less than twenty miles a day or many hours of golf or other games.'[17] However, it should be noted that many of the Scottish patients in my sample were already too advanced in the disease, once institutionalised, to be able to exercise or work.

Good nursing in suitable surroundings was seen to be essential. Great care was to be exercised in handling a general paralytic, 'as he not only bruise[d] readily, but his bones [were] very brittle'.[18] The annual reports of Gartnavel throughout the 1920s, backed up by the reports of the Commissioners, are full of references to the caring nature of the institution. Commissioner Sturrock of the Board of Control reported: 'The nursing care is of an excellent description. The staff generally give the impression of being alert, kindly and well-trained.'[19] One of the commonest concerns in the care of paralytics was the prevention of bedsores. This was reportedly achieved by taking great care to keep the patient clean by changing soiled clothes and providing daily ablutions. Still, in spite of the care of skilled nurses and attendants, bedsores often arose on parts subjected to pressure. In the bedridden and final stage of GPI, a water or air bed was viewed as desirable. The case notes of James F. of Rosslynlee, a 32-year-old single miner, admitted in March 1896, recorded that he had 'some very bad bedsores, in spite of [the use of a water bed]'.[20]

According to contemporary physicians, the bowels also required careful attention and continual care. Both constipation and retention of urine were common symptoms. The most useful medicine for constipation was a dose of castor oil, to be repeated as occasion demanded. Robert S., a 37-year-old married quarryman, admitted in August 1889, had his bowels moved with Croton Oil.[21] William D., a 32-year-old single labourer, admitted in April

1904, had an enema and castor oil to ease his pronounced constipation.[22] Alexander D. of Gartnavel, a 40-year-old married store owner, was a large eater and required 'laxative medicines'.[23] James S., a 36-year-old widowed mattressmaker, admitted to the REA in December 1882, had his '[b]owels moved well by a hotwater enema'.[24] In contrast, diarrhoea was an occasional complication of the last stage of GPI. Antacids, chalk and aromatics were considered useful against it, while half drachm doses of dilute sulphuric acid were said sometimes to check it.[25]

Finally, great care was to be taken to see that demented patients or patients suffering from seizures did not have a full bladder. Where necessary, a sterilised catheter was to be passed. As the neuropathologist Frederick Mott cautioned: 'This warning seems hardly necessary, but I have seen a demented paralytic fall out of bed in a seizure and rupture his distended bladder.'[26] In the four asylums, a catheter was frequently employed in the care of these patients. In Woodilee, Robert O., a 49-year-old married iron moulder '[r]equire[d] catheterisation every day' because his bladder was fully distended.[27] William F. of Rosslynlee, a 38-year-old married labourer admitted in February 1900, had his catheter treatment described in more detail: 'This morning it was found that his bladder was distended, and he was unable to pass his water, so reporter passed a no.9 rubber catheter, and drew off nearly a chamber [pot] full of urine.'[28]

The decades after 1850 saw an increased emphasis upon diet and regimen by physicians, including a vogue for using alcoholic beverages as stimulants. Thomas Clouston saw diet as crucial to the treatment of insanity. His 1881 annual report noted that all acute mental diseases and most nervous diseases 'tend[ed] to thinness of body', thus any foods, medicines and treatments that fattened should be an integral part of treatment. Clouston preached 'the gospel of fatness' to his assistants, nurses and patients as a 'great antidote to the exhausting tendencies' of mental disease, and considered that it would be 'well if all people of nervous constitution would obey this gospel'.[29] For Clouston, a combination of milk and eggs 'in the shape of liquid custards' was to be given frequently 'when everything else was refused'.[30]

This ethos seems to have spread quickly to other asylums. Thus, in 1892, John A. of Rosslynlee, a 40-year-old married dairyman/farmservant, was said to 'take very little food' and 'is now on custards'.[31] Margaret D., a 31-year-old married housewife, was placed on a special diet 'consisting of eggs, brandy, milk and bread. Tends to take form of: 4 Eggs, 3ozs Brandy, 2.5 Pints of Milk, Milk diet for dinner, Bread and Milk at 7pm.'[32] Alexander U. of Gartnavel, a 40-year-old married coal salesman, admitted in July 1898, was 'not looking well' and was therefore 'ordered extras'.[33] James M., a 45-year-old married spirit merchant, admitted in September 1902, was found 'to have lost considerably in weight so at present he is being kept in bed and is getting plenty of food'.[34]

It was, however, at the REA that 'feeding up' was most prevalent. A number of patients were said to require an extra nourishing diet due to their thin state. They were generally put on extra custards, or two custards daily. Robert U., a 41-year-old married physician, admitted in August 1897, received a 'liquid diet milk and eggs and a gregory' upon admission.[35] Notably, as with the three other institutions, such food treatments ended *circa* 1905, with none being prescribed after Robertson succeeded Clouston as Physician-Superintendent of the REA in 1908. This 'gospel of food' regimen was specific to the writing of Clouston, so it is unclear why the other institutions also ended this form of treatment around the same time.

Careful dieting and feeding were also necessary 'owing to the liability of general paralytics to choke, both on account of their greediness and of the defective powers of deglutition.'[36] 49-year-old William E. of Rosslynlee had 'to be hand fed, getting good fluid nourishment' due to his difficulty in swallowing.[37] Elizabeth O., a 55-year-old married housewife, admitted in January 1924, had to be fed rectally because she was hardly able to swallow.[38] Even more unpleasantly, other patients had to be force fed. At Gartnavel, John U., a 36-year-old married clerk, had to be tube fed 'as he refused to swallow, [and] there was no obstruction or difficulty in passing the tube'.[39] Similarly, at Rosslynlee, Alexander I., a 63-year-old married housepainter, had to be forceably fed because he refused food.[40] James I., a 40-year-old widowed 'low life' – his occupational label in the case notes – admitted in August 1927, was said to have 'good nourishment by being forcibly fed'.[41] Such force feeding was presumably made necessary through such patients having delusions of persecution.

Certain published authorities stated categorically that all alcohol was forbidden for general paralytics.[42] However, the use of alcohol as a stimulant was fairly widespread in this period, and quite a number of general paralytics in Scotland received alcohol in some form during their asylum stay. Thus, at Rosslynlee, William A., a 40-year-old single dairyman/farmservant, was given brandy because he was very weak and restless.[43] John R., a 48-year-old married labourer, got wine 'as his strength is failing', followed four months later by brandy four or five times a day, 'but he often spits it up'.[44] Interestingly, both of these patients were admitted with a diagnosis of melancholia rather than of the neurosyphilis family, so that this might still be compatible with the 'alcohol forbidden' rule. However, this was not true of others, such as Alexander U. of Woodilee, a 52-year-old single labourer, who received whisky daily due to '[d]yspnoea with a feeble irregular pulse';[45] or James J., a 42-year-old married draper, admitted to Gartnavel in June

1891, who received 'two glasses of whisky by day and night' because he was said to be 'sinking pretty rapidly'.[46]

Another prominent physical symptom associated with GPI was extreme restlessness. As one physician noted, '[t]here is nothing that calls for greater tact than having to regulate the exuberant spirits of the general paralytic in the early stages. With physical fatigue, every symptom from which he suffers will become exaggerated.'[47] When there was insomnia, hypnotics were to be given, and general restlessness required sedation. Asylum physicians had recourse to numerous drugs with which to calm and sedate their patients. Those employed in the nineteenth century included bromides, chloral hydrate, hyoscine, paraldehyde and sulfonal. Popular in the Scottish asylums, chloral was said to promote a deep sleep with no toxic effects and no after-effects the following day. Clouston's drug of choice was paraldehyde. He found it to be 'so valuable, so reliable, and so free from risks near or remote, that I think it cannot be too widely known by the profession.'[48] On the other hand, he believed that sulphonal could not 'be said to be perfectly and always satisfactory, or even safe'.[49] Sulphonal was generally believed to be slower in action and left dullness the next day. In fact, its continuous employment was believed to be injurious, aggravating the disease by its pernicious influence on the blood. Calomel was also used for the restlessness of GPI, as in the treatment of mania, although more rarely.

The most common method of sedation at the four Scottish asylums was a combination of paraldehyde, sulphonal and chloral, although sedatives were often simply referred to as 'draughts'. From the case notes sample, 35 Rosslynlee patients (19 per cent) were noted to have received some form of sedation during their stay. William E., a 49-year-old patient, admitted in January 1924, required regular sedation:

> While in bed patient had a violent outburst of excitement, raving incoherently and struggling. He was with difficulty controlled – and after a dose of paraldehyde which he took under the impression that it was alcohol he went asleep.[50]

Twenty-six Woodilee neurosyphilitics (12 per cent of my sample) received sedation, and 64 at Gartnavel (40 per cent). John U., a 45-year-old married hotel keeper and inmate of Woodilee, was '[v]ery restless and refusing to lie in bed' so that a draught was administered 'with some difficulty... which soon put him to sleep'.[51] At Gartnavel, Alexander I., a 37-year-old married warehouseman, admitted in September 1894, was reported as having '[f]or the last four or five days... small doses of sulphonal, with marked beneficial effect. It ha[d] subdued the excitement and made him more tolerable to live with.'[52] James E., a 39-year-old married mine manager, admitted in March 1919, was '[n]oisy, excited and destructive.

Nearly every night he ha[d] to receive an hypnotic of some kind or another.'[53] 42 REA patients (12 per cent) received some form of sedation, such as Margaret I., a 39-year-old married housewife, admitted in October 1905, who required sedation to 'subdue her dangerous excitement'.[54]

Mercury

Mercury had in the past been used as an ointment for diseases characterised by skin eruptions such as leprosy and scabies. First used on syphilis in the late fifteenth century, the popularity of mercurial treatment waxed and waned over the next three centuries, largely because of the dire effects of the heroic dosages customarily administered. However, by the eighteenth century, mercury had become the linchpin of treatment for all but a few venereologists, and it enjoyed an extraordinary vogue in early nineteenth-century therapeutics.

Mercury treatment appeared effective because physicians and patients wanted the venereal sores and eruptions to clear up, and with mercury they did. The copious involuntary salivation that it induced was seen as further proof that the drug was exerting an 'alternative' effect, that is, altering the fundamental balance of forces and substances which constituted the body's ultimate reality.[55] Though other drugs, most prominently arsenic and iodine, were believed able to exert such an effect, mercury seemed particularly useful because of the seemingly unequivocal relationship between varying dosage levels and its consequent action. Mercury was, in this sense, the physician's most flexible and powerful weapon for treating ailments in which active intervention might mean the difference between life and death.

While many believed mercury to be genuinely effective, there had always been a vocal minority who insisted that it was useless. At best, they asserted, mercury relieved some of the symptoms of syphilis and left the infection 'simmering... so that the disease was constantly progressing towards the stage of tertiary manifestations'. At worst, mercury treatment greatly aggravated the destructive effects of syphilis. In fact, it could not be clear 'which of the... symptoms of treated patients were due to syphilis and which to mercury intoxication'.[56] After all, mercury was a poison which disturbed human metabolism and produced side-effects ranging from nausea and pain to disorders of the skin, colon and kidneys. Prolonged exposure to mercury could produce mental and neurological disturbances, and at any time an overdose could kill. In fact, the estimated 'curative' dose was perilously close to the 'lethal' dose. Nonetheless, given the recognised dangers of syphilis, these effects were often portrayed favourably and typically accepted as necessary to combat the disease.

If mercury was so ineffective in syphilitic infection, why then did it remain the most popular remedy for centuries? Brandt asserts that mercury held favour regardless of a particular physician's theoretical perspective.[57] Although there was considerable debate about the mechanism of mercury's cure, there was broad consensus that with the salivation and profuse sweating induced by the drug, poison or pox 'virus' was expelled from the body. Furthermore, the punitive nature of mercury treatment reconciled therapy with moral norms regarding the causes of syphilis, as Chapter 6 will discuss. Finally, with the premise that serious disease required serious treatment, mercury certainly met the criteria. Established wisdom was summarised by the French virologist Philippe Ricord, who said that it was possible to cure syphilis only as long as the patient had the courage to go through with the treatment and the doctor had the courage to treat the disease properly.[58]

As a therapeutic agent, mercury was also used extensively in the treatment of insanity long before GPI was recognised as a disease entity. Benjamin Rush, the eminent American physician, claimed that mercury acted upon insanity 'by abstracting morbid excitement from the brain to the mouth'.[59] This therapy was subsequently administered in relation to GPI, even though the disorder's syphilitic origins were not yet suspected. Ironically, mercury's ineffectiveness was actually used as an argument *against* the syphilitic origin of GPI for a time. After all, if GPI was caused by syphilitic infection, surely mercury – the drug of choice for treating syphilis – would also cure GPI.

During the period from 1880 to 1930, there is no record of Rosslynlee physicians giving mercury to their neurosyphilitic patients, while Woodilee appears to have used it in the treatment of only one general paralytic, and the REA for only three. In all four cases, mercury was administered in combination with potassium iodide. William O., a 39-year-old married labourer, had mercury and potassium iodide administered on the same day, 20 March 1922. However, the treatment was unsuccessful, the patient dying in Woodilee on 24 June 1923.[60] Robert I., a 30-year-old single engineer, received mercury and potassium iodide treatment on 4 November 1889. He died in 1916, having been resident in the REA for twenty-seven years, yet received no subsequent treatment except 'urinary antiseptics, passing fluid and mild stimulants'.[61] Susan U., a 24-year-old single barmaid, was admitted to the REA in January 1899 with acute mania/syphilitic insanity. The physicians felt that the cause of her disorder, '[i]f not alcoholic, may be syphilis. She will thus be given a course of... [mercury and potassium iodide]', which she received one week after admission. She was discharged 'recovered' on 1 March 1899.[62]

Mercury proved a little more popular at Gartnavel, physicians treating nine (six per cent of my sample) neurosyphilitics in this manner, and in combination with a variety of other therapies. Alexander D., a 46-year-old single manager of a silk manufacturing business, received mercurial ointment in July 1903 and again in March 1904. He died on 18 January 1906.[63] James A., a 41-year-old married custom house officer, similarly received a mercury inunction on 5 January 1915. That and potassium iodide were tried 'but without any mental improvement'. He was thus transferred 'not improved' to Riccartsbar Asylum on 27 February 1915.[64] Robert O., a 40-year-old married marine engineer, was under inunctions of mercury during December 1919. He was transferred to Fulton Asylum in Yorkshire, in May 1920, due to the fact that his wife resided in England.[65] William O., a 45-year-old married grain weigher, was given mercurial inunctions in August 1922 because he was found to be 'Wassermann positive'. He died in November 1925.[66] Finally, Jane S., a 39-year-old married housewife, received malaria and quinine followed by a mercury inunction in January 1931. She died the following month.[67]

The iodides

For most of the nineteenth century, the importance of iodides to the treatment of syphilis was second only to that of mercury. Iodine was discovered in 1811 by a French chemist, Bernard Courtois, while potassium iodide was introduced by Charles Coindet, of Geneva, in 1820. However, this therapy gained general acceptance only as a result of the work of William Wallace, of Dublin, during the early 1830s. He first investigated the kinetics of iodine and iodides in dogs. Then, in a series of experiments which began in 1832, he showed that after oral administration, iodides were present in many body fluids, including the milk of nursing mothers. In 1836, he described the successful treatment of 139 cases of post-primary syphilis, and his results were soon confirmed by others.[68] Thereafter, it gained widespread acceptance for treating secondary and tertiary syphilis, in conjunction with mercury for the primary stage of the disease.

The iodides were usually prescribed as iodide of potassium, sodium or ammonium, or as a combination of all three. They were not, as a general rule, to be used for more than fourteen consecutive days, after which an interval of one week was to be allowed to pass. There were further considerations. In order for iodide of potassium to be 'well tolerated, and productive of benefit', the tongue was to be 'clean, the appetite good, and the nutritive and assimilative processes in fair working order'.[69] Despite their side effects – principally coryza and skin rashes – iodides retained their place in the treatment of late syphilis and, in combination with mercury, arsenicals or penicillin, were used well into the twentieth century. In fact, one writer hailed iodide of potassium 'the therapeutic magician', able to conquer syphilis in any of its stages, although he added that this drug did not possess in his hands 'that illimitable potency which many have ascribed to it'.[70]

The iodides were given more frequently to Scottish asylum patients than mercury and usually in the form of potassium iodide. The first of the thirty-three REA patients to be treated with iodide was Elizabeth O., a 39-year-old single slipper maker, in July 1880, a month after her admission.[71] Subsequently, according to my sample, this form of therapy was employed in the REA for the treatment of neurosyphilitics up to 1922. At Gartnavel, fifteen neurosyphilitics received iodide treatment, the first being John E., a 42-year-old single clerk, admitted in March 1887.[72] James H., a 53-year-old married mason, admitted in July 1897, had an ulcer on his leg which looked 'very suspicious of syphilis but no other evidence [could] be obtained of this'. However, no chances were taken, and the patient was treated with potassium iodide.[73] At this asylum, the use of iodide continued beyond 1930. About half of these iodide-treated patients received it in conjunction with mercury.

Moving to the parochial asylums, only 3 out of 210 Woodilee-based neurosyphilitics in my sample received iodides, while in Rosslynlee 7 out of 181 patients received this form of treatment. The first of these Woodilee patients to receive iodide was Robert E., a 32-year-old married mason, admitted in April 1889. The following month, he was prescribed 5gr of potassium iodide thrice daily 'in view of his syphilitic condition'.[74] William F., a 37-year-old married boilermaker, admitted in March 1911, '[could not] voluntarily raise the right eyelid' and so was also put on potassium iodide. However, as the potassium iodide 'had no apparent effect on the eye condition it was stopped.'[75] The first neurosyphilitic patient recorded to have received iodide treatment in Rosslynlee was John O., a 49-year-old single labourer, in August 1895.[76] This treatment was then given in the asylum throughout the first three decades of the twentieth century, usually three times daily, and usually in combination with some form of sedation. All patients who received it were male paupers, five of whom received the treatment just after their admission.

Bismuth

Due to the obvious disadvantages of mercury in treating late syphilis, the search for a replacement continued throughout the late nineteenth century. Numerous compounds were marketed during the 1880s – at one time there was a choice of 113 – but eventually intramuscular injections of metallic bismuth or one of its insoluble salts were favoured. Various compounds containing bismuth were first tried in the treatment of syphilis in 1889, but at that time they were abandoned. Attention returned to them in 1916, but it was only in 1921 that bismuth was introduced by two Parisian physicians, Robert Sazerac and Constantin Levaditi, when experiments in humans were undertaken.[77] Bismuth soon became an accepted adjunct to arsenical treatment and within a short time had replaced mercury in many quarters.

Soon, confidence in bismuth compounds was such that they also largely replaced potassium iodide in the treatment of tertiary gummas.

Clinically, there was a mass of evidence to show that bismuth favourably influenced the course of syphilis in all of its stages. In fact, the drug was believed to have a special reputation in the treatment of the neurosyphilis disease group, Levaditi recording an amelioration of symptoms in tabes dorsalis and GPI, 'possibly because many of these cases have become resistant to treatment by the arylarsonates'.[78] Once again, however, the same types of results were recorded: some remission of symptoms, modifications in the laboratory findings, but no hint of an unmistakeably curative agent. It seems that bismuth, like the many forms of treatment already considered, was to be relied upon 'more as a therapeutic ally than as a specific cure'.[79]

Bismuth was very rarely documented in the case notes of the Scottish neurosyphilitics. No patient in Rosslynlee or Gartnavel appears to have received such a treatment, while only one patient in both Woodilee and the REA received bismuth, both female. On 2 November 1905, Margaret J., a 40-year-old married domestic, admitted in September 1905, received some form of bismuth treatment, in addition to being put onto a milk diet for dyspepsia and vomiting. Having been resident in the asylum for forty-four days in total, she died ten days after the treatment.[80] Susan O., a 44-year-old married housewife, received bismuth injections following a course of two intramuscular injections of malaria and then 12gr of tryparsamide. Admitted on 16 April 1928, she was discharged 'relieved' on 2 March 1930.[81]

Surgery

In the spring of 1889, John Batty Tuke and Thomas Claye Shaw independently performed the operation of trephining upon general paralytics in an attempt to overcome cerebral congestion.[82] This was in response to Shaw's belief that one of the most prominent causes of the demented state that general paralytics often presented in the early stage was pressure. This, it was argued, if long continued, must cause atrophy of the cells followed by effusion of fluid. Tuke thus concluded:

> We are all witnesses to the relief afforded by depletion, such as strong purgatives; and I have little doubt that the loss of blood following the large incision that is advisable in operations for trephining is in itself a source of relief. Why not, then, in this early stage, before pressure has had time to cause destruction, provide a means more directly than can be done by any other method, of returning it?[83]

The propriety of surgical interference in GPI was said to rest on general and special grounds: general, in relieving pressure and draining off the fluid that had accumulated; and special, 'in the hope that it [would] afford a new system of nutrition for the brain, and another channel for the elimination of waste products'.[84]

Given the feeling of hopelessness that physicians experienced in the treatment of GPI, any means of relieving some of its symptoms was deemed worthy of consideration and trial. Trephining was considered to be 'a safe operation in skilful hands' which did 'not subject the patient to unfair risk, and that even in its present state [could] be shown to have conferred advantages'.[85] However, Shaw had some difficulty in persuading others to follow his lead, and to allow 'surgical interference' to 'be admitted within the circle of allowable remedies'.[86] He wished to stress that, in embarking upon this operation, he shared the opinion of more than one eminent neurologist. By 1895, John MacPherson, senior assistant physician at the REA, was claiming that cerebral surgery had become as thoroughly established as surgery of the abdomen had been during the previous decade.[87] Significantly, it was around GPI that the chief interest in the surgical treatment of insanity lay.

Scottish asylum records document a certain amount of experimentation in this technique. Batty Tuke and Shaw had performed the operation of trephining for the relief of GPI in Edinburgh and Stirling respectively. Of Batty Tuke's three cases,[88] the first had two trephine openings made, one on each side of the head a little above and in front of the parietal eminence. For five days after the operation a marked change in the mental condition of the patient was reported: his mind was clear, his manner calm. The hallucinations from which he had previously suffered disappeared, as did his severe headache. However, the improvement was apparently not permanent, as the disease soon resumed its progressive march. Worse still, the second patient saw his old symptoms return immediately after the closing of the wounds, and he died several months afterwards. Case three had a double trephine opening made in the Rolandic area. There was a distinct layer of fluid felt under the pia arachnoid membranes, which were opened and a small drainage tube inserted. However, the wound healed in five days and could not be kept open longer. On the second day after the operation, the pupils were found to be equal and the headache had disappeared. Three weeks after the operation the patient felt well, with no headache, a steady walk, and no tremulousness in his speech. He left the Royal Edinburgh Infirmary – where all three operations had been performed – on the fortieth day after the operation, completely cured. He remained well for three months, but reportedly gave way ultimately to drink and died in delirium tremens from exhaustion.

Shaw's cases met with similar results.[89] Case one had the dura mater opened, and a considerable quantity of CSF escaped. Four months after the operation, Shaw reported that the patient's general condition was much

165

improved and that, in his opinion, the patient was no longer insane. However, the motor symptoms were not relieved by the operation and seven months after the operation the patient died during convulsive seizures. Two more cases died, one during convulsions suffered thirteen months after the operation, and another from gradual exhaustion. A further five cases were under Shaw's care in Stirling Asylum. One died three months after the operation, one died eighteen months after the operation as the disease ran its usual course, and three were alive three years after the operation and with an arrest of the motor symptoms, although mental symptoms remained. Only one case was recorded as 'cured', and the last report upon this patient was made at too early a period after the operation (five months) to be conclusive. Thus, as the article summed up, a review of these twelve cases was hardly encouraging. A trawl of the literature has found no other record of surgical therapy in relation to the neurosyphilis family of diseases. Moreover, although this form of treatment was clearly known and to a limited extent employed in Scotland, if not elsewhere in Britain, no mention is made of it in the case notes and annual reports of any of the four asylums under study here.

Sera

In the same decade, serum therapies and anti-toxins aroused much interest. They consequently found their way into the treatment of syphilis, with the aim being to produce a serum that would vanquish the disease. In fact, with the discovery of the syphilitic spirochaete and the fact that it could be produced in apes, increasing research was conducted for the production of a syphilitic serum. Ilya Ilyich Mechnikov and Emile Roux had undertaken a series of experiments in order to manufacture a serum from monkeys, but were rewarded with little success.[90] Monkeys were chosen not only because they were inoculable with syphilis, but because they could furnish a serum which had very little haemolytic action on human red blood corpuscles. Dr Finger employed human sera obtained from patients with tertiary syphilis, from cases of secondary syphilis successfully treated by mercury, and from infants with hereditary syphilis. Charles Robert Richet and Jules Héricourt made a further modification by using the serum of animals previously inoculated with human serum obtained from cases of primary and secondary syphilis. George Tarnowski injected serum from horses mercurialised by injections of calomel.[91]

Within Scotland, W. Ford Robertson, the Edinburgh pathologist and Director of the Scottish Asylums' Pathological Scheme, was instrumental in the development of sera to treat the neurosyphilis diseases.[92] In 1901, he suggested that GPI was a disease caused directly by the toxins of bacteria, the point of attack being the alimentary tract. Two years later, he first announced his theory of *bacillus paralyticans* as a cause of GPI. In 1905, Ford Robertson and G. Douglas McRae, assistant physician at the REA, reported the presence of the diphtheroid bacilli in the genito–urinary tract in GPI and tabes dorsalis. Two years later, the same authors discussed the treatment of GPI and tabes by vaccines and anti-serum.[93] Such therapy could be administered by mouth, nose or hypodermic. Although initial experimentation with vaccines was undertaken, they were to place their reliance on the anti-serum.[94]

This method of combating GPI was given a trial. Ford Robertson described the symptoms in one of the cases which improved after two courses of this treatment.[95] The patient was a 41-year-old married man with no history of insanity. Three weeks after his third injection, a marked physical improvement was noted. However, his weight was only 8st 8lb as compared with 9st 4lb on admission. Within another month he had gained 6lb and was able to walk and even run. Co-ordination and pupil reflexes had returned to normal and mentally he was said to be much improved. Four months later his mental and physical improvement was noted to be well marked – he had gained another 6lb and was now working on a farm. About seven months after admission, he was being considered for discharge to his wife's care. However, two months later he had dropped to 8st 4lb in weight, become faulty in habits, and so bad on his legs that he had to be sent back to bed, to all appearances well advanced in the third stage of GPI. A second course of serum was given, after which he showed some improvement, but died soon after. Despite the hope with which serum therapy was heralded, it soon became evident that another treatment would have to be found as this cure could boast no long-term success.

Sera were not utilised by the physicians of Gartnavel, Woodilee or Rosslynlee, according to the case notes of their neurosyphilitics. However, the REA alienists made some use of this form of therapy, presumably due to the personal influence of Ford Robertson. Ten patients received some form of serum treatment in this institution during the period between August 1896 and August 1911. The first of these, James E., a 45-year-old married waiter, was treated with an anti-syphilitic serum on 1 August 1896. He died on 26 August 1897.[96] There is then a substantial gap of nine years before this treatment is mentioned again in the sample of neurosyphilitic case notes. The next patient to be similarly treated, this time with immune serum, was Mary I., a 34-year-old married housewife who was admitted in May 1906. This patient was said to be 'always more excited after injection but... more coherent and lucid'. However, she died on 26 July 1906.[97] Also in 1906, Elizabeth L., a 46-year-old married housewife, received 20cc of sheep serum on 5 December 1906, but died two days later.[98] Susan I., a 39-year-old married housewife, received serum treatment intraspinally during 1907, and again in October 1909. By January 1908, she was said to have: 'Greatly improved as result of serum treatment and vaccine.' However, she died in November 1910.[99] In most cases, there was no discussion about the rationale behind patient selection for this therapy. One exception was Jane I., a 45-year-old married housewife, who was treated with serum for a week in November 1909, but showed no improvement. The case notes record that she was chosen for this therapy 'as she was in such a poor mental and physical state of health'. She died in August 1910.[100]

This mode of treatment was only slightly more successful in the remaining five patients. Robert U., a 39-year-old married rubberworker, was 'the subject of experimentation with Ford Robertson's injections' in September 1906. He was transferred 'relieved' to Bangour District Asylum on 22 September 1906.[101] Jane E., a 28-year-old married housewife, was under serum treatment in 1906. By September 1907 she had 'to all intents and purposes recovered' yet was discharged merely 'relieved' in December 1907.[102] William D., a 43-year-old single gentleman farmer, had an injection of serum on 20 July 1907, with no reaction recorded in the following weeks.[103] Margaret A., a 53-year-old single domestic servant (cook), was given four serum treatments during 1907, on 28 April, and 7, 14 and 24 May. The course was given despite the first dose causing a reaction of 'drowsiness and pain all over her body'. She was transferred 'not improved' to Rosslynlee on 30 July 1907.[104] Mary C., a 38-year-old married housewife, was given anti-sera in September 1907. She reacted only slightly to the therapy, 'though she expresse[d] herself as stronger after each dose' and was discharged 'relieved' in December 1907.[105]

Twentieth-century therapies

Salvarsan

In 1909, the immunologist Paul Ehrlich (1854–1915) announced the discovery of dioxydiamide-arsenobenzol-dihydrochloride as a chemo–therapeutic cure for syphilis.[106] It was a yellow powder containing about thirty-one per cent of arsenic, kept sealed in ampoules containing a neutral gas, such as nitrogen, on account of its liability to form a poisonous compound upon exposure to air.[107] It was to be administered intravenously because of the extreme pain and even necrosis that followed its injection intramuscularly or subcutaneously. Ehrlich's discovery soon came to be known as 'salvarsan', and is widely held to have marked a fundamental breakthrough in the history of modern medical science: for the first time, a specific chemical compound had been demonstrated to kill a specific micro-organism. Ehrlich called the substance – the 606th arsenical he had synthesised in his chemotherapeutic institute, founded three years earlier – a 'magic bullet', a drug that would seek out and destroy the mark.[108] He posited that the world of twentieth-century bioscience would be the elucidation of such magic bullets to cure disease. Ehrlich received many honours, culminating in a Nobel prize for medicine in 1908, which he shared with the Russian Mechnikov for their contribution to immunology.[109]

Upon its launch, there was widespread agreement as to the remarkable effect that salvarsan, or '606', produced on syphilitic manifestations. Physicians worldwide wrote to Ehrlich eagerly seeking supplies of the drug, in order to replace the heavy metals previously used to treat the greatly feared disease, and triumphantly reported miraculous recoveries. The Glasgow-based pathologists Carl Browning and Ivy MacKenzie quickly asserted that 'in this drug we have by far the most active anti-syphilitic or anti-spirochaetal remedy yet discovered'.[110] As MacKenzie, first Director of SWARI, further proclaimed:

> There is already sufficient evidence to prove that one dose of No.606 can accomplish more than a prolonged course of the ordinary treatment, and that, too, without subjecting the tissues to a continuous saturation with drugs. During the past eight months about 8,000 cases have been treated, and if the hopes which this experience has raised, be realised, Ehrlich's most recent discovery will mark an epoch-making stage in the advance of scientific therapy.[111]

The compound was also used in cases diagnosed as syphilitic brain disease.[112] In fact, George Robertson, Physician-Superintendent of the REA, appears to have been the first physician in Britain to use this treatment in relation to GPI.[113] He discussed his belief that this new drug, 'owing to the large quantity of arsenic in its composition, is strongly germicidal, and a wonderful tonic in disorders of the blood', and that it might ultimately prove to be of value in the treatment of other forms of mental disease.[114] Landel Oswald, Physician-Superintendent of Gartnavel, claimed that it was thanks to Ivy MacKenzie that Scottish physicians were 'among the first' to treat GPI with this compound. As he further noted, '[t]he results [had] been encouraging, but a prolonged period must elapse before a definite opinion of the value of this treatment [could] be arrived at.'[115] The following year, Oswald provided further details:

> The treatment of general paralysis by means of Salvarsan was continued, and two cases derived so much benefit that they were discharged, and when last heard of were doing well. Remembering, however, that remissions to the extent of apparent recovery occur spontaneously in this disease, it cannot absolutely be stated that the improvement was due to the use of the drug.[116]

At the REA, George Robertson similarly commended MacKenzie in his cautious praise of the compound's effects on GPI:

> Through the kindness of the Director of the Glasgow Asylums' Research Institute, we were supplied with the drug before it was for sale, and since then we have purchased more. We have treated a good many cases without apparent benefit, but one patient, who was one of the first to be treated, made, almost at once after the injection, the best apparent recovery of any case of undoubted general paralysis I have yet seen. It is two months since this happened, and the patient still keeps well, but I will not yet commit myself to any definite opinion as to whether the progress of the disease has been checked or not.[117]

Henry Carre, Physician Superintendent of Woodilee, simultaneously published his results of treatment in seven cases of GPI. In four patients, the salvarsan was 'undoubtedly beneficial', patients showing marked improvement both in their physical and mental symptoms after the injection. Two of these had no recurrence of symptoms, but the others suffered a relapse, their initial symptoms reappearing in around twelve months.[118] Moreover, not only among Scottish doctors and pathologists was this new treatment received with such hope. News of this therapy was quickly disseminated, so that it became known by the general public that salvarsan offered hope for those afflicted with syphilis. Thus, the case notes of James T. of Gartnavel, admitted in February 1912, state that he was 'anxious that something should be done to "cure" him. He has evidently heard of salvarsan injections.'[119]

However, not all reports on salvarsan were so positive. Indeed, Ehrlich had himself advised caution, and tried in vain to restrict supplies of '606'.[120] His 'magic bullet' had its shortcomings. Salvarsan was toxic, difficult to administer, and required an extensive regimen of treatment of up to two years. Even when administered properly, the therapy could have all kinds of unpleasant side-effects, including headaches, chills, fever, itching and nausea. Only twenty-five per cent of patients received the full complement of injections as, not surprisingly, it was difficult to get patients to endure the entire course of treatment.[121] In addition, many considered themselves cured when they were relieved of the symptoms of infection. Patients could not understand why doctors insisted that they get so many injections, especially when each was so costly.

Despite the optimism with which the larger Scottish asylums – Gartnavel and the REA – received salvarsan, results do not appear to have lived up to initial hopes. As early as 1913, Oswald found that salvarsan had:

[S]o far had no good result when injected into the blood in cases of General Paralysis, this manifestation of the Syphilitic virus not appearing till many years after the original infection. The prevention of this protean and inevitably fatal disease therefore depends on the prevention of Syphilis, or on its early cure, although possibly benefit may result in the later stages when some means are discovered of killing the parasite by bringing the drug into more actual contact with the brain substance, the local seat of the disease.[122]

Similarly disappointing results were soon recorded by R. Dods Brown, senior assistant at the REA, who noted that he had taken the opportunity to treat cases of GPI with salvarsan given intravenously and with salvarsanised serum administered intrathecally. He concluded that 'definitely favourable results were not obtained by these methods of treatment', and that 'remissions which occurred in these cases did not exceed in number those of spontaneous remissions'.[123] In fact, so disappointing were the results recorded in studies of salvarsan that Mott was moved to declare in 1914: 'Candidly, I do not think any measure of success has attended any of the methods of treatment so far employed for General Paralysis.'[124]

For several years after its release, Ehrlich was bombarded by doctors and patients with requests for supplies of the drug and advice on its use, and he allegedly took it upon himself to investigate personally each and every complaint of adverse reaction. Despite this, and due to the difficulties connected with the preparation of '606' for injection, he managed to bring out his 914th compound, a modified salvarsan called 'neosalvarsan' which could be administered by intramuscular rather than intravenous injection. It was a yellow powder which contained twenty per cent of arsenic and was very soluble in water, in which it formed a neutral solution. However, it was much more liable than its predecessor, '606', to become toxic upon exposure to air so that, after dissolving it, there could be no delay over its injection. Although this compound was not as effective, it reportedly produced less severe reactions in patients and did not require such high precision in technique as salvarsan. Yet there still remained many adherents to '606'.

Despite the optimistic rhetoric which accompanied the release of salvarsan and the fact that Scottish clinicians were among the first to make use of it in the British context, very little use was made of it within the four Scottish asylums. No neurosyphilitic patients in Rosslynlee appear to have received it, and only one of my REA sample. Robert D., a 33-year-old single manufacturer, admitted in July 1911, received an intravenous injection of salvarsan on admission, after which his private medical attendant described him as being 'more alert and responsive than he ha[d] been for some time'. He received a further 15cc injection of salvarsan serum a fortnight later. However, there was noted to be very little reaction to this second injection, so that he was tried on Ford Robertson's anti-diptheroid serum instead. He was ultimately discharged 'relieved'.[125]

Three neurosyphilitics in the Woodilee sample received this form of therapy. The first of these, Elizabeth E., a 42-year-old married housewife, received 3gr of salvarsan by intramuscular injection on 8 January 1913. She died nine months later.[126] However, the two other patients to receive this form of therapy are recorded to have made a recovery. William O., a 41-year-old married shoemaker, received 4gr of neosalvarsan intravenously on 13 March 1913. He was discharged 'recovered' on 7 December 1914.[127] John T., a 41-year-old married railway clerk, received a rigorous course of neosalvarsan because '[h]is blood show[ed] a strong positive reaction to the Wassermann test'. He received intravenous injections in varying doses between October 1925 and January 1926. He also received malarial therapy and quinine in mid-1926, resulting in his swift discharge 'recovered' on 2 July 1926.[128] In both of these cases, it will be noted that treatment was by the modified version of salvarsan rather than the original agent.

Finally, four Gartnavel neurosyphilitics received this form of therapy between December 1910 and September 1922. Alex P., a 44-year-old married master mariner, admitted in October 1910, had three intravenous injections of '606'. After the first, in December 1910, administered by Ivy MacKenzie, '[n]o ill effects were got, no sickness, no rise of temperature and no disturbance of any kind were observed.' One month later, another injection was given without bad effect. However, '[a]lthough Mr [P.] had no nausea after this injection, today it was noticed that there were signs of thrombosis in the vein,' so that he did not receive another injection until 31 March 1911, when a half dose was given intravenously. This patient was discharged 'relieved' on 15 May 1911.[129] James Y., a 52-year-old married chandler, received a half dose of salvarsan in April 1911 with a resulting 'rise of temperature to 102 otherwise he is very well, talks sensibly and is in good health.' By October 1911, the verdict on his course of salvarsan was that it 'seems to have had the effect of staying the progress of his trouble, and mental and physical symptoms are stationary.' However, receiving no other treatment while in the asylum, Mr Y. died in July 1913.[130] Robert T., a 54-year-old single marine engineer, received 6gr of salvarsan on 5 November 1913, but to no avail, the patient dying on 11 January 1914.[131] Similarly, William O., a 47-year-old married public house manager, received six injections of '914' in 1922, but died three years later.[132]

Although very few patients appear to have obtained salvarsan treatment, it seems to have been considered for a number of patients but rejected on the grounds that they were 'not suitable' to receive it. The rationale behind such a decision is not entirely consistent. The 'not suitable' label does not appear to be gender or age-related, nor related to the fees which a patient could afford. The duration of the disorder is, however, important. Five of the Gartnavel patients were noted to have been insane less than twenty-seven weeks prior to admission, and they were the only ones to receive any treatment. Treatment was rarely given to anyone who had been insane for over a year prior to admission. However, some patients were recorded only to have been insane for a few days yet received no treatment. In such cases, it seems that their medical condition determined whether they were suitable to undergo any form of 'heroic' therapy, some being deemed too weak or irritable to withstand it. Admitted to Gartnavel in October 1910, 58-year-old John T.'s neosalvarsan was 'stopped on account of his nervous and depressed condition combined with a suicidal tendency'.[133] Bodily condition on admission was also considered. Alexander T. had no symptoms of organic disease on admission and thus received 6gr of salvarsan. However, James A., a 35-year-old single colliery salesman, admitted in March 1926, was described as a 'poorly developed young man' on admission and received only sedation and no other treatment during his five-year stay.[134]

Tryparsamide

Research based on Erlich's theories continued to produce important results. Further experiments with organic arsenic compounds yielded another valuable drug, tryparsamide. This new pentavalent arsenical, a sodium salt of n-phenyl-glycineamid-p-arsenic acid, was first synthesised by Walter A. Jacobs and Michael Heidelberger at the Rockefeller Institute in 1915. A white, amorphous, crystalline salt, freely soluble in water, it could be given intravenously, intramuscularly or subcutaneously. First tried on humans in 1921 to treat African sleeping sickness, it was put to the test in cases of syphilis in the following year.

Although it appeared to have little or no direct action on the spirochaete, and although found to be relatively useless in the early stages of syphilis, tryparsamide was sold as having a remarkable therapeutic efficiency in cases of neurosyphilis, most probably due to its power of penetrating the nervous system through the meninges. Practitioners reported that the most salient features which made it so useful in the treatment of neurosyphilis were that the drug possessed a marked affinity for the tissues of the central nervous system; there was no known substance with an equal degree of spirochaeticidal action that possessed the same high power of penetrability; the drug had a remarkable stimulating effect; and it was capable of reinforcing the natural processes of resistance and of promoting recuperation.[135]

Indeed, tryparsamide quickly proved successful in producing remissions in up to thirty per cent of general paralytics.[136] The first publication on its use in neurosyphilis appeared on 26 May 1923, when William F Lorenz and

Arthur S. Loevenhart reported very favourably on a series of 180 neurosyphilitics who had been under treatment for two years.[137] They concluded that tryparsamide was more effective than any other form of treatment presently available, and that both clinical and serological improvement was striking. Further reports appeared to confirm these results, although subsequent trials of this drug seemed to vary considerably in their level of success.

Clinically, the effects of the drug were encouraging for the patient. American workers noticed that the skin became clearer and the general bodily condition improved.[138] The Edinburgh surgeon and lecturer David Lees found that the first and most striking effect of the drug was the marked improvement in the patient's general well-being.[139] The weight of the patient was well maintained, and toxic symptoms such as headache, malaise and irritability often disappeared rapidly under its use. While the drug appeared to exercise no great effect on the Wassermann test, it apparently decreased very markedly the cell count of the CSF. In addition, it reduced the amount of globulin present and, in the majority of cases, favourably influenced the colloidal gold curve. Central to its superiority over alternative methods of treatment for syphilis of the nervous tissues was its ease of administration, incurring little discomfort to the patient and few side-effects. It was also pointed out that both clinical and serological improvement could continue for some time after the completion of a course of injections.[140] The condition of the patient at the end of treatment and the reactions of his fluids were not to be accepted as the final result, the drug continuing to exert a beneficial effect for some weeks afterwards.

Further European literature on the treatment of general paralysis by tryparsamide found that complete remissions ranged from fourteen to sixty per cent. A clinical remission with considerable recovery of 'economic efficiency' characterised about thirty-five per cent of these cases.[141] Those studies which found the drug to be of value usually conceded that, although short-term findings were good for tryparsamide, 'judgment must be suspended until a longer series of cases ha[d] been observed over a prolonged period'.[142] In fact, the general consensus of opinion advised that a preliminary course of tryparsamide followed by malarial injection was the most rational method of treatment, particularly in the debilitated type of early paralytic.

It was said to be '[t]hrough the kindness of Sir Frederick Mott' that a supply of tryparsamide from the Rockefeller Institute reached the Maudsley Hospital in London early in 1924 and became available for the treatment of 'suitable cases' of GPI and tabes dorsalis.[143] The number of cases treated initially was small, but nonetheless it was thought worthwhile to publish the results, and a preliminary report was sent to the Medical Research Council.

The Council judged that, while several GPI cases appeared to have their course arrested, in no case in this series was any result produced that was not achievable by the administration of other arsenic compounds. They concluded that it remained unproven whether tryparsamide was really more potent than other arsenicals, but deemed the drug worthy of further trial, it being easy to administer and not toxic in the doses used.[144]

In Scotland, the trials of Dr T. Davie, assistant physician at the REA, produced mixed findings. In October 1925, he commenced investigations at Gartloch Mental Hospital near Glasgow by placing seventeen cases of GPI under tryparsamide treatment.[145] Two deaths occurred before the course was completed and in both instances the patients were of the slowly dementing, apathetic type with no other psychotic symptoms. After treatment was concluded, two months were allowed to pass and then further clinical and laboratory investigations were carried out. Only two cases failed to benefit. Speech, tremor and gait all improved, especially the latter, and this was one of the first changes to be manifested. Another study found that, of sixteen patients treated in two (unspecified) Scottish asylums, six recovered or obtained a full clinical remission; two were greatly improved; three moderately improved; in two the condition appeared to be arrested; in one it progressed; and two died. Five of those in full remission were discharged, and three of these discharged patients returned to their previous occupation.[146]

Only one patient in Woodilee received tryparsamide, and none at all in Rosslynlee. Margaret D., a 44-year-old married housewife, received a course of tryparsamide in April 1929. Resident in Woodilee for five and a half years, she was discharged as merely 'relieved' in December 1933.[147] In Gartnavel, six patients received this therapy from April 1928 onwards. However, it was the REA physicians who were first to introduce tryparsamide into their therapeutic regime. Seven patients of the sample received the therapy after February 1924. Robert T., a 57-year-old married solicitor, admitted in March 1927, received six tryparsamide treatments within one month. However, after each injection, he 'became exceedingly confused, restless and dirty in his habits'. As his confusion reportedly worsened with each injection, the treatment was stopped.[148] William V., a 41-year-old widowed tracer, admitted in November 1923, received fourteen separate intravenous tryparsamide injections over a two-year period. During the latter weeks of the treatment, he:

[B]ecame decidedly more alert. He used to walk about slowly and displaying little interest. Now he walks briskly and is very helpful in the ward. His speech is unaltered. There is still the very noticeable slurrings. Neurological findings remain the same. He is still euphoric but since he has always

175

expressed himself as feeling perfectly well it is difficult to ascertain how he does feel at present. At any rate he has been toned up and is decidely improved.[149]

Furthermore, this improvement resulting from the tryparsamide treatment was noted as being maintained five months later. However, of the seven REA patients who received this treatment, only one was discharged 'relieved' and one 'recovered', with the remainder dying.

While some were quick to celebrate any successful discharge which treatment with tryparsamide allowed, another more dramatic story was simultaneously unfolding, and one which was to curtail further developments in relation to salvarsan and tryparsamide, the so-called 'specific' therapies. Just at the critical stage when tryparsamide was being released for widespread distribution, early reports on the potential of malarial treatment began to surface. Such reports soon directed attention away from the arsenical compounds, with the result that further research on the experimentation of tryparsamide was inhibited.

Malarial therapy

At the end of the nineteenth century, there seems to have been a general awareness amongst physicians of the therapeutic use of fever that extended back to Antiquity. Julius von Wagner-Jauregg, an Austrian alienist, began to experiment with this form of therapy whilst working at the Asylum of Lower Austria in Vienna during the 1880s.[150] He employed a variety of fever-producing agents, including Robert Koch's tuberculin and dead cultures of staphylococci, which he used on all types of asylum patients, including schizophrenics, manic–depressives and general paralytics. However, it was only his use of malaria upon general paralytics that apparently met with a significant degree of success.

This therapy took time to spread, due partly to Wagner-Jauregg's arduous institutional duties and to the inadequacy of the facilities at his disposal.[151] However, World War One allowed further opportunities for the alienist to refine his experimentation, and malaria therapy was widely adopted soon after, spreading rapidly throughout Europe and North America. During 1920, several German institutions experimented with malaria, including the Hamburg Clinic for Nervous Diseases. By 1921, malarial therapy had been introduced to the Netherlands and South America; by 1922, it had spread to Britain, Czechoslovakia and Italy; and by 1923, its use was being reported in Denmark, France, Russia and the United States.[152] Whittingham in Lancashire was the first British asylum to employ malarial treatment in July 1922. Dr R.M. Clark inoculated a general paralytic with malaria supplied by J.W.W. Stephens, Professor of Tropical

Medicine at Liverpool University. In the same year, alienists at the City of London Asylum ran trials of this therapy, followed closely by doctors at six other London asylums, as well as Rainhill, Cardiff and Winwick.[153] In Scotland, W.M. McAlister, Consultant in Psychiatry at Edinburgh Royal Infirmary, inoculated his first patient at the REA in March 1923.

Constraints and challenges

In contrast to previous remedies such as tryparsamide that were believed to have a specific anti-treponemal effect, malarial therapy acquired the designation 'non-specific' as it was considered to act through more general physiological mechanisms. Broadly speaking, researchers proposed four explanations for the efficacy of fever therapy. Some believed that the high temperatures killed the syphilitic spirochaete throughout the body, while others suggested that malarial infection increased antibody formation and hence increased immunity against the spirochaete. Yet others looked to the vaso–motor system for an explanation, believing that in some cases a condition of anaemia of the brain was cured by the fever. A final and popular explanation focused upon the specific effect of protein that the disintegrating malaria parasite delivered into the blood. No consensus could be reached on this issue, however, since no one factor seemed completely to account for the efficacy of malaria's therapeutic application to GPI.

Aside from theoretical disagreements on how the therapy actually worked, there were a number of practical difficulties which had to be overcome in order to implement it. Two basic schools of thought prevailed as to how the treatment should be conducted: the blood-to-blood school and the mosquito school. The most common method for inducing malaria was the former, by inoculating a general paralytic with 1–3cc of malaria blood obtained from another patient who was undergoing this treatment.[154] There were three methods here: subcutaneous, intravenous and intramuscular. The most popular was an intravenous injection, and Gartnavel physicians seem generally to have favoured this method. It was, however, in the method of intramuscular inoculation that relapses were found to be the least frequent, and this was the method that the staff of the REA tended to employ.

A series of logistical hurdles had to be overcome in order to obtain suitable blood. First, the proper strain of malaria had to be obtained, as the wrong species of malaria could be deadly.[155] Secondly, and more generally, this was a period in which the knowledge of blood types was very primitive, so that it was not well understood which potential medical complications might result from using the blood of one paretic to infect another, although there was some rudimentary fear about the compatability of donor and recipient blood.[156] It is unknown what proportion of malaria-treated patients were affected adversely by such incompatible blood transfusions, and the Scottish records make no mention of this problematic aspect of treatment.

Thirdly, it was not always possible to have suitable malarial blood available exactly when required. For many years, Scottish physicians appear to have struggled to find and maintain suitable malarial blood. In Edinburgh, a delay in getting such an experiment under way was due precisely to the difficulty of obtaining an uncomplicated case of benign tertian malaria. As the alienists of the REA complained: 'We ransacked the whole of Edinburgh and even applied to the School of Tropical Medicine in London in a vain effort to get a suitable case.'[157] However, they soon had 'the good fortune to admit a young man suffering from Dementia Praecox', from whose blood 'in the course of a paroxysm' they were able to isolate the tertian organism. Before proceeding with the inoculations, they had their diagnosis confirmed by Colonel Marshall, Lecturer on Tropical Diseases at Edinburgh University. Such strains of malaria could be maintained for long periods by repeated sub-inoculations from paralytic to paralytic, such as in Bangour District Asylum in Edinburgh, where GPI cases were 'inoculated one from the other, so as to keep the organism alive as long as possible'.[158] However, it was said to be extremely difficult to keep a strain going in more remote areas where demand was very small. Such difficulties were mitigated to some extent by improving methods of transportation. As one physician put it: 'Few places were more remote from civilisation than Western Argyll, yet malarial blood had been conveyed successfully down there, a thermos flask being used.'[159] By the 1940s, by which time there was an increasing and more constant demand within Scotland, a Central Register was being maintained by the Board of Control in order to simplify the procedure for the Physician-Superintendents of the Scottish asylums.[160]

As an alternative to the inoculation method, physicians might induce malaria with the bite of infected mosquitoes. The Scottish Board of Control recommended that this method be used, possibly because in certain private asylums exception was taken to the injection of blood from one patient into another.[161] The special department of the Ministry of Health, which maintained a supply of mosquitoes, offered to send a few on application to any hospital which required them.[162] However, this method was also problematic. There was the difficulty of obtaining and feeding the mosquitoes, who did not make good travellers and often died in transit. The incubation period could also vary widely, even when two patients were 'fed' at the same time and from similar mosquitoes. In addition, when pyrexia developed, the first and second rigors were often unsatisfactory, rarely reaching more than 102°F.

The case notes of the Gartnavel paralytics who received malarial treatment often mention their inoculation method. John P., a 28-year-old patient, and Mary T., a 39-year-old married housewife, both admitted to Gartnavel in late 1930, received malarial blood that had been taken from a patient undergoing a rigor.[163] Jane O., a 40-year-old married housewife, and Elizabeth C., a 26-year-old married ropeworker, both admitted to Gartnavel in early 1930, each received malarial blood from Hawkhead, an asylum located on the outskirts of Glasgow.[164] However, suitable blood was not always available so close by. The case notes of James T., a 31-year-old married stationer, admitted in January 1930, mention that his Gartnavel physician was forced to travel 'through to Edinburgh today' in order to obtain 10a of citrated blood from the Infirmary. The blood was noted to have been taken from the vein of a patient at 7.15pm, that patient having had a rigor for fifteen minutes 'before the blood was taken off'.[165]

Even once malarial infection had successfully occurred, it was acknowledged that the therapeutic use of malaria could have serious complications and was in fact a potent factor in the GPI mortality rates.[166] Side-effects were well documented, and ranged from muscle pain and jaundice to convulsions and cardiac failure. Indeed, as late as World War Two, experts considered the state of malaria control to be 'in a well-nigh primitive condition', with the decision as to when to end the febrile attacks by quinine treatment the chief cause of anxiety to the practitioner.[167] Yet, when weighed against the grave prognosis for untreated GPI, the risk seemed acceptable to many physicians.[168]

In addition to such practical difficulties, there were clear ethical concerns. As one Glasgow-based physician noted, many objected to the use of malaria 'on the ground that an actual living organism [was] used', since the introduction of a virus capable of multiplying in the body of the individual until there was no possibility of estimating the dose to which he had been subjected was clearly 'not desirable'.[169] David Henderson, Physician-Superintendent of Gartnavel, claimed similarly that his use of this treatment met with fierce opposition in certain quarters, stating 'we were threatened, if our malarial treated patients died, that criminal proceedings would be instituted against us'.[170] However, the benefits derived from malarial therapy were said to have stifled any 'criticism and opposition', and patients of all classes in Scotland appear to have received the therapy.

The attitude of British physicians to the considerable risks this therapy involved were by no means straightforward. Some betrayed a rather cavalier attitude to their patients and dispensed with the practice of obtaining family consent;[171] whilst others claimed that they always attempted to obtain consent, which was almost always readily given.[172] Scottish practice in this regard is difficult to assess, since there was rarely any indication in the case notes. Unusually, the case notes of Margaret C., a 26-year-old married ropeworker, admitted to Gartnavel in April 1930, record: 'No history has as yet been obtained from husband, whose permission for malaria will also require to be obtained.'[173] This would suggest that consent was generally obtained from the patient's family before treatment would commence. Certainly, there are no recorded incidences in the records of these Scottish asylums of malarial treatment having been withheld due to lack of consent. Thus, while occasional ethical misgivings were expressed, such concerns do not seem to have impeded the institutionalisation of malarial therapy. A combination of pragmatism and desperation in all likelihood prevented the majority of practitioners from treating ethics as a serious obstacle to practice.

The application of malarial therapy

Despite the divergence of beliefs concerning malaria transmission, a basic protocol was soon developed throughout Britain.[174] Having been infected with malaria, and after an incubation period of about two weeks, the patient would typically develop recurring febrile attacks accompanied by delirium and rigors, during which time he would be put on a four-hourly temperature chart, cold-sponged to prevent excessive temperature rises and subjected to daily blood examinations. After between eight and twelve of these paroxysms, he would be treated with quinine to arrest the disease. Following such treatment, the patient would be 'generally exhausted and anaemic', and would gradually be built up again with tonics and a nourishing diet – sometimes to receive further infections at intervals.[175]

Due to the combination of potential complications and a shortage of malarial blood, alienists were generally very selective as to whom they treated. Gender does not seem to have been a significant consideration. Age rarely proved a barrier to treatment either. The Scottish physician J. Steel set a barrier of sixty-eight to seventy, provided the patient was in a moderate state of health. He reported that one of his discharged patients had been 'inoculated a fortnight after his 65th birthday, and has since been doing very well at home, and has resumed to some extent his occupation as a hawker'.[176] However, the various forms of GPI seem to have been of significance here. Although patients with all forms of the disease were exposed to malarial treatment, the classical grandiose and exalted type of GPI was reported to give the best results, while the depressed and apathetic type often recovered more slowly and steadily. The 'galloping' type, senile and juvenile cases were noted to have the least hopeful prognosis.

Nonetheless, the matter of greatest importance to physicians was the physical condition of the patient. Any prolonged and severe attack of malaria would tax the patient's strength considerably. Thus, it was seen as 'courting disaster' to treat advanced semi-bedridden cases, obese patients or cases in which there was some serious heart lesion.[177] Allied to this was the relation of the onset of the disease to the time of commencement of treatment. The ideal was considered to be to treat the patient as early as possible, as it was found that the highest percentage of remissions occurred in those cases treated in the early stage of GPI.[178] Unfortunately, as the Glasgow-based physician T. Paton bemoaned, physicians were:

> [S]eriously handicapped by the fact that many cases, indeed most cases, that arrive in mental hospitals, do so when their social activities and mental stage necessitate segregation from their fellows. By then, their condition has progressed beyond a phase when a complete return to their status quo is possible.[179]

David Henderson's rationale for selecting patients for malarial treatment was that, 'with few exceptions', any patient suffering from GPI would benefit from such treatment 'provided that he [was] in a fair state of health, and [was] not too advanced in years.[180] Robert O., a 56-year-old widowed chemical worker, admitted in September 1928, received an inoculation of malaria and was said to have 'stood the strain well'.[181] However, the first of the twelve Gartnavel patients to receive malarial therapy was William S., a 56-year-old single buyer in a drapery warehouse, admitted in February 1927. After having malarial blood injected into him on 16 March 1927, his treatment was 'stopped as in the opinion of the Medical Staff he has had as much as he can stand'. He died in December 1928.[182] Yet, Susan O., a 48-year-old married housewife, admitted in November 1923, was deemed inappropriate for this form of treatment: 'Dr Henderson stated that the question of giving her something in the way of treatment would have to be considered, but that at present she was not fit for much physically.'[183] This was despite the fact that the asylum staff had already 'asked her husband's permission' in relation to the malarial therapy.

Any attempt to gauge the efficacy of this treatment within the asylums of Scotland must first acknowledge that there is a range of problems in interpreting the results of malarial treatment. Contemporary evidence ranged between extremes of dismissive pessimism and triumphant optimism, but few studies acknowledged the remissive character of GPI and the need, therefore, to delay findings sufficiently to rule out this explanation. However, within the Scottish context, both David Henderson and W.M. McAlister, Deputy Physician-Superintendent of the REA, urged caution in interpreting clinical results owing to the fact that it was 'impossible to distinguish clinically natural remissions from those produced artificially'.[184]

The REA appears to have been the first Scottish asylum to employ malarial therapy. Within my patient sample, the case notes of ten REA patients refer to them having received the treatment. The first was 54-year-old John U., who was inoculated with 2cc of benign tertian malarial blood on 16 April 1923.[185] A week later he suffered 'a typical attack of malaria which continued at regular intervals until he had about a dozen attacks'. His temperature 'rose to 105' and, as he 'looked very ill', quinine was administered and the attacks thereupon ceased. As his case notes concluded, '[f]ollowing this he was soon his old self again, but no material benefit resulted from the malarial treatment'. According to the REA annual reports, twelve general paralytics were inoculated with malarial blood in 1923 alone. Three of the twelve were dead within two years, although it was claimed that no patient actually died from the malaria.[186] While none of the remaining nine patients was completely restored as a result, their general physical condition was said to have witnessed a small improvement, and their mental condition a more obvious improvement. In 1930, forty-five GPI patients were noted to have been treated with malaria in this institution during the previous twelve months. Over thirty per cent of these patients were reported subsequently to be well, both physically and mentally, and able to return to work.[187]

The case notes and annual reports would appear to indicate that the physicians of Rosslynlee did not employ malarial therapy, while Woodilee physicians seem to have administered this treatment to only three patients within my sample. The first, Alexander O., a 53-year-old married mechanic, admitted in July 1925, began a course of malaria in December 1925.[188] The physicians of Gartnavel seem to have been a little later in adopting this treatment. In 1926, the annual report reveals that William Whitelaw, successor to Ford Robertson as Director of the SWARI pathological laboratory, treated two cases of GPI with malaria. David Henderson, Physician-Superintendent of Gartnavel, found that one of these cases quickly began to show a certain amount of improvement, but he concluded that 'far more cases [would] have to be treated, and a much longer time... elapse, before any definite statement of results [could] be made'.[189] The annual report for 1927 reported the continuation of treatment, but concluded that '[t]he results of this work ha[d] not been entirely satisfactory'.[190]

In 1930, Henderson wrote much more positively that continued treatment of general paralysis with malaria had, 'in many instances', resulted in 'astounding and beneficial results never previously attained', so that he would 'advocate malaria therapy in every patient suffering from general paralysis who show[ed] a reasonable chance of betterment'.[191] However, the following year's annual report conceded that it was only in 'a minority of cases' that the course of the disease had been 'ameliorated and lengthened', and 'a return to home and employment' made possible.[192] In a series of twenty cases treated at Gartnavel in 1931, ten patients were claimed to have been discharged 'recovered', or so far relieved as to be cared for under home conditions. Six more were 'improved', while four had died. In a series of thirty-four cases which were not treated, only four were claimed to have been discharged 'recovered' or 'relieved', while twenty-six died. Thus the death-rate in malaria-treated cases was noted to be approximately 20 per cent, as compared to seventy-six per cent in the non-malaria treated cases.[193] Nonetheless, the Gartnavel case notes reveal the widely differing results actually obtained. Upon receiving malarial treatment, James J. 'was practically his old self', while Jane O. managed a spontaneous remission after an intravenous injection of malarial blood.[194] In contrast, after having received a malarial inoculation, William U. soon underwent a pronounced deterioration, 'constantly raving during wakeful hours and frequently requiring sedative'.[195]

By the late 1920s, studies began to emerge which suggested that it would be more effective to combine malaria with other types of therapy, particularly tryparsamide or bismuth. Many British institutions began to combine tryparsamide with malarial therapy, or to supplement fever therapy with arsenicals, although this tendency towards combined therapy posed difficulties in the appraisal of malarial therapy. Within Scotland, T. Dymock, the Glasgow-based physician, used a combination of malarial, tryparsamide and bismuth therapy, with an alleged recovery rate of sixty-seven per cent. A further seventeen per cent of his cases supposedly had their disease arrested, and no deaths occurred.[196] The physicians of Woodilee did not combine malaria with tryparsamide, giving one or the other to their neurosyphilitics, whereas in the REA, tryparsamide and malaria could be given separately *or* together. In Gartnavel, on the other hand, tryparsamide was only ever used in combination with malaria. Unfortunately, from the surviving case notes it is not possible to be certain as to why practices varied between asylums.

In 1931, the Lunacy Board published a report into malarial therapy in Scotland, which compared the total number of cases of GPI admitted to Scottish asylums during the years 1922 to 1931 with the proportion of those treated by induced malaria or other methods. Table 5.2, overleaf, reveals that there was a steady rise in the numbers being treated by this method, but also that the majority of general paralytics were still being treated by other means. From the returns received from all Scottish asylums during the decade ending 31 December 1931, 403 general paralytics were discharged, 116 after treatment by induced malaria and 287 after another form of treatment. Of these patients, 110 (including 40 after malarial treatment) were discharged 'recovered', 99 (including 48 after malarial treatment) were discharged 'relieved', and 194 (including 28 after malarial treatment) were discharged 'not improved'. The Board concluded that a discharge rate of fifteen per cent was proof that malaria did induce at least a partial 'remission'. There appears to have been similar ambivalence to this therapy south of the border. By 1930, despite the Board of Control speaking of

Table 5.2

Methods of Treatment for GPI Patients in the Scottish Asylums, 1922–1931

Year	Total No. of GPI Patients	Malaria Only	Other Methods
1922	201	-	48
1923	182	5	50
1924	172	8	62
1925	150	18	57
1926	156	24	53
1927	169	36	51
1928	175	28	54
1929	186	43	82
1930	180	34	74
1931	161	43	84

Source: *Eighteenth Board of Control for Scotland Annual Report*, 1931, NHSGGCA13B/14/72, xxiii.

malarial therapy as an 'established and proven treatment', almost half of English asylums were still not making use of it within their therapeutic arsenal, for a variety of ideological and practical reasons.[197]

The advent of penicillin in the mid-1940s signalled the beginning of the end for malarial therapy. This safer alternative was quickly noted to impact significantly upon both the frequency and morbidity of syphilis in its various stages. However, penicillin was not immediately accepted. As one authority observed in the early 1950s, while penicillin had 'produced worth-while results in treating general paresis', it had been 'no more satisfactory than fever therapy'.[198] In Scotland, malarial therapy was still being employed by the Western and Northern Regional Hospital Boards as late as 1959. Elsewhere in Scotland it had been gradually abandoned in favour largely of intensive penicillin therapy, although pyrexial treatment using the inductotherm – a device which artificially produced fever by means of electromagnetic induction – was still employed in resistant cases of GPI.[199] The 'final curtain' did not come down on malarial therapy in Britain until the 1970s,[200] although occasional medical authors still speculate today on its potential usefulness in the treatment of infectious disease.[201]

Non-treatment

It has to be noted that, despite the publicity surrounding GPI treatments throughout the period under study, and particularly during the 1920s with the substantial coverage which malarial therapy attracted in both the medical and popular press, the vast majority of GPI patients in Scottish asylums in fact received no treatment at all. Many of even the long-stay patients received no treatment except occasional nursing. This was true of nearly half of the neurosyphilitics admitted to Gartnavel between 1880 and 1930: 47 per cent received no treatment except nursing during their stay. This proportion rises to 75 per cent for the REA sample, 77 per cent for Rosslynlee, and 83 per cent for the sample of Woodilee neurosyphilitics. Obviously, each incidence of treatment is not always noted in the case notes, so that the percentages are possibly not as pronounced as those noted. Nonetheless, this is a remarkably high rate, given the continuous advances made in syphilitic and neurosyphilitic treatment during the period from 1880 to 1930.

Curiously, having analysed the social and medical characteristics of these patients, there are no outstanding factors which explain why these particular patients received no treatment. Age is certainly not a factor – in Woodilee, patients aged from seventeen to sixty received no treatment. Neither is it gender, as both males and females were given the various forms of treatment, or no treatment at all, except in Woodilee, where none of the forty-one females resident appear to have received any treatment. Clearly class is not the issue, as the four asylums cover the spectrum of the very poor to the very wealthy, and there is no apparent distinction between them in relation to treatment. Equally, length of stay does not appear to have been a significant factor. Although patients often received treatment soon after their admission, some of these patients had been insane a long time prior to admission, while others were only recently deemed insane. In the REA, for example, some patients were there for in excess of six years yet received no treatment whatsoever, including Elizabeth E., a 49-year-old single tailoress, admitted in January 1905, and John T., a 41-year-old single grocer, admitted in April 1915.[202]

The only variable which seems to have significantly affected the likelihood of treatment was the pre-existing health of the patient. It was made clear that, if a patient was not in decent bodily health, tryparsamide or malaria would not be risked. Thus, patients like Alexander U. of Rosslynlee, a 59-year-old married labourer, admitted in February 1924, was 'in a low state of health' and received no treatment whatsoever.[203] This might be of particular relevance to Woodilee's low treatment rate. As Chapter 2 discussed, quite a number of these patients had been transferred to Woodilee from another institution, so it is just possible that their disease was more advanced than those general paralytics residing in the other three Scottish asylums. On the other hand, patients such as James H., resident in 1926 when several means of treatment were available and judged to be in good physical condition, received no treatment according to his case notes.[204] Thus, even this factor does not fully explain the rationale behind the treatment regimes of the four Scottish asylums.

It might be considered whether some of those patients who were physically able to withstand treatment yet left untreated formed part of an experiment into the nature and progress of untreated neurosyphilis. However, although at least one such experiment had been conducted, that carried out in Oslo between 1891 and 1910,[205] it seems unlikely that this was true of the Scottish experience. This was an era in which charitable hospitals and asylums had to be careful to respect public sentiments and to please their subscribers. Non-treatment was never justified in either the case notes or printed literature which emanated from these four asylums, which would suggest that the inhibitor was the perceived dangers or general ineffectiveness of these remedies rather than any desire to experiment upon these patients, as seen later elsewhere in the notorious Tuskegee experiment.[206]

The results of neurosyphilitic treatment in the Scottish asylums

Finally, it remains to chart the efficacy of all of these potential treatments and non-treatments within the four Scottish asylums. At the outset, such an analysis has clearly to acknowledge that the definitions used present a problem to the historian. Terms such as 'cured' and 'in remission', for example, were often used interchangeably, despite the fact that temporary remissions were a common and natural characteristic of GPI. In the medical institutions of Edinburgh, a patient was said to be considered 'cured' if he was able to resume his life without supervision and to carry on a similar occupation. This could be in spite of positive serological tests. To be 'improved', the patient had to show very striking physical and mental improvement, no longer require institutional care or strict supervision, and be able to resume his former occupation and mode of life.[207] Thus, in general terms, a 'good remission' involved a degree of mental and physical recovery which enabled the patient to become a normal citizen again. A 'partial recovery' covered those unable to obtain or retain regular employment. More slippery was the term 'relieved', which covered a multitude of improvements, however minor, relating to bodily or mental health, or merely to habits. 'Not improved' was a term applied to those patients who were deemed unable to be kept at home, and tended to be reserved for only the most chronic patients.

Table 5.3

Results of Asylum Stay for Scottish Neurosyphilitic Patients, 1880–1930

Result	1880-1910 (%)	1911-1930 (%)
Recovered	4	5
Relieved	13	13
Died	8	8
Not Improved	75	72
Unknown	0	2
(n)	(557)	(354)

Source: *Four Asylum Case Notes*, 1880–1930, LHSA LHB7/51/34–120, LHSA LHB33/12/5–36, NHSGGCA13/5/62–67 & 123–148, NHSGGCA13/5/98–122 & 149–194, NHSGGCA30/4/1–63, and NHSGGCA30/5/1–61.

Despite the exciting developments charted in neurosyphilitic treatments in the post-1910 period, we find remarkably little difference in terms of the efficacy of treatments for the Scottish patients. As Table 5.3 illustrates, in the period from 1880 to 1910, only about four per cent of patients were reported to have recovered, and for the following two decades the proportion is only slightly higher at five per cent. Equally significantly, in the period from 1880 to 1930, only forty-three patients in my sample recovered, and of the four patients to be discharged 'recovered' from Rosslynlee, not one of them had received any treatment while resident in the asylum. According to their case notes, the three males and one female, aged 21, 24, 43 and 45 respectively and resident between 57 and 529 days, did not even receive sedation. Only in one of these cases was there any suggestion that their GPI diagnosis may have been erroneous. It was recorded upon her admission in August 1923 that 24-year-old Jane H. suffered from adolescent insanity, later altered to GPI, and there might therefore have been doubt initially over her neurosyphilitic status.[208] The Woodilee records reveal rather more recoveries in this fifty-year period, with thirteen patients falling into this category. Significantly, these were all male general paralytics, with only two receiving any form of neurosyphilitic treatment. Robert O., a 41-year-old married shoemaker, received 4gr of neosalvarsan in March 1913;[209] while William T., a 41-year-old married railway clerk, received a course of neosalvarsan, followed by malaria and quinine between October 1925 and June 1926.[210] Both were treated immediately upon admission.

The physicians of Gartnavel discharged six patients as 'recovered' during the period from 1880 to 1930. Two of these, admitted in 1908 and 1917 respectively, received no treatment. The third, John A., a 35-year-old single colliery salesman, received only sedation during his stay despite being resident in the asylum from March 1926 to January 1931.[211] However, the remaining three patients received a combination of therapies. Alexander P., a 28-year-old patient, admitted in July 1930, received an extensive regimen of sedation, malaria, quinine, and eight separate tryparsamide treatments over a period of just four months.[212] Susan O., a 40-year-old married housewife, received sedation, malaria and quinine treatment during her six-month stay between March and September 1930.[213] Finally, James K., a 34-year-old married mason, received malaria, quinine and seven tryparsamide injections within the space of four months in late 1930.[214]

The REA case notes reveal a more impressive record of twenty recoveries within the sample of neurosyphilitics over the period from 1880 to 1930. Eight of these patients received no treatment, while a further eight received iodide only, and two received a combined therapy of mercury and potassium iodide. Mary E., a 36-year-old married housewife, admitted in November 1897, received only quinine during her stay, although it is possible that she received this as part of malarial therapy.[215] Only Robert O., a 56-year-old widowed chemical worker, received anything more substantial, being subjected to sedation, malaria, quinine and tryparsamide over a three-month period upon admission in September 1928.[216]

The evidence would suggest that the vast majority of the few patients who were recorded as recovered had in fact received no treatment whatsoever during their asylum stay. Nor was their diagnosis questioned or altered upon recovery. Those given one or more therapies rarely, in fact, made a full recovery. If we focus upon the 'relieved' patients, not one of the nine Rosslynlee patients discharged 'relieved' had any form of treatment. Even more significantly, only one of the thirty-nine patients discharged 'relieved' from Woodilee had received treatment, in this case malarial therapy. The Gartnavel neurosyphilitic case notes record that twenty-two patients were discharged 'relieved', of which two received potassium iodide treatment, one received three courses of salvarsan over a three-month period, one received malaria, and two received combined tryparsamide and malaria. For the REA, of forty-six 'relieved' neurosyphilitics, eight received potassium iodide, one received serum, one salvarsan and one malaria, while one patient received a combination of malaria, tryparsamide and bismuth. The remaining thirty-four, according to their case notes, received no treatment.

Furthermore, the majority of those patients who did receive treatment died. Within Rosslynlee, of the five patients who received iodide treatment, four died and one was transferred to the REA 'not improved'. Of those receiving salvarsan in Woodilee, two recovered and one died, although one of those to recover also received malarial therapy. The patient to get tryparsamide was discharged 'relieved', while of the three patients who received malarial therapy, one died, one was 'relieved' and one 'recovered'. For the REA, the one patient to receive salvarsan was discharged 'relieved'. Of the seven to receive tryparsamide, four died, one was 'relieved', and one 'recovered', with the remaining outcome of treatment recorded as 'unknown'. Finally, of the ten patients who received malaria, one was discharged 'recovered', two 'relieved' and seven died. Indeed, the REA case notes also contain a heading 'prognosis' from 1912 onwards. In this column, all of the REA neurosyphilitic cases had either 'hopeless', 'helpless', 'poor', 'bad' or nothing at all recorded. Not a single patient had a positive comment written underneath this heading.

What stands out from this analysis is the marked contrast between rhetoric, as evidenced in the published medical literature, and clinical practice, as gleaned from the case notes. Such were the changes and perceived advances that took place in the treatment of the neurosyphilis disease group, particularly GPI, over the period after 1880, and particularly during the two decades before 1930, that the literature contains many reflections on the significance of this period. George Robertson, Physician-Superintendent of the REA, remarked that in the 1880s, two-thirds of the males admitted to asylums between the ages of thirty-five and fifty suffered from GPI, with no known cause and no form of treatment to check its fatal course. Fifty per cent of those afflicted died within one year, and ninety per cent within three years of its recognised onset.[217] By 1930, in marked contrast, physicians claimed that they knew its cause, could predict its development and, by treating it in the early stages, could stay its course and return the patient to work. Yet, if we compare such rhetoric with the figures contained in Table 5.3, as with the findings of Chapter 4 on the diagnostic capabilities of the laboratory, the published comments of physicians on the efficacy of these therapies lie in stark contrast to the case-note findings. Even in the latter half of the period under study, when a range of therapies were available in these Scottish asylums, the outcomes of treatment were virtually identical to those found for the earlier decades, and in fact it was those patients left untreated who were most likely to recover to any significant degree.

Notes

1. J. Mickle, *General Paralysis of the Insane*, 2nd edn (London: H.K. Lewis, 1886).

2. T. Austin, *A Practical Account of General Paralysis, its Mental and Physical Symptoms, Statistics, Causes, Seat and Treatment* (London: John Churchill, 1859), 207.

3. *74th Royal Edinburgh Asylum Annual Report*, 1876, Lothian Health Services Archive (LHSA), LHB7/7/8, 17.

4. G. Robertson, 'The Morison Lectures, 1913 – General Paralysis of the Insane', *Journal of Mental Science*, 59 (1913), 185–221: 216.
5. Table 5.1 charts the number of patients receiving each therapy, *not* the number of times each therapy was used. Any patient receiving more than one of each course of therapy is counted as just one incidence of that treatment. If a patient received more than one form of treatment, such as mercury combined with potassium iodide, each type is recorded once under its appropriate category.
6. *Royal Edinburgh Asylum Case Book*, LHSA LHB7/51/42/70.
7. *Ibid.*, LHSA LHB7/51/96/305.
8. *Glasgow Royal Asylum Case Book*, NHS Greater Glasgow and Clyde Archives, NHSGGCA13/5/183/370.
9. *Midlothian and Peebles District Asylum Case Book*, LHSA LHB33/12/34/121.
10. Mickle, *op. cit.* (note 1), 206.
11. H. Solomon, 'General Paresis: What it is and its Therapeutic Possibilities', *American Journal of Insanity*, 2 (1922–3), 623–46: 630.
12. Cited in *Ibid.*
13. *Ibid.*, 640.
14. W. Godding, 'Active Treatment of General Paralysis of the Insane', *British Medical Journal*, 2 (1897), 1407–9: 1407.
15. W. Barker, *Mental Diseases: A Manual for Students* (London: Cassell, 1902), 108.
16. M. Craig, *Psychological Medicine: A Manual on Mental Diseases for Practitioners and Students* (London: J. and A. Churchill, 1917), 252.
17. *Ibid.*
18. *Ibid.*, 253.
19. *113th Glasgow Royal Asylum Annual Report*, 1926, NHSGGCA13B/2/224, 54.
20. *Midlothian and Peebles District Asylum Case Book*, LHSA LHB33/12/14/133.
21. *Ibid.*, LHSA LHB33/12/9/467.
22. *Ibid.*, LHSA LHB33/12/19/389.
23. *Glasgow Royal Asylum Case Book*, NHSGGCA13/5/130/438.
24. *Royal Edinburgh Asylum Case Book*, LHSA LHB7/51/40/166.
25. Austin, *op. cit.* (note 2), 222.
26. F. Mott, 'General Paralysis of the Insane', in D. Power and J. Murphy (eds), *A System of Syphilis*, Vol. IV (London: Oxford University Press, 1910), 290.
27. *Barony Parochial Asylum Case Book*, NHSGGCA30/4/4/302.
28. *Midlothian and Peebles District Asylum Case Book*, LHSA LHB33/12/16/249.
29. *79th Royal Edinburgh Asylum Annual Report*, 1881, LHSA LHB7/7/8, 18.
30. T. Clouston, *Unsoundness of Mind* (London: Methuen, 1911), 303.
31. *Midlothian and Peebles District Asylum Case Book*, LHSA LHB33/12/10/73.

32. *Ibid.*, LHSA LHB33/12/17/401.
33. *Glasgow Royal Asylum Case Book*, NHSGGCA13/5/132/149.
34. *Ibid.*, NHSGGCA13/5/134/319.
35. *Royal Edinburgh Asylum Case Book*, LHSA LHB7/51/7/209. Gregory's mixture consisted of a compound powder of rhubarb.
36. Barker, *op. cit.* (note 15), 108.
37. *Midlothian and Peebles District Asylum Case Book*, LHSA LHB33/12/33/121.
38. *Ibid.*, LHSA LHB33/12/26/20.
39. *Glasgow Royal Asylum Case Book*, NHSGGCA13/5/145/479.
40. *Midlothian and Peebles District Asylum Case Book*, LHSA LHB33/12/9/33.
41. *Ibid.*, LHSA LHB33/12/35/37.
42. See, for example, Craig, *op. cit.* (note 16), 253.
43. *Midlothian and Peebles District Asylum Case Book*, LHSA LHB33/12/10/73.
44. *Ibid.*, LHSA LHB33/12/11/84.
45. *Barony Parochial Asylum Case Book*, NHSGGCA30/4/18/111.
46. *Glasgow Royal Asylum Case Book*, NHSGGCA13/5/126/408.
47. Craig, *op. cit.* (note 16), 252.
48. T. Clouston, 'On the Use of Hypnotics, Sedatives, and Motor Depressants in the Treatment of Mental Diseases', 1889, LHSA GD16, 4.
49. T. Clouston, 'Sulphonal – Its Advantages and Disadvantages', 1895, LHSA GD16, 481.
50. *Midlothian and Peebles District Asylum Case Book*, LHSA LHB33/12/33/121.
51. *Barony Parochial Asylum Case Book*, NHSGGCA30/4/6/21.
52. *Glasgow Royal Asylum Case Book*, NHSGGCA13/5/129/96.
53. *Ibid.*, NHSGGCA13/5/146/269.
54. *Royal Edinburgh Asylum Case Book*, LHSA LHB7/51/88/33.
55. M. Vogel and C. Rosenberg, *The Therapeutic Revolution* (Philadelphia: University of Pennsylvania Press, 1979), 9.
56. J. Walkowitz, *Prostitution and Victorian Society: Women, Class and the State* (Cambridge: Cambridge University Press, 1980), 53.
57. A. Brandt, *No Magic Bullet: A Social History of Venereal Disease in the United States since 1880* (Oxford: Oxford University Press, 1985), 565.
58. Cited in J. Cassel, *The Secret Plague: Venereal Disease in Canada, 1838–1939* (Toronto: University of Toronto Press, 1987), 51.
59. Cited in G. Zilboorg and W. Henry, *A History of Medical Psychology* (New York: Norton, 1941), 548.
60. *Barony Parochial Asylum Case Book*, NHSGGCA30/4/52/64.
61. *Royal Edinburgh Asylum Case Book*, LHSA LHB7/51/6/63.
62. *Ibid.*, LHSA LHB7/51/74/9.
63. *Glasgow Royal Asylum Case Book*, NHSGGCA13/5/134/425.
64. *Ibid.*, NHSGGCA13/5/142/580.
65. *Ibid.*, NHSGGCA13/5/147/19.

66. *Ibid.*, NHSGGCA13/5/182/295.

67. *Ibid.*, NHSGGCA13/5/190/839.

68. See J. Oriel, *The Scars of Venus: A History of Venereology* (London: Springer-Verlag, 1994), 87.

69. *Ibid.*, 58.

70. T. Dowse, *The Brain and its Diseases, Volume 1: Syphilis of the Brain and Spinal Cord* (London: Baillière, Tindall and Cox, 1879), 57–8.

71. *Royal Edinburgh Asylum Case Book*, LHSA LHB7/51/5/168.

72. *Glasgow Royal Asylum Case Book*, NHSGGCA13/5/124/525.

73. *Ibid.*, NHSGGCA13/5/131/248.

74. *Barony Parochial Asylum Case Book*, NHSGGCA30/4/2/365.

75. *Ibid.*, NHSGGCA30/4/29/29.

76. *Midlothian and Peebles District Asylum Case Book*, LHSA LHB33/12/13/425.

77. Cassel, *op. cit.* (note 58), 57.

78. Cited in E. Duff, 'Modern Conceptions in Syphilology with Special Reference to Serological Diagnosis and Treatment by the Arylarsonates and Bismuth', MD thesis, University of Edinburgh (1935), 103.

79. N. Macleod, 'General Paralysis of the Insane with Special Reference to its Treatment by Malaria', MD thesis, University of Edinburgh (1928), 21.

80. *Barony Parochial Asylum Case Book*, NHSGGCA30/5/12/36.

81. *Royal Edinburgh Asylum Case Book*, LHSA LHB7/51/117/937.

82. Tuke was the owner of a private asylum in Edinburgh and succeeded Skae as an extra-mural lecturer. Shaw was Lecturer in Psychological Medicine at St Bartholomew's Hospital, London.

83. Cited in T. Claye Shaw, 'Surgical Treatment of General Paralysis of the Insane', *British Medical Journal*, 2 (1891), 581–3: 583.

84. *Ibid.*, 581.

85. *Ibid.*, 582.

86. *Ibid.*, 583.

87. J. MacPherson, 'Surgical Treatment of Insanity', 1895, LHSA GD16, 495.

88. *Ibid.*, 524.

89. *Ibid.*, 525–6.

90. See T. Rankin, 'Syphilis', MD thesis, University of Glasgow (1909), 196.

91. *Ibid.*

92. In fact, Ford Robertson also produced these sera to treat other types of insanity, including dementia praecox.

93. W. Ford Robertson and D. McRae, 'Observations on the Treatment of General Paralysis and Tabes Dorsalis by Vaccines and Anti-Sera', *Review of Neurology and Psychiatry*, 5 (1907), 673–85.

94. Anti-serum was obtained from immunised sheep which had been inoculated with dead cultures of the *bacillus paralyticans-longus* isolated from the brain

of a general paralytic. After two months' treatment of the sheep, the serum was judged to be fit for use.

95. Ford Robertson and McRae, *op. cit.* (note 93), 677.

96. *Royal Edinburgh Asylum Case Book*, LHSA LHB7/51/7/145.

97. *Ibid.*, LHSA LHB7/51/9/143.

98. *Ibid.*, LHSA LHB7/51/88/325.

99. *Ibid.*, LHSA LHB7/51/88/33.

100. *Ibid.*, LHSA LHB7/51/90/757.

101. *Ibid.*, LHSA LHB7/51/84/781.

102. *Ibid.*, LHSA LHB7/51/88/621.

103. *Ibid.*, LHSA LHB7/51/86/569.

104. *Ibid.*, LHSA LHB7/51/90/237.

105. *Ibid.*, LHSA LHB7/51/90/401.

106. Paul Erhlich coined the term 'chemotherapy'. At the most simple level this involved the synthesis of a series of compounds. Their chemical structure was modified and the compound which was found to be most active against the pathogen and least toxic to the host was selected. This signified a marked departure from the nineteenth-century extractive tradition of pharmaceutical production.

107. L. Harrison, *The Diagnosis and Treatment of Venereal Disease in General Practice*, 2nd edn (London: Hodder and Stoughton, 1919), 350.

108. See A. Brandt, 'The Syphilis Epidemic and its Relation to AIDS', *Science*, 239 (1988), 375–80: 375.

109. He was nominated for a further Prize in 1912 and 1913 for his work on arsphenamine but, because of the War and his death in 1915, this was never awarded.

110. C. Browning and I. MacKenzie, *Recent Methods in the Diagnosis and Treatment of Syphilis* (London: Constable and Company, 1911), xiv.

111. I. MacKenzie, 'Joint Communication on Syphilis: Recent Methods of Diagnosis and Treatment', *Glasgow Medical Journal*, 5 (1910), 335–49: 349.

112. Indeed, salvarsan was used to treat other types of mental disease, including dementia praecox, delusional insanity, acute mania and acute melancholia.

113. See Macleod, *op. cit.* (note 79), 19.

114. *98th Royal Edinburgh Asylum Annual Report*, 1910, LHSA LHB7/7/12, 20.

115. *97th Glasgow Royal Asylum Annual Report*, 1910, NHSGGCA13B/2/223, 17.

116. *98th Glasgow Royal Asylum Annual Report*, 1911, NHSGGCA13B/2/223, 22.

117. *98th Royal Edinburgh Asylum Annual Report*, 1910, LHSA LHB7/7/12, 19–20.

118. The three remaining cases showed no change in their condition after injection, but they were said to have only come under observation in the later stages of the disease. See *Barony Parochial Asylum Annual Report*, 1911, NHSGGCA30/2/15, 12.
119. *Glasgow Royal Asylum Case Book*, NHSGGCA13/5/145/479.
120. See Oriel, *op. cit.* (note 68), 92.
121. Brandt, *op. cit.* (note 57), 573.
122. *100th Glasgow Royal Asylum Annual Report*, 1913, NHSGGCA13B/2/223, 18.
123. D. Brown, 'Some Observations on the Treatment of Mental Diseases', *Edinburgh Medical Journal*, 36 (1929), 657–77: 673.
124. Cited in D. MacKenzie, 'The Evaluation and Differentiation of Mental Disorders associated with Syphilis of the Nervous System', MD thesis, University of Glasgow (1950), 8.
125. *Royal Edinburgh Asylum Case Book*, LHSA LHB7/51/91/757.
126. *Barony Parochial Asylum Case Book*, NHSGGCA30/5/32/46.
127. *Ibid.*, NHSGGCA30/4/34/44.
128. *Ibid.*, NHSGGCA30/4/57/32.
129. *Glasgow Royal Asylum Case Book*, NHSGGCA13/5/139/530.
130. *Ibid.*, NHSGGCA13/5/139/522.
131. *Ibid.*, NHSGGCA13/5/142/334.
132. *Ibid.*, NHSGGCA13/5/181/284.
133. *Ibid.*, NHSGGCA13/5/186/592.
134. *Ibid.*, NHSGGCA13/5/190/848.
135. See, for example, Macleod, *op. cit.* (note 79), 22.
136. D. Leigh in C. Thompson (ed.), *The Origins of Modern Psychiatry* (Chichester: John Wiley and Sons, 1987), 222.
137. See M. Brown and A. Martin, 'The Treatment of General Paralysis by Tryparsamide', *Journal of Mental Science*, 73 (1927), 225–33: 226.
138. W. Dawson, 'The Treatment of General Paralysis and Tabes by Tryparsamide', *Archives of Neurology and Psychiatry*, 9 (1927), 1–8: 7.
139. D. Lees, *Practical Methods in the Diagnosis and Treatment of Venereal Diseases* (Edinburgh: E. and S. Livingstone, 1927), 277.
140. Dawson, *op. cit.* (note 138), 7.
141. Brown, *op. cit.* (note 123), 672.
142. W. Dawson, 'Review', *Journal of Mental Science*, 71 (1925), 613.
143. Dawson, *op. cit.* (note 138), 1.
144. *Ibid.*, 8.
145. Cited in Brown and Martin, *op. cit.* (note 137), 227.
146. Brown, *op. cit.* (note 123), 672.
147. *Barony Parochial Asylum Case Book*, NHSGGCA30/5/59/51.
148. *Royal Edinburgh Asylum Case Book*, LHSA LHB7/51/116/77.

149. *Ibid.*, LHSA LHB7/51/112/201.
150. Wagner-Jauregg (1857–1940) qualified in medicine at the University of Vienna in 1880. He had success in the fields of goitre and cretinism research, but it was his work on malarial therapy which earned him the Nobel Prize for Medicine and Physiology in 1927, the first such honour to be awarded in psychiatry. For a full account of his life, see M. Whitrow, *Julius Wagner-Jauregg, 1857–1940* (London: Smith-Gordon, 1993).
151. *Ibid.*, 153.
152. J. Braslow, *Mental Ills and Bodily Cures: Psychiatric Treatment in the First Half of the Twentieth Century* (Berkeley: University of California Press, 1997), 77.
153. J. Hurn, 'The History of General Paralysis of the Insane in Britain, 1830 to 1950', PhD thesis, University of London (1998), 203.
154. W. Bruetsch, 'Neurosyphilitic Conditions', in S. Arieti (ed.), *American Handbook of Psychiatry* (New York: Basic Books, 1974), 144.
155. Three species of human malaria were available for therapeutic use in the 1920s: *P. malariae* (quartan), *P. vivax* (benign tertian), and *P. falciparum* (malignant tertian). The most commonly used was benign tertian, though quartan was noted to be more useful for those patients who had developed immunity to the former by residence in the tropics.
156. Braslow, *op. cit.* (note 152), 76. The Nobel Prize in Physiology or Medicine was awarded in 1930 to Karl Landsteiner for his discovery of human blood groups.
157. Letter from Royal Edinburgh Asylum to General Board of Control, 11 June 1923, The National Archives (TNA), Public Record Office, MH51/697.
158. *Ibid.* Once the blood was obtained, it could be carried in the syringe from one ward to another, wrapped in cotton wool that had been dipped in water at about 100°F. See G. Fleming, 'The Present Status of the Malarial Inoculation Treatment for General Paresis', *Journal of Mental Science*, 71 (1925), 605–8: 606.
159. Discussion, 'General Paralysis', *Journal of Mental Science*, 75 (1929), 271–97: 288.
160. Letter from General Board of Control for Scotland to Superintendents of Mental Hospitals and Medical Officers of Health, 10 January 1944, TNA MH51/538.
161. J. Steel, 'Malarial Therapy in General Paralysis of the Insane', MD thesis, University of Edinburgh (1926), n.p.
162. These mosquitoes were delivered in small glass jars whose open tops were covered with gauze of fairly wide mesh. The skin of the patient's thigh was gently warmed with a hot water bottle before the mouth of the jar was applied to it. The mosquitoes fed through the gauze and the jar was only removed when several were seen to be gorged. See N. Macleod, 'General

Paralysis of the Insane with Special Reference to its Treatment by Malaria',
MD thesis, University of Edinburgh (1928), 42–3.

163. *Glasgow Royal Asylum Case Books*, NHSGGCA13/5/189/814 and
NHSGGCA13/5/190/839.

164. *Ibid.*, NHSGGCA13/5/189/799 and NHSGGCA13/5/190/817.

165. *Ibid.*, NHSGGCA13/5/189/769.

166. See, for example, R. Ironside, 'On the Treatment of General Paralysis by
Malaria Inoculation', *Journal of Venereal Disease*, 1:1 (1925), 60–1; E.
Meagher, 'General Paralysis and its Treatment by Induced Malaria', *Journal of
Mental Science*, 75 (1929), 714–17: 716; B. Reid, 'Malarial Therapy in
General Paralysis', MD thesis, University of Glasgow (1932), 155–6.

167. G. Harrison, *Mosquitoes, Malaria and Man: A History of the Hostilities since
1880* (London: John Murray, 1978), 208.

168. Since few institutions were equipped to handle the complexities of the
parasites, special treatment and research centres were soon established. The
best known of these were the Horton Laboratory in Epsom, England; the
Syphilis Division of the Johns Hopkins Hospital, Baltimore, Maryland; and
the Station for Malaria Research in Tallahassee, Florida. Horton increasingly
yielded research into malaria itself, thus also gaining a reputation as Britain's
leading research centre for malariology.

169. J. McCully, 'Non-Specific Therapy in the Treatment of Neuro-Syphilis', MD
thesis, University of Glasgow (1930), 14.

170. D. Henderson, *The Evolution of Psychiatry in Scotland* (Edinburgh: E. and S.
Livingstone, 1964), 235.

171. See, for example, Letter from Keen to Board of Control, 11 June 1923, TNA
MH51/697.

172. See, for instance, Letter from Clarke to Board of Control, 13 June 1923,
TNA MH51/697.

173. *Glasgow Royal Asylum Case Book*, NHSGGCA13/5/190/817.

174. W. Nicol, 'The Treatment of General Paralysis by Malaria', *British Journal of
Venereal Diseases*, 5 (1929), 85–101.

175. *Ibid.*, 91.

176. Steel, *op. cit.* (note 161).

177. W. Nicol, 'The Relation of Syphilis to Mental Disorder and the Treatment of
General Paralysis of the Insane by Malaria', *Journal of Venereal Disease*, 9
(1933), 224–34: 226. However, pregnancy was not classed as a contra-
indication.

178. Macleod, *op. cit.* (note 79), 45.

179. T. Paton, 'Therapeutic Malaria in General Paralysis of the Insane', MD
thesis, University of Glasgow (1933), 2.

180. *118th Glasgow Royal Asylum Annual Report*, 1931, NHSGGCA13B/2/225,
23.

181. *Royal Edinburgh Asylum Case Book*, LHSA LHB7/51/115/873.
182. *Glasgow Royal Asylum Case Book*, NHSGGCA13/5/187/612.
183. *Ibid.*, NHSGGCA13/5/184/420.
184. W. McAlister, 'The Role of Infection in the Treatment of General Paralysis', *Journal of Mental Science*, 70 (1924), 76–81: 81.
185. *Royal Edinburgh Asylum Case Book*, LHSA LHB7/51/108/53.
186. W. McAlister, 'The Results of the Treatment of General Paralysis by Malaria', *Journal of Mental Science*, 71 (1925), 236–40: 237.
187. *Annual Report of the City of Edinburgh Public Health Department*, 1930, LHSA LHB16/2/12, 75.
188. *Barony Parochial Asylum Case Book*, NHSGGCA30/4/57/12.
189. *113th Glasgow Royal Asylum Annual Report*, 1926, NHSGGCA13B/2/224, 26.
190. *114th Glasgow Royal Asylum Annual Report*, 1927, NHSGGCA13B/2/224, 25.
191. *117th Glasgow Royal Asylum Annual Report*, 1930, NHSGGCA13B/2/224, 23.
192. *118th Glasgow Royal Asylum Annual Report*, 1931, NHSGGCA13B/2/225, 23.
193. *Ibid.*
194. *Glasgow Royal Asylum Case Books*, NHSGGCA13/5/190/844 and NHSGGCA13/5/184/420.
195. *Ibid.*, NHSGGCA13/5/187/632.
196. T. Dymock, 'A Review of the Treatment of General Paralysis', MD thesis, University of Glasgow (1933), 96.
197. Hurn, *op. cit.* (note 153), 195.
198. W. Sadler, *Practice of Psychiatry* (London: Henry Kimpton, 1953), 499.
199. R. Davidson, *Dangerous Liaisons: A Social History of Venereal Disease in Twentieth-Century Scotland* (Amsterdam: Rodopi, 2001), 277–8. During the 1930s, it became clear that it was not the malaria *per se* but the fever that produced the improvement, presumably because the high temperature and some aspect of the body's reaction to the heat combined to destroy the spirochaete. Thus, devices began to be developed which could artificially heat patients in order to obviate some of the risks of malarial therapy. See, for example, 'Pyrexia in the Treatment of GPI', *Lancet*, 2 (1932), 406–7: 406.
200. Anon, 'A Final Curtain', *British Medical Journal*, 1 (1975), 578.
201. As one example, Morton and Rashid have recently considered whether induced fevers could have a place in the treatment of HIV. See R. Morton and S. Rashid, 'Role of Fever in Infection: Has Induced Fever any Therapeutic Potential in HIV infection?', *Genitourinary Medicine*, 73 (1997), 212–15.

202. *Royal Edinburgh Asylum Case Books*, LHSA LHB7/51/85/345 and LHB7/51/98/173.

203. *Midlothian and Peebles District Asylum Case Book*, LHSA LHB33/12/33/133.

204. *Ibid.*, LHSA LHB33/12/183/366.

205. The Norwegian syphilologist, Caesar Boeck (1845–1913), initiated a long-term study in which he abstained from treating two thousand patients with primary and secondary syphilis in order to see whether they might progress just as well if left untreated. He claimed afterwards that only twenty-five per cent of these patients relapsed into the secondary stage, and only ten per cent developed full neurosyphilis.

206. The Tuskegee study was unquestionably the most controversial study of the course of untreated syphilis ever conducted and probably the longest non-therapeutic clinical experiment ever undertaken. In July 1972, the story broke that for forty years the United States Public Health Service had been conducting a study of the effects of untreated syphilis on black men in Macon County, Alabama – 399 who had tertiary-stage syphilis and an additional 201 who were disease-free and were chosen to serve as controls. Written informed consent was not obtained from any of the participants. For detailed accounts of this experiment, see J. Jones, *Bad Blood: The Tuskegee Syphilis Experiment* (New York: The Free Press, 1993); and S. Reverby (ed.), *Tuskegee's Truths: Rethinking the Tuskegee Syphilis Study* (Chapel Hill: University of North Carolina Press, 2000).

207. R. Lees, 'The Treatment of General Paralysis of the Insane', MD thesis, University of Edinburgh (1938), 75.

208. *Midlothian and Peebles District Asylum Case Book*, LHSA LHB33/12/33/93.

209. *Barony Parochial Asylum Case Book*, NHSGGCA30/4/34/44.

210. *Ibid.*, NHSGGCA30/4/57/32.

211. *Glasgow Royal Asylum Case Book*, NHSGGCA13/5/190/848.

212. *Ibid.*, NHSGGCA13/5/189/814.

213. *Ibid.*, NHSGGCA13/5/189/799.

214. *Ibid.*, NHSGGCA13/5/190/844.

215. *Royal Edinburgh Asylum Case Book*, LHSA LHB7/51/68/541.

216. *Ibid.*, LHSA LHB7/51/115/873.

217. 'Mental Treatment: Progress in Asylum Methods', *Royal Edinburgh Asylum Presscuttings Book*, Vol. VII, 1926, LHB7/12/7, 404.

6

Aetiology and Social Epidemiology

The late nineteenth and early twentieth centuries arguably constituted the critical period in medical conceptualisations of GPI's causation, during which time the disease was being reframed as a consequence of social and scientific change. Despite the fact that, by the early 1910s, scientific proof had been obtained which appeared to establish that syphilis was the definitive cause of GPI, the Scottish asylum case notes reveal that there was in fact much resistance to the syphilitic hypothesis. Instead, alienists developed and then clung to a complex and multi-causal concept of GPI which drew heavily on issues of blame and respectability, and on the wider Victorian medico–social concepts of civilisation and degeneration. The broader social concerns and sexual politics of the *fin de siècle* will therefore be outlined, and it will then be established to what extent these concerns were reflected in the Scottish clinical records and in Scottish alienists' epistemologies of causation.

The broader aetiological debate

The idea of a necessary and specific cause, generally considered to be essential in order for one to have a defined disease entity, is noticeably absent from published accounts of GPI throughout much of this period. The range of causation factors suggested was quite diverse, so it is interesting that GPI was widely believed to be a definite disease entity *without* a definite single or dual causation. The American alienist Arthur Hurd listed the 'comparatively small' number of causes assigned to GPI as syphilis (acquired or inherited), alcohol, mental stress and worry, heredity, cerebral traumatism, sunstroke and lead poisoning.[1] Thomas Clouston listed a similar range of triggers: 'brain exhaustion, irritation, excesses in drinking, sexual excess, over-work, over-worry, syphilis or injuries'.[2] George Wilson, REA assistant physician, might therefore be excused for exclaiming: 'A course of reading on the aetiology of general paralysis would incline one to believe that there is no evil under the sun that may not sufficiently account for the onset.'[3] While there does indeed seem to be a bewildering array of causes proposed for GPI in this period, most alienists in fact combined shared notions of debauchery and strain in their aetiological explanations of this disease. Alienists like Hurd acknowledged that it was in fact the hierarchy of causal factors that could not be agreed upon and that the divergence of possible causes should not be allowed to mask this fact.

From the mid-nineteenth century until the early decades of the twentieth century it was widely noted that most general paralytics had 'loose' ways or immoral habits, and indulged in the consumption of both alcohol and tobacco and in promiscuous sexual intercourse. As Wilson summarised, a 'busy, immoral life culminated in' general paralysis.[4] Alcohol was particularly widely cited as a cause, not just of GPI, but of insanity more generally. Within Britain, the majority of alienists seem to have shared Clouston's belief that 'if alcohol is taken in sufficient excess there is no brain whatever, even the strongest, that can resist some bad mental effects, although they may not take the form of technical insanity'.[5] Such beliefs concurred with wider European views, most notably those of Kraepelin and Bayle.[6] Tobacco was discussed much less in relation to insanity, particularly in Scotland. However, Richard von Krafft-Ebing, the world-renowned Austro–German alienist, was much cited by British alienists in stating that the smoking of ten to twenty Virginia cigars might produce GPI.[7]

It appears that from the time GPI began to be discussed as a clinical entity distinct from other diseases, syphilis was regarded as a possible aetiological factor. Although he did not include it as a 'predisposing' cause, the French physician Antoine-Laurent-Jesse Bayle – who was credited with establishing the disease as a definite pathological entity, as detailed in Chapter 3 – did give this factor some consideration, and noted that about a fifth of the patients he had observed had 'indulged in venereal excesses and often… contracted syphilitic maladies'.[8] However, syphilis was not seen as a significant specific cause during the nineteenth century. In 1883, Clouston reflected the view of most alienists when he emphasised that there was no proof that GPI was syphilitic in origin.[9] Four years later, during a Medico–Psychological Association discussion, he met with little opposition when he insisted that there was no connection between the two diseases. Whilst the historian Margaret Thompson has suggested that this denial – 'in face of mounting evidence' – was due to his being 'raised in the heyday of Victorian prudery' and was a result of his strict Calvinist upbringing,[10] Clouston's declared reason was pragmatic – a lack of statistical evidence to support what was at that time a major reformulation of the syphilitic domain. Indeed, evidence would support Allan Beveridge's view that Thompson is very much overstating this point, and that Clouston was in fact representative of the majority of *fin-de-siècle* alienists in this regard.[11] Most alienists were suggesting a multitude of causes for GPI in this period, and Clouston's speculations appear no more 'inaccurate' than do those of his contemporaries. After all, until the early twentieth century there were few related statistical surveys, no diagnostic tests to identify syphilis, and no findings of the spirochaete in the brain of general paralytics. Furthermore, Clouston did recognise that syphilis could predispose one to GPI.

Indeed, this tendency to regard syphilis as a predisposing factor in GPI rather than an actual cause was shared by other physicians. For example, David Yellowlees, Physician-Superintendent of Gartnavel and Clouston's west-coast counterpart, stated that he fully agreed with the neuropathologist Frederick Mott's view that syphilis was not an essential and invariable cause of GPI, but only a frequent cause.[12] By the close of the nineteenth century, as Clouston's successor as REA Physician-Superintendent, George Robertson, noted, syphilis was starting to be seen as constituting 'the most important aetiological factor' though 'not an absolutely essential factor'. Robertson insisted that 'there must be some other factor introduced to account for the phenomena of the disease'.[13] Similarly, Yellowlees' successor, Landel Oswald, argued that syphilis was the most common cause of GPI but rarely the sole cause.

A significant development in the widespread recognition of the aetiological importance of syphilis was the 'parasyphilis' concept developed during the late nineteenth century by the French dermatologist Jean Alfred Fournier (1832–1914). He published evidence which favoured the hypothesis that syphilis was a cause of both GPI and tabes dorsalis, yet hesitated to suggest a firm link because he considered the figures of antecedents unconvincing, since such conditions proved resistant to mercury treatment, and due to the lengthy interval between initial syphilitic infection and the onset of GPI.[14] The term 'parasyphilis' – or 'metasyphilis', as German physicians preferred to call it – was thus intended to convey Fournier's belief that such late manifestations were syphilitic in cause but not in nature, and were only indirectly caused by the syphilitic spirochaete. In addition, Fournier encouraged physicians to use the term 'pseudo-GPI' in those patients whose tertiary syphilis imitated GPI, thus separating 'true' GPI from 'syphilitic pseudo-GPI', the so-called 'duality' theory. Such prefixes as 'para' and 'pseudo' therefore allowed physicians tentatively to relate syphilitic infection to GPI and tabes without having to commit fully to syphilis as the definitive or single cause.

A further development in the gradual acceptance of the link between syphilis and GPI was the 'toxin' theory. Developed in the early years of the twentieth century, this theory postulated that a microbe or bacillus was the cause of GPI. It is particularly important within the Scottish context because the key figure involved in developing this theory was the Edinburgh Pathologist and Director of the Scottish Asylums' Pathological Scheme, W. Ford Robertson. Based upon experiments conducted in 1902, he advanced the hypothesis that general paralysis was:

[T]he result of a chronic toxic infection from the respiratory and alimentary tracts, permitted by general local impairment of the defences against bacteria and dependent upon the excessive development of various bacterial forms, but especially upon the abundant growth of a diptheroid bacillus which gives the disease its distinctive character.[15]

At Gartnavel, Yellowlees expressed great interest in this possible bacterial origin of GPI but was not initially disposed to accept it in the face of clinical evidence. However, Clouston expressed more fulsome confidence in the theory. He explained that 'modern medicine had lately discovered' that human bodies were 'subject to be invaded by all sorts of microbes and by many kinds of poisons that [were] adverse to the general health and to the brain soundness.' He continued: 'We, at Morningside at least, now believe that General Paralysis – that most terrible of all brain diseases we have to treat – is caused by poisons and microbes.'[16] The toxin theory chimed with Clouston's belief in the organic nature of insanity, for he expected such toxins to be the bodily cause of certain delusions and hallucinations in his patients.

In general, Ford Robertson's Edinburgh colleagues seem to have been keen to support and incorporate the pathologist's findings into their epistemologies of GPI's causation. The toxin theory also found its way into aetiological conceptions of GPI in geographical areas where laboratory work was available to investigate it. The alienists of both Bangour District Asylum and Crichton Royal Institution in Dumfries received Ford Robertson's investigations enthusiastically. The latter's 1903 annual report concluded that this theory was 'one of the most important contributions to our knowledge of nervous pathology that has been made during the year.'[17] Indeed, a rash of newspaper articles around 1903 reported on the pathologist's findings and claimed that considerable interest had been aroused by his work. Clouston's public support must have helped, as must that of his successor George Robertson, who 'was very pleased to be able to say he could confirm, right up to the hilt, Dr Ford Robertson's original theory that general paralysis was associated with a diphtheroid organism'.[18]

Nonetheless, this causation theory was incorporated into existing aetiologies of GPI, rather than replacing them wholesale. Clouston argued that GPI was caused by a microbe that acted upon brains which had been previously weakened by dissipation and alcoholic poisoning – or 'physical degeneration' originating from the 'vicious degraded life of the slums'. The microbe, 'even if... shown to be immediately responsible', was not 'the original cause'.[19] Similarly, George Robertson 'did not wish anyone to go off with the idea that he believed that organism to be the cause of general paralysis of the insane'.[20] Furthermore, Ford Robertson himself sought, in the discussions which followed his presentations, and which were reported in the *Journal of Mental Science*, to deny the point alleged by a number of speakers that he attached little or no importance to syphilis in the aetiology of GPI. On the contrary, he maintained that syphilis was by far the most important aetiological factor. He only wished to make clear that it was not an absolutely essential factor and to insist that there must be some other factor introduced to account for the phenomena of the disease.[21]

However, based mainly on the fact that the micro-organism was not found uniformly in all GPI cases examined, Ford Robertson's conclusions were received with scepticism and outright criticism in certain quarters. Similar investigations were carried out in London, with the results said to be by no means convincing. Furthermore, it was argued that Ford Robertson had found the diphtheroid bacillus in only nine out of twenty-three cases of GPI, which was not considered sufficient to 'support the theory – though it may lend colour to it – that the presence of the micro-organism in question was actually the cause of the malady'.[22] If the bacillus was the cause of the disease, then it ought to be found in all cases of GPI, which it was not. Moreover, the bacillus ought not to be found in healthy people, yet it was. By 1906, Ford Robertson's theory was being subjected to much adverse criticism as support grew for the syphilitic hypothesis.[23]

It was the decade which followed Kraepelin's 1904 statement that 'syphilitic infection is an essential for the later appearance of paresis' which was to prove the most significant period for the categorical establishment of GPI's aetiology.[24] For decades, asylum pathologists had sought to discover the answer to GPI at post mortem in the brain of its victims. The syphilitic spirochaete was, instead, identified in the blood by two German laboratory researchers, Fritz Richard Schaudinn and Paul Erich Hoffmann, who in 1905 demonstrated the causal agent of syphilis to be a small spiral bacterial micro-organism known as the *Spirochaeta pallidum*. In the following year, August von Wassermann, the German bacteriologist, discovered that in the blood of patients suffering from syphilis there occurred changes which were detectable by laboratory methods, the Wassermann test, discussed in Chapter 4. This method of serum diagnosis was said to place the diagnosis of syphilis, as well as the so-called 'parasyphilitic' affections of GPI and tabes, upon a much more certain basis, with physicians no longer reliant upon clinical observation. In 1907, Felix Plaut extended Wassermann's method to the examination of the CSF.

The final textbook proof of GPI's syphilitic aetiology came in 1913 when Hideyo Noguchi (1876–1928), the Japanese bacteriologist, demonstrated the presence of *Spirochaete pallidum* in the brain of a patient who had died of GPI. Noguchi and J.W. Moore announced that in fourteen out of seventy cases of GPI they had been able to isolate *Treponema pallidum* within the brain cortex, the bacteria that they believed produced syphilis.[25] However, once again, the syphilitic hypothesis did not necessarily replace previous epistemologies of causation. By the 1920s, the consensus of opinion within European and American venereology and psychiatry appeared to favour the hypothesis of syphilis plus 'other determining factors such as alcohol, head trauma and various other aspects of the swirl of civilisation'.[26] Such conceptions of GPI relied on the action of syphilis upon a nervous system weakened by the stresses of civilisation, as captured by Krafft-Ebing's oft-quoted phrase 'syphilisation and civilisation', a phrase which originated at the Moscow Congress back in 1897.[27] These multiple causal pathways would explain the fact that only a small proportion of syphilitics went on to develop GPI, and that GPI was rare in uncivilised countries while syphilis was not. Indeed, there were still many qualified observers who, as late as 1927, stated that GPI could occur quite independently of any syphilitic infection – for instance, from head injury, alcoholism or an erratic mode of life.[28] Thus, whilst the syphilis link lent new associations to GPI, it does not appear to have represented a wholesale revolution in causal ideas. Rather, it was incorporated into the traditional nineteenth-century framework, with multiple causal explanations for GPI employed well after the link with syphilis had been established statistically.

The city as a pathogen

The structure of debate on the aetiology and social epidemiology of GPI link directly to broader discussions and concerns of this period, and reflect, in particular, contemporary fears relating to urbanisation and degeneration. The theme of excess was a common pre-occupation of Victorian alienists, and was clearly a potent element within the conceptualisation of GPI. Alcohol and sexual excess, routinely mentioned in connection with many forms of insanity in this period, played a significant part within the perceived aetiology of GPI. Such evils featured in wider discussions of degeneration and racial decay, as will be discussed below, but they also contributed heavily to debates over urbanisation and the potential dangers of 'civilisation'. Syphilitic infection and alcoholism were identified as steadily increasing conditions, whilst overwork was claimed widely to have intensified over the later-nineteenth century. Since modern urban life was seen to have enhanced promiscuous sexual behaviour, the temptations and supply of alcohol, and the perceived stresses and demands of life and work, the perceived risks of all three elements were increasingly attributed to the dangerous influence of the urban environment and the deleterious effects of civilisation. As one *Lancet* contributor summed up, 'the refining influences of civilisation had not been altogether an un-alloyed boon'.[29]

The concept of 'diseases of civilisation' appears to have been first discussed during the eighteenth century. The rapid industrial and urban processes of late eighteenth-century Britain focused greater attention on the interface between sickness and society. The spread of big city life was feared to be making populations more vulnerable, not merely to 'filth diseases', but to new modes of ailment created by modernity itself: hysteria, hypochondria, chlorosis and their nineteenth-century neuropathological successors such as neuralgia and neurasthenia.[30] Indeed, it was in the nineteenth century that the 'diseases of civilisation' notion attained its greatest credibility and induced the greatest fear. This was partly because certain disorders which fell under the epithet's umbrella appeared to grow more deadly. Above all, tuberculosis – one of the classic diseases to be associated with the unwholesome metropolitan environment – reached its height around the mid-nineteenth century and accounted for up to a quarter of all urban deaths in north-western Europe. 'The growth of civilisation', as *The Times* in London noted in 1868, meant 'the growth of towns', which effected 'a terrible sacrifice of human life' and created 'the materials for an immense hotbed of disease'.[31] The historian Charles Rosenberg notes that such perceptions of the inherent dangers of urban life were widespread by the mid-nineteenth century throughout America, Britain and the Continent.[32]

Within psychiatry specifically, 'civilisation' was a prominent factor in debates throughout the later-nineteenth and early twentieth centuries. As one American alienist argued, this era of inventions, electricity, rapid means of communication and business competition had 'called forth more and more mental exertion and struggle'.[33] Such deleterious effects of the urban environment were commonly noted in Scottish asylum annual reports of this period. Clouston showed particular concern for this theme in his writings. It was his stated opinion that the continual process of too sudden an adaptation to new environments and new conditions constituted one of the great causational factors of both criminality and insanity.[34] As more and more people moved to the cities, 'where the brain cells' were 'continually being stimulated and new impressions being made on them every minute of life', more rest was needed 'than in the old quiet country life'.[35] Clouston argued that, since mental disease was 'largely the penalty of the faults of civilisation, as it unquestionably is', it was 'the clear duty of that civilisation to apply its best resources to undo and mitigate the evil that has mingled with its good.'[36] Indeed, asylum treatment for the insane was based fundamentally on the notion that the insane could be healed if they could be separated from the damaging influence of their environment. Thus, to Clouston, public asylums constituted 'one of the recognised parts of our complicated modern civilisation'.[37]

GPI and neurasthenia were generally cited as the prime examples of these psychiatric disorders of civilisation.[38] During the *fin de siècle*, GPI was widely conceived to be caused, or at least exacerbated, by the realities of urban industrial society. In fact, Clouston held it to be 'the most terrible of all the modern diseases of modern life'.[39] Both in Scotland and elsewhere its geographical and racial distribution was believed to throw light upon its aetiology. GPI appeared to prevail in some places and amongst some races but to be entirely unknown in others. Both the 'Asiatic' and the 'savage' were claimed to be 'free from it', whilst 'the Irishman and Scotch Highlander need[ed] to come to the big towns or to go to America to have the distinction of being able to acquire it'.[40] The disease appeared to be quite rare among the uncivilised races and rife in the highly civilised nations, with large towns and manufacturing centres furnishing the majority of cases. Physicians therefore constructed GPI as a disease of the city, with its occurrence said to be 'very closely connected with modern developments of civic life'.[41]

Moreover, its favoured habitat was seen as strongly corroborative of its moral origin. Clouston referred to GPI as the disease 'most closely connected with the special overwork and with the special vices of our modern civilisation'. It was argued that 'when the Highlander and the Irishman come to Glasgow and Edinburgh, and work hard, eat flesh meat, have too little fresh air, drink much impure liquor, and live a bad life', they became subject to the disease 'just as readily' as the Englishman or Scottish Lowlander.[42] In 1896, the General Board of Commissioners noted that the mortality rate from GPI in the Scottish asylums varied markedly depending on the location of the asylum. This rate was claimed to vary from between 19.8 and 28.2 per cent of all asylum deaths in the large urban asylums of Gartnavel and the REA respectively, to 12.0 in Murray's Royal Asylum and 20.2 in Rosslynlee, institutions which drew their population chiefly from smaller urban communities and mining districts, and dropping to 5.8 and 7.9 in the rural asylums of Inverness District and Elgin District respectively.[43] Such statistics were said to 'throw a lurid sidelight on some of the dangers of city life'.[44] Inverness District Asylum boasted the fewest paralytics of all the Scottish asylums during the later nineteenth century. As its 1888 annual report stated with pride, the infrequency of GPI constituted a 'remarkable' feature in the institution's history. This disease had 'not been found in patients who ha[d] never left their native glens, but only in those who ha[d] resided in large towns, and been exposed to the vices of civilisation.'[45]

Between 1880 and 1930, a noticeable pattern emerged in the admission figures to the Scottish asylums. The number of GPI diagnoses appeared to be increasing throughout Britain, but particularly in its urban centres, most notably Edinburgh and Glasgow. This increase was a source of significant interest and concern to Scotland's Lunacy Commissioners, and received specific and detailed analysis in their annual reports for the years 1875, 1895, 1901, 1906 and 1912. Whilst the Commissioners felt it desirable to 'suspend judgment upon such increase... until further experience' had thrown 'more light on the subject',[46] others were quick to posit possible explanations for this trend. It was widely claimed that the increase in GPI admissions reflected the fact that Britain had become more urbanised and prosperous in recent years and that its citizens were therefore more vulnerable to the 'emotional volatility' of civilised life. Alienists also drew a relationship between GPI and the strength of the economy, and could fairly neatly correlate economic booms with rises in GPI admissions, despite later assertions that – with syphilis found to be the main causal agent – initial infection would often take ten or even twenty years to progress to the tertiary stage.

Thomas Clouston was, as ever, one of the most vocal alienists to attempt to explain these peaks and troughs in GPI admissions. He claimed that the first five years of his Physician-Superintendency, from 1873 to 1877, were 'mostly years of plenty and inflation of wages', during which time 115 (or 7.3 per cent) out of 1580 total admissions to the asylum were diagnosed with GPI. In the later years 1881 to 1885, 'years of dull trade, and little money to squander', the proportion of GPI admissions was only 75 (or 4.5 per cent) out of 1667.[47] The Edinburgh alienist attributed this decrease to the 'enforced sobriety and better living of the present unprosperous years, as compared with the [earlier] years of plenty and inflated wages'. By the turn of the century, the disease was documented to be on the rise again, both in proportion to the population and absolutely in numbers, which Clouston held as 'a bad sign of our ways of life'.[48] It is possible that at least part of this increase could be explained by improved diagnostic methods, more honest reportage by patients, families and doctors, and a greater willingness in families to institutionalise their afflicted, rather than any actual increase in incidence. Whatever the reason, REA physicians noted the rise with particular concern, perhaps due to the fact that this institution had the highest proportion of general paralytics of any Scottish asylum.

Degeneration and heredity

Although associated originally with the French alienist Bénédict-Augustin Morel (1809–73), the classic clinical description of degeneracy is generally taken from his fellow countryman Valentin Magnan (1835–1916), who in 1895 defined it to be:

[A] pathological state of the organism which, in relation to its most immediate progenitors, is constitutionally weakened in its psycho-physical

207

resistance and does not realize but in part the biological conditions of the hereditary struggle for life. That weakening, which is revealed in permanent stigmata, is essentially progressive, with only intervening regeneration; when this is lacking, it leads more or less rapidly to the extinction of the species.[49]

This 'constitutional weakness' was believed to lower the resistance of the victim's will and thereby expose him to a wide variety of dangers, both biological and social. The degenerate was understood to tend towards extinction since their progeny would exhibit a progressive moral and physical deterioration, a medicalised notion of the 'fall from grace'.[50] Nineteenth-century sociologists appear to have found degeneration theory indispensable in their work. It effectively accounted for the terrible human costs of modernisation which was expressed in the perceived growth of 'urban' diseases such as alcoholism, crime, insanity and suicide, and resolved the apparent paradox of these miseries amidst the growing plenty of vigorous industrial life.[51]

The 'richly eclectic, though savagely negative, worldview'[52] that degeneration entailed has been defined in very broad terms within the historiography as a European reaction to urbanisation, industrialisation, and the democratisation of political life, embedded within a medical model of cultural crisis.[53] The historian Daniel Pick argues that its generalised discourse transcended national and professional boundaries, and was 'never successfully reduced to a fixed axiom or theory'.[54] Yet, the theory was important less for its verifiable content than for its capacity to articulate diffuse belief in cultural decadence, and alarm at the social forces that seemingly threatened the delicate mental and physical health of *fin-de-siècle* Europeans.[55] Moreover, it seems to have been precisely because of its power to express anxieties about the political future and to resolve them by recasting them in less traumatic naturalistic terms that the theme of degeneration persisted well into the twentieth century.[56] Racial stereotypes increasingly became a convenient place for the projection of new social anxieties, with racial degeneration contributing to a more general theory of 'morbid anthropology'.[57]

Related but distinct from such degenerationist modes of thought, Social Darwinism has been portrayed as constituting one of the major intellectual changes of the late nineteenth and early twentieth centuries. While there were many varieties within this species of thought, the historian Greta Jones has detailed two of the most crucial aspects as the pre-occupation with external racial and national competition, and fears over the proliferation of the working class at the expense of the better stocks.[58] The concept of a race hierarchy with the white man at the top had emerged long before Darwin popularised his evolutionary theory, with Europeans having almost invariably assumed that they were biologically superior to the races they were subjugating with the assistance of their military technology. Darwin's theories merely supplemented and further justified such attitudes. Paradoxically, much Victorian fear both stemmed from and was propagated by warfare.

Famously, the alarmingly poor physique of large numbers of potential British army recruits during the Boer War of 1899 to 1902 caused great concern about the physical condition of the national stock, fears that were further augmented by the mass mobilisation of World War One. Whilst Social Darwinism argued that nations and races were locked in a struggle for survival which would penalise weakness, and that nature tended to eliminate the unfit through sterility, disease, war and poverty, the fear grew that the interbreeding of 'misfits' and 'profligates' would lead to the swamping of the healthy by the 'genetically suspect' residuum over the generations,[59] since it began to be widely assumed that such degenerates were driven by perverted sexual appetites and lacked self-control and would thus breed disproportionately.[60] Within this context, a number of 'social' diseases – particularly alcoholism, feeble-mindedness, and venereal disease – became depicted as racial poisons and specific threats to national health, and potential eugenic solutions flourished.[61]

An integral part of such degenerationist and evolutionary debates was the relative importance of heredity, which became a prominent element of medical and psychiatric discourse by the second half of the nineteenth century. From the work of Bayle onwards, the influence of hereditary predisposition upon the causation of GPI received much attention. The nineteenth-century alienists of the REA appear to have ascribed it a particularly important role. The REA physician George Wilson emphasised the importance of inherited tendencies when he advanced his 'diathesis' – meaning 'predisposition to' – hypothesis that general paralytics were 'born, not made'.[62] To make his case, he highlighted the enormous number and variety of alleged causes associated with this disease, as well as the absence of any assignable cause in some cases. He also drew attention to the 'trifling nature of many of these causes' in comparison with 'the fatally progressive nature of the disease', which left him wondering whether 'such conditions [could] possibly be held to account for the overthrow of a human brain were it of anything like a normal constitution'.[63]

A further argument in support of Wilson's theory was said to come from a fairly large number of cases in which he deemed the disease to be a manifestly 'family affair'. Wilson noted that several cases of this kind had been resident at the REA, drawing particular attention to the 'remarkable case' of GPI diagnosed in twin brothers recorded by Clouston and George Savage (1842–1921), Physician-Superintendent of the Bethlem Asylum and one of the most enthusiastic British degenerationists. Clouston explained that there had been a strong family history of insanity here, and that both men were of 'the same temperament and disposition, viz., sanguine and keen, both being of very active habits, both indulging to great excess in wine and women, both following a similar occupation – an exciting one – and both being affected by the disease within a year of one another.' He argued that such a clinical history showed 'conclusively that the heredity may predispose to the disease'.[64]

These Edinburgh-based alienists seem to epitomise those contemporary physicians who portrayed the disease – and particularly its juvenile form – as constituting a disease of degeneracy because it combined immoral behaviour with parental hereditary taint. Even where the hereditary element was not noted to be significant, and despite the fact that it was predominantly associated with acquired rather than inherited syphilis, the association between GPI, mental dissolution, sexual excess and syphilis converged easily within the nebulous framework of degeneracy. Concerns over this apparent relationship between GPI and urban or racial degeneration did not just coincide with contemporary discourses surrounding urban degeneracy and heredity but were actively shaped by them.

In this regard, physicians used dramatically evocative language to describe the onset of the neurosyphilitic disorders. Thus, tabes dorsalis was described as 'a slow process of decay and death of the intra-spinal portion of the sensory protoneurones', while Frederick Mott described GPI dramatically as the 'smouldering destruction of neural elements, the latter conflagration often fanned into flames by circulatory disturbances'.[65] At the turn of the century, as rates of GPI were perceived to be rising out of proportion to the other forms of insanity in both sexes, such apocalyptic images were applied increasingly to it. Indeed, in 1896, R.S. Stewart, the Scottish alienist and deputy Medical Superintendent of Glamorgan County Asylum, published one of the most negative accounts of the disease written, in which he suggested that the rise of GPI represented 'a reversion to a lower and more hopeless form of brain disease, a diminishing vitality, a lessening power of resistance, and an increasing tendency to premature and rapid racial decay.'[66] Although Stewart noted that hereditary influences were less prominent in GPI than in other insanities, his broader view of degeneration enabled him to blame drunkenness, sexual excess and moral decadence for a reduction in racial resistance, of which GPI was said to be a prime manifestation. Indeed, he argued that the individual history of the illness provided an appropriate metaphor for the deterioration of society: 'The opening chapter is moral decadence; the closing acutely rapid physical and intellectual degeneration and premature extinction.'[67]

Historians have turned to this shared stock of ideas about morality, sexuality and degeneration that both syphilis and insanity suggested to Victorian observers, and have portrayed the disease similarly as constituting the classic Darwinian disease.[68] Roy Porter speaks of 'the late nineteenth-century obsession with GPI', which was conditioned to a large extent by growing fears of the consequences of unbridled sexuality. He notes: 'Sooner or later... all who had committed youthful sexual indiscretions would pay the price by growing demented.'[69] In her study of Clouston, Thompson suggests that his ideas about GPI, as 'an irrevocable consequence of "dissipated habits"', came from the same stock as his ideas about syphilis, despite his non-acceptance of syphilis as the cause of GPI.[70] As Clouston himself stated, 'one must know that General Paralysis practically means certain forms of immorality'.[71]

However, the majority of British alienists seem, in fact, to have been reluctant to place GPI within the framework of hereditary neuropathy, and seem generally to have deemed heredity no more significant to GPI than to any other form of insanity. As just one example, Maurice Craig, the London physician, argued that hereditary propensity to madness did not play an important part in GPI's causation since 'a large percentage of these patients' had 'no special history of nervous instability in their immediate relatives'.[72] Contemporary physicians appear to have been less likely than historians to conceptualise GPI as an actual disease of degeneration. Until the turn of the century, few accounts of degeneration made any mention of GPI. Indeed, lack of heredity in GPI was perceived to add to the cruelty of the disease. As the 1902 annual report for Woodilee noted, GPI 'rob[bed] the community of men and women in the prime of life untainted as a rule by predisposition to nervous and mental breakdown.'[73]

The moral agenda of aetiology

It could be argued that the hypotheses advanced in order to explain the aetiology of GPI tell us much not just about the disease itself but about the more general concerns of the alienists. This seems particularly true of the period before syphilis became accepted as the definitive cause of this disorder. Lacking a uniform understanding of its aetiological agent, contemporaries appear to have framed a picture of GPI that sought to reduce its threat of randomness whilst simultaneously articulating their own social and cultural values. Thus, GPI became related to an immoral lifestyle decades before the syphilis link became widely accepted.

Although the medical profession has been bound by oath to relieve suffering wherever possible, the historiography of venereal disease demonstrates quite clearly that willingness to do so can be modified by feelings rooted in more moral considerations, as doctors consciously or unconsciously absorb prevailing values into their medical judgements.[74] Judith Walkowitz asserts that the treatment of gonorrhoea and syphilis conformed to moral and sexual attitudes prevailing among the dominant classes of nineteenth- and early twentieth-century society. The pain associated with mercury applications made it 'an appropriately punitive method of treating syphilitics', while cauterisation 'served a similar punitive and deterrent function'.[75] Alienists of the period found themselves in the position of men whose society regarded venereal disease as just punishment for promiscuous sexuality as well as a metaphor for social decay.

Thus, doctors were placed in the difficult, even anomalous, role of curing the patient without passing moral judgment on his behaviour or sexual conduct, and yet sin and sexuality were inextricably linked in the Scottish consciousness. Typical of many asylum case notes in this period, descriptions of patients, their symptoms and behaviour were imbued with a moral tone of disapproval or outright disgust rather than what we ourselves might consider to be factual and scientific language. It is interesting to note the judgemental attitudes inherent in case-note phrases like 'he masturbates frequently, often shamelessly and continuously' or 'he does not obey the calls of nature and is wet and dirty in his habits'. Patients could be described as 'filthy', 'wretched' or even 'an animal'. Such phrases illustrate vividly the conflation of medicine and morality. While such judgemental phraseology was used to describe patients diagnosed with other disorders in this period, GPI appears to have particularly entangled alienists in moral issues due to its strong associations with the excesses of alcohol, tobacco and active sexuality.

Such negative associations led some alienists explicitly to adopt an additional role as moral arbiter in their discussions of, and dealings with, such patients. Thomas Clouston epitomises this stance. From his arrival at the REA in 1873, Clouston stressed that good mental health was dependent on adherence to Victorian standards. He sought to distinguish between harmful or self-destructive behaviour and that which was prudent and prophylactic, encouraging patients 'to live according to physiological and moral law' in order to 'lessen materially in civilised societies the total amount of the great nervous disturbances'.[76] Excessive study was specifically advised against in the young, and the dangers of 'deviance' were preached to all: dissipation, sexual excess and self-abuse. The exercising of 'self-control' was particularly encouraged, referred to by Clouston as 'the practical and important side of morals and religion'.[77] Whilst willing to accept that factors such as urbanisation had an adverse effect on health, his published belief was that if the individual reacted to this by engaging in dissipated behaviour, he alone was responsible for the results. Hence GPI, 'like alcoholic insanity, must be regarded as a largely preventable scourge of humanity.'[78]

Marriage was portrayed as a significant and responsible prophylactic measure.[79] Clouston's *Before I Wed* was a polemic aimed at young men which warned of the irrevocable relationship between sexuality and madness.[80] He stressed the importance of monogamous sexual relationships and virtuous marriage, and warned that if men indulged in masturbation, the habit would lead to drunkenness, liaisons with prostitutes, syphilis and ultimately insanity.[81] Clouston echoed wider European views in this regard. At the international Brussels conference on syphilis in 1902, Professor Burlureaux declared marriage 'the most secure shelter against the venereal peril'. In France, Alfred Fournier, a leader of the French movement to regulate and control prostitution, used the risk of syphilitic infection as 'a perfect excuse to preach marital fidelity and family devotion'.[82] Fournier demanded that all extramarital relations should be made illegal, for if 'humankind returned to the golden age of innocence, the days of syphilis would be numbered.'[83] Nonetheless, within the British context, Clouston's open preaching on such matters as sexual relationships and alcohol consumption appears to have stood in marked contrast to the majority of alienists. The comparative silence of Gartnavel's physicians on such matters is particularly noticeable. Even so, as we shall see, the contents of the asylum case notes – a more private source of medical perceptions – suggest that there was much sympathy for Clouston's views amongst the Scottish alienists. Good mental health, it seems, demanded strict adherence to the Victorian moral values of continence and self-control, with GPI epitomising this most clearly.

Indeed, religion was mentioned explicitly on occasion within those medical texts on both insanity and venereal disease. The fall of man was a particularly potent image, as this Glasgow-based physician's writing illustrates in relation to syphilis:

> God has fixed our being beneath stern yet beautiful laws, which ever bear their testimony to the obedience of virtue, and their witnessing judgment to the disobedience of vice. The man who walks in fellowship with the laws of virtue, will not only have the testimony of his conscience within him, but the witness of purity in his flesh, by the sweet harmony which will run through his physical constitution, holding in healthy balance all the functions of his body. But if he depart therefrom, discord and disunion will be set up in his system, with all the miseries of disease.[84]

Through their original sin, Adam and Eve brought disease and death into the world as punishments for disobedience. If we see medicine within this context of the Fall of man, then disease becomes man's punishment. In this regard, Clouston's significantly titled 'Lay Sermon' of 1903, and his comment that doctors were 'priests of the body', seem particularly relevant.[85] As a scientist, Clouston felt himself able to discern nature's purpose and

Table 6.1

REA Predisposing and Exciting Causes of GPI, 1880–1930

	Predisposing		Exciting	
Unknown	**194**	**(60%)**	**160**	**(50%)**
Syphilis	31	(10%)	30	(9%)
Alcohol	**16**	**(5%)**	**50**	**(16%)**
Heredity	44	(14%)	1	(0%)
Physical Disease	**9**	**(3%)**	**15**	**(5%)**
Brain Disease	7	(2%)	28	(9%)
Shock/Grief/Stress	**20**	**(6%)**	**24**	**(7%)**
GPI	0	(0%)	13	(4%)

n=321

Source: *Royal Edinburgh Asylum Case Books*, 1879–1931, LHSA LHB7/51/34–120.

therefore to advise mankind on the subject of healthy living in order to ensure the 'hygiene of mind'. As he warned with specific reference to GPI, the early twentieth-century increase in the incidence of the disease was due to the fact that 'the lives of some classes' were 'more immoral than they used to be'. He continued: 'The social reformer, the clergy, and the educationalist have an uphill fight with human nature, and as yet not an altogether successful one.... Let science now step in to their aid.'[86]

In the last third of the nineteenth century, disease boundaries were being expanded to include behaviour patterns that might have been dismissed as immoral or criminal by earlier generations, due partly to the perceived alarming increase in the number of insane and partly to the contemporary prestige of somatic models.[87] Alcoholism and moral insanity became potential diagnoses rather than culpable failures of willpower. A growing secularism paralleled and lent plausibility to this framing in medical terms of matters that had been previously construed as essentially moral. Physicians like Clouston appear to have believed that science should replace theology as the arbiter of such questions. Alienists were thereby assuming a wider social role during this period, in replacing the priest or judge as the appropriate guardian of the rights and morals of both society and the individual.

Causation factors according to the Scottish case notes

Disease causation within psychiatry was generally conceived as an interplay between 'predisposing' (longstanding) and 'inducing' or 'exciting' (more recent or aggravating) factors. The REA and Woodilee asylum case notes reflect this basic division by separating causation into separate 'predisposing' and 'exciting' columns, although their alienists were never explicit in explaining how exactly it was decided whether a causal factor was predisposing or inducing to the onset of GPI. On the other hand, the case notes of Gartnavel and Rosslynlee are more simplistic in having one single causation column, so that a uniform comparison of all four asylums is not possible.

Table 6.1 displays the main recorded causes of GPI admissions to the REA in the period from 1880 to 1930 and divides these into 'predisposing' and 'exciting' causes in order to replicate the structure of the case notes. It can be seen that the majority of general paralytics in this asylum were assigned a cause of 'unknown' upon admission. The next most significant predisposing factors recorded were 'heredity' and 'syphilis'. However, it was alcohol that was deemed the most significant exciting cause, followed by syphilis and brain disease.

Tables 6.2 and 6.3, overleaf, break this data down in order to allow a comparison of the pre-1910 and post-1910 recorded causes of GPI. The most significant finding to note here is that, despite the supposedly growing acceptance of the syphilitic hypothesis and the professed impact of the Wassermann test on diagnosis, a far greater number of cases were in fact allocated an 'unknown' cause in the later period. The recording of syphilis as a cause of GPI within the REA case notes actually diminishes over the period, as does alcohol and heredity. It is difficult to explain this phenomenon. Perhaps it relates simply to a practical apathy in completing that section of the document rather than an intellectual weakness. However, the other sections of the case notes do not exhibit this 'negligence', so it would seem that something more complex is going on here. Each of these causation factors will be discussed more fully below.

In addition to the division between predisposing and inducing factors in the case-note causation column, which was completed by the admitting physician, the process of recording causation was further complicated by the fact that a cause or causes were generally assigned separately to new patients in the admission register. Such information was probably recorded prior to the filling-in of the case notes and appears to have been elicited from the patient, his family or family physician where he could afford one. Most significantly, causation is often found to differ between the two sources. For general paralytics admitted to Gartnavel, Rosslynlee and Woodilee, the aetiology is recorded in the admission registers, and such information is tabulated in Table 6.4 alongside the corresponding case-note data.[88] Clearly, 'unknown' is again a significant aetiological factor for general paralytics admitted to these three asylums, in both their admission registers and case notes (seventy-eight per cent and fifty-five per cent respectively), although

Table 6.2

REA Predisposing and Exciting Causes of GPI, 1880–1910

	Predisposing		Exciting	
Unknown	117	(51%)	75	(33%)
Syphilis	22	(10%)	28	(12%)
Alcohol	14	(6%)	47	(20%)
Heredity	44	(19%)	1	(0%)
Physical Disease	9	(4%)	15	(7%)
Brain Disease	7	(3%)	28	(12%)
Shock/Grief/Stress	17	(7%)	23	(10%)
GPI	0	(0%)	13	(6%)

n=230

Source: *Royal Edinburgh Asylum Case Books,* 1879–1910, LHSA LHB7/51/34–94.

the asylum physicians appear more likely to have ascribed a cause to the illness than those who accompanied the patient upon admission.

There are several other differences to observe between the two sources. In particular, 'syphilis' was noted in the case notes far more frequently than in the admission registers. The much greater tendency of the asylum physicians to ascribe GPI to syphilis could be partly accounted for by the use of the Wassermann test in the asylums from 1909 onwards, plus the growing acceptance of syphilis as a factor of causation in GPI, which may have motivated and enabled alienists to look more rigorously for proof of syphilis. While their families might genuinely be unaware that their relative had syphilis, admitting physicians were more able to recognise the signs or diagnose it through the laboratory. They may also have been looking for such evidence, which the family in all likelihood would not have been. There is also the possibility that the patient or family were aware of the syphilitic infection but were too ashamed to admit it to the asylum officials, or that a family doctor was protecting their virtue. The family or doctor might have been more likely to impart this information once the extent of the patient's illness had become clear upon admission. Similar factors may explain the fact that alcohol was also noted somewhat more often by alienists than in the admission registers. One final cause in need of explanation is 'GPI'. Although this was clearly a diagnostic label, the admission register and case-note causation columns included 'GPI' as a cause as well as a diagnosis in a number of cases. Surprisingly, the more specialised asylum physicians were twice as likely to utilise this as non-specialists employed outside the asylums. The remaining factors were fairly constant between the two sources.

Table 6.3

REA Predisposing and Exciting Causes of GPI, 1911–1930

	Predisposing		Exciting	
Unknown	77	(86%)	85	(94%)
Syphilis	9	(9%)	2	(2%)
Alcohol	2	(2%)	3	(3%)
Heredity	0	(0%)	0	(0%)
Physical Disease	0	(0%)	0	(0%)
Brain Disease	0	(0%)	0	(0%)
Shock/Grief/Stress	3	(3%)	1	(1%)
GPI	0	(0%)	0	(0%)

n=91

Source: *Royal Edinburgh Asylum Case Books,* 1911–1931, LHSA LHB7/51/91–120.

Once again, we can break this data down into the pre-1910 and post-1910 periods in order to ascertain whether or not the supposed proof of syphilitic causation in the early twentieth century made any noticeable impact. As expertise and knowledge of GPI developed over time, one would at least expect physicians in the latter period to be more likely to ascribe a specific cause to GPI admissions, whether or not that cause was syphilis. Certainly, as Tables 6.5 and 6.6 reveal for Gartnavel, Rosslynlee and Woodilee, there is a drop of eighteen per cent in those GPI case notes that were ascribed an 'unknown' cause. On the other hand, the admission registers exhibit a slight increase in those cases with an 'unknown' cause. In comparison with the REA case notes, the increase in those GPI admissions ascribed to syphilis in the case notes of the three other asylums is significant, rising from three per cent before 1910 to thirty per cent in the two decades afterwards. The admission registers exhibit a much smaller increase in those cases of GPI ascribed to syphilis. The remaining causes appear to have remained fairly stable throughout the period as a whole.

As revealed above, syphilis was never commonly noted in the REA case-note sample throughout the period from 1880 to 1930. It was, in fact, one of the district asylums that appears to have been quickest to accept the syphilitic hypothesis for GPI. From 1914 onwards, syphilis became much more significant in Woodilee's case-note causation columns than it had been before. The Gartnavel records reveal the same trend from 1918 onwards, in which year syphilis became far more frequently mentioned in the GPI case notes. This could partly be accounted for by the fact that this was the same year that service patients began to arrive at the asylum, and soldiers were

Table 6.4

Admission Register and Case-Note Causes of GPI in Gartnavel,
Rosslynlee and Woodilee, 1880–1930

	Predisposing		Exciting	
Unknown/Not Given	427	(78%)	298	(55%)
Syphilis	13	(2%)	89	(16%)
Alcohol	17	(3%)	39	(7%)
Heredity	6	(1%)	7	(1%)
Physical Disease	15	(3%)	21	(4%)
Brain Disease	12	(2%)	29	(5%)
Shock/Grief/Stress	35	(6%)	38	(7%)
GPI	26	(5%)	55	(10%)

n=546

Source: *Glasgow Royal Asylum Registers of Lunatics,* 1871–1963, NHSGGCA13/
6/78–80; *Glasgow Royal Asylum Case Books,* 1880–1930, NHSGGCA13/5/62–194;
Registers of Discharges and Removals, 1874–1942, LHSA LHB33/5/1–2; *Rosslynlee
Case Books,* 1880–1930, LHSA LHB33/12/5–36; *Barony Parochial Asylum Registers
of Admissions,* 1875–1957, NHSGGCA30/10/1–4; *Barony Parochial Asylum Case
Books,* 1880–1930, NHSGGCA30/4/1–63 and NHSGGCA30/5/1–61.

often linked to these diseases and to the debauched lifestyle that was
generally held to accompany them. However, these were not the only
patients to have this cause ascribed to them, for private patients were also
admitted with syphilis as a cause of their insanity. Despite being a district
asylum, the Woodilee physicians appear to have accepted the syphilis
hypothesis more quickly and uniformly than the other Scottish asylums, and
often listed syphilis alone as the cause of GPI unlike the usual 'multiple
causes' approach of most institutions in this period. Although the reason for
this is unclear, it provides some further support both for Woodilee's
importance within the history of Scottish psychiatry, and for the possibility
that the district asylums were quicker to incorporate new theories and
activities into their regimes.

Another factor that is perhaps particularly worthy of mention is heredity.
The REA case notes contain a significant number of general paralytics whose
disease was ascribed to heredity: forty-four patients (nineteen per cent) of
my sample between 1880 and 1910, as Table 6.2 reveals. This ties in with
Clouston and Wilson's, his assistant, published comments on the
importance of the 'diathesis' hypothesis. A comparison of Tables 6.2 and 6.3
suggests that Clouston's successors were far less likely to ascribe a cause of

Table 6.5

*Admission Register and Case-Note Causes of GPI in Gartnavel,
Rosslynlee and Woodilee, 1880–1910*

	Predisposing		Exciting	
Unknown/Not Given	211	(74%)	179	(63%)
Syphilis	2	(1%)	9	(3%)
Alcohol	13	(5%)	21	(7%)
Heredity	6	(2%)	3	(1%)
Physical Disease	5	(2%)	10	(4%)
Brain Disease	7	(3%)	19	(7%)
Shock/Grief/Stress	17	(6%)	18	(6%)
GPI	20	(7%)	27	(9%)

n=280
Source: See Table 6.4.

heredity to GPI admissions. The other three Scottish asylums – Gartnavel, Rosslynlee and Woodilee – appear to have been more consistently representative of the national picture over the period from 1880 to 1930, for in each of these institutions the factor of heredity appears to have been considered marginal to the onset of GPI, as attested by Table 6.4.

However, the 'causation' section of the case notes for these institutions contained a further heading – 'HP', or hereditary propensity to madness – and this section reveals a noticeably higher proportion of heredity in the general paralytics than the causation section of their case notes. In Gartnavel, 33 GPI patients (21 per cent) were noted to have an hereditary propensity (to insanity or alcoholism), and 25 (14 per cent) in Rosslynlee. The general paralytic samples for Woodilee and the REA reveal that 20 (10 per cent) and 59 (16 per cent) respectively were noted to have an hereditary propensity.

The fact that this information was rarely copied into the causation section of the case notes suggests that the Scottish asylum physicians, despite rigorously noting this information in the records, did not conceive it to be relevant to the onset of GPI. Yet, the language used in this part of the case notes is noteworthy, exhibiting a fairly judgemental tendency. For example, rather than simply writing 'no HP', a common comment was 'denied' or 'none admitted', as though the patient and his family were trying to conceal a shameful secret. Such language suggests that the admitting physician doubted the veracity of the patient and suspected him to have indulged in behaviour that was morally or medically objectionable.

Table 6.6

Admission Register and Case-Note Causes of GPI in Gartnavel, Rosslynlee and Woodilee, 1911–1930

	Predisposing		Exciting	
Unknown/Not Given	216	(81%)	119	(45%)
Syphilis	11	(4%)	80	(30%)
Alcohol	4	(2%)	18	(7%)
Heredity	0	(0%)	4	(2%)
Physical Disease	10	(4%)	11	(4%)
Brain Disease	5	(2%)	10	(4%)
Shock/Grief/Stress	18	(7%)	20	(8%)
GPI	6	(2%)	28	(11%)

n=266
Source: See Table 6.4.

However, a lack of such information in some case notes seems to have resulted merely from a lack of knowledge in the patient or whoever accompanied him to the asylum, rather than signalling any deliberate attempt to deceive the physicians. For example, it was noted of Robert N., a 39-year-old married labourer, admitted to Woodilee in February 1922: 'There is no history of insanity on either side of his family but this is from ignorance of the informant.'[89] Particularly in the case of pauper patients or patients who had no family or friends accompany them upon admission or visit them during their asylum stay, their recorded history was either short or entirely absent. This is true, for example, of William H., a 48-year-old single twister, admitted to Woodilee in May 1911, who was noted to have 'no friends' as an explanation for his almost completely blank case-note admission pages.[90] Indeed, it is a possibility that the royal asylums registered a higher rate of hereditary propensity in their patients because their greater proportion of private patients meant that their patient histories were more likely to be comprehensive.

Moving to the qualitative data contained within the case notes, we can attempt to build a more thorough picture of how physicians perceived the aetiology of GPI. As with the published medical literature, there appears to have been a prevalent and consistent belief throughout the late nineteenth and early twentieth centuries that excessive use of alcohol and tobacco could produce this disease. John T., a 40-year-old married joiner, admitted to Rosslynlee in October 1892, was noted to be 'fond of a dram', while Alexander I., a 45-year-old single labourer, admitted in February 1894 that he was 'drunk every pay night'.[91] William N., a 37-year-old partner in a steam laundry company, admitted to Gartnavel in April 1918, was said to have 'drunk heavily for several years' prior to admission.[92] The case notes of James N., a 33-year-old married marine engineer, admitted in February 1908, record that he was 'a very heavy cigarette smoker, consuming as many as 100 cigarettes a day: in fact the steward had to be induced not to supply him with tobacco'.[93] It was noted that Elizabeth S., a 39-year-old married housewife, admitted in September 1930, was 'teetotal but smoked about fifteen cigarettes a day until two years ago when she gave it up'.[94]

Such behaviour was often linked to a more generally degenerate lifestyle. Thus, the case notes of Captain James O., a 44-year-old married master mariner, admitted to Gartnavel in October 1910, record that he 'smoke[d] a good deal, and became notorious in Dover for "misconducting himself" with two of his nieces'.[95] Case-note histories, particularly those of the poorer male patients, often depict a more general lifestyle of debauchery in describing a history of such excesses as alcohol, tobacco, or sexual promiscuity. Robert M., a 32-year-old married solder, admitted in April 1892, was: 'Given to drink and women (own statement)'.[96] William N., a 43-year-old married fireman, admitted to the REA in February 1899, 'drinks a bit. Has apparently lived a fast and free life.'[97] William B., a 33-year-old married labourer, admitted in July 1891, was '[a]lcoholic [and] idle'.[98] Alexander H., a 63-year-old married housepainter, admitted to Rosslynlee in May 1888: 'Married a strong young woman when he was 50 years of age. Excessive sexual indulgence is very probable in this case.'[99] Excess could even take the form of tea drinking or atheism. James G., a 38-year-old married bottle blower, admitted to Woodilee in October 1913, 'was a great tea drinker, drinking it to excess'.[100] Although Robert G., a 67-year-old single silversmith, admitted in November 1924, was said to be only a moderate drinker: 'He has always been rather an agnostic.'[101]

As we have seen, it was principally as a result of these perceived dangers of excess that the urban environment was constructed as the prime location for this disease. As the REA annual report for 1900 argued, the person most at risk of GPI was 'the vigorous city worker, making more money in good times than his education and social requirements [could] utilise for his legitimate enjoyments'.[102] The temptations of the city – excess, fast living and the resulting mental strain – were, in fact, the professed causes in the majority of GPI cases admitted to the four Scottish asylums between 1880 and 1930. Phrases like 'degraded life', 'debauchery' and 'sins of youth' were frequently employed to describe these patients. Such terms were not explicitly sexual in meaning, but tended to refer more generally to a debauched or socially unacceptable history. In fact, broadly speaking, there was a fundamental case-note division between 'steady' and 'unsteady' patients with 'faulty' or 'correct' habits. Those with 'correct' habits were usually temperate, married non-smokers, who generally fitted a particular social profile – female or middle class. Those with 'faulty' habits constituted a much more numerous group, and commonly referred in their admitting consultations to an excess of some form, most notably alcohol, tobacco or sexual intercourse. Such patients were likely to be a working-class male or female prostitute.

Those general paralytics who were described as 'steady' and respectable include John E., a 39-year-old married labourer, admitted to Rosslynlee in December 1895, who was noted to be '[s]teady at work and sober'.[103] Similarly, Robert I., a 48-year-old married ex-sergeant in the police force, admitted to Gartnavel in October 1918, 'was a teetotlar [*sic*], steady and well behaved'.[104] John I., a 43-year-old married baker, admitted to the REA in September 1883, was recorded to be '[s]teady and regular, fond of literature (reading)', while Alexander D., a 41-year-old married newsagent, admitted in April 1890, was described as '[t]emperate and industrious'.[105] Mary E., a 40-year-old married housewife, admitted to Woodilee in March 1913, was claimed to be: 'Non alcoholic. Clean in her habits.'[106] In fact, underneath a 'disposition' heading in the REA case notes, the majority of GPI admissions were described as bright and cheerful, sociable, quiet, intelligent and hardworking, perhaps reflecting the more middle-class nature of that institution's general paralytics. For those patients considered to be 'steady' in character, the typical designated causes of their GPI were worry, stress, fright, organic brain disease or injury.

A more statistically significant group of general paralytic patients within the four Scottish asylums were labelled as 'unsteady' or 'faulty in habits'. William D., a 43-year-old married wholesale supply agent, admitted to Rosslynlee in March 1928, combined a number of 'debauched' elements. He was a:

> Fairly heavy smoker – cigarettes. When younger he was a heavy drinker up till marriage. He had some thick times with his pals. His habits have been pretty wild apparently.... As regards women very probably he indulged himself in this direction as he did on alcohol but brother does not know definitely.[107]

Robert H., a 36-year-old single miner, admitted to Gartnavel in June 1900, had 'always lived a fast life both as regards drink and girls'.[108] John T., a 60-year-old married unemployed male, admitted to the REA in March 1895, was simply '[w]ild, dissipated, drunken &c',[109] while Alexander D., a 30-year-old single sailor and labourer, admitted in September 1898, had led a '[l]oose intemperate sailor life'.[110]

There were also those patients whose case-note history indicated that their previously steady character had undergone a rapid deterioration only recently. The clinical records of Alexander I., a 42-year-old married spirits salesman, admitted in May 1898, record that: 'His general mode of life was good up to the last twelve months when he has been drinking heavily'.[111] More dramatic was the case of John N., a 38-year-old miner, admitted to the REA in October 1904. His wife reported that '[h]e was always a steady worker, a temperate and most respectable man. Total abstainer for many years lately.' However, following a pit accident, his conduct, physical and mental health appeared to have deteriorated rapidly '[e]ver since the accident he was slightly depressed', and would 'come back in the evening and tell his wife without any sense of shame that he had been with half a dozen prostitutes.' His wife claimed that he seemed to have 'lost all sense of decency and talked in the silliest fashion about his relations with the prostitutes.'[112]

More rare were those patients whose case-note history indicated an opposite behaviour trajectory. For example, it was recorded of James N., a 56-year-old married teacher, admitted in February 1907, that '[i]n early life he drank heavily but has not taken any kind of drink for over six years.'[113] Similarly, it was noted of Robert R., a 33-year-old single bricklayer, admitted in October 1911, that '[u]ntil about a year ago patient was a constant tippler, dating from time of accident. Has stopped entirely for the last year. No sexual disorders'.[114] The fact, however, that at the time of admission these patients were 'correct' and 'steady' in their habits might be reconciled by REA Physician-Superintendents David Skae and Thomas Clouston's shared belief that 'the seeds of the disease were sown many years before its actual development, and that the man in his prime suffered for the sins of his youth.'[115]

A number of the case notes of general paralytics within the Scottish asylums contain more lengthy family statements or letters which provide a more complete account of the patient's life and how their family believed them to have succumbed to illness. Such accounts might incorporate the events that had occurred in either the patient's long-term or immediate past, or even both, but generally related to a particularly stressful incident which the patient had endured. They also display a tendency to reflect positively on the patient's kind or industrious character. Two examples will suffice where the patient's family located their relative's ill-health within such a web of stressful events and processes. First, the son of Jane O., a 61-year-old widow, admitted to the REA in February 1903, explained that 'his family always date[d] the starting point of his mother's disease from a great strain she went through seven years ago. She nursed her daughter suffering from' rheumatic fever.[116] Secondly, the family of William D., a private 49-year-old widowed

223

retired sea captain (ship master), admitted to Gartnavel in June 1892, wrote that his illness dated 'from the time of his shipwreck off the coast of S. America' when 'his vessel was run down and foundered quickly, and the patient lost his wife and three children who were on board and himself was rescued after having been some hours in the water.' Afterwards it was claimed that he was 'worried by litigation resulting from the loss of his vessel, and an attempt to prove that the accident was due to his negligence, which is said to have been in no way the case.'[117]

A body of literature explains this use of narrative by patients and their families in order to explain the seeming randomness of disease. In matters of illness, it has been noted that the patient and his family often find inadequate meaning in the medical view, and so elaborate reconstructions of their experience in such a way that illness can be given a sensible or meaningful place within it.[118] Specifically in psychiatric cases, the patient's history or 'story' tends to be accorded less significance or status, due to their limited memory and coherence, and a relative or close friend often assumes the role of telling the patient's story and making sense of the illness.[119]

Perhaps unsurprisingly, syphilis figured only rarely in the accounts of either patients or their families. Although rarely given as the *sole* cause, there are some examples where syphilis was noted as *a* cause of GPI, particularly by the twentieth century. John D., a 50-year-old single managing director, admitted to the REA in March 1902, had '[s]yphilis (his own confession) eight years ago.'[120] Similarly, William I., a 34-year-old married mason, admitted to Gartnavel in September 1930, 'talk[ed] freely of having had syphilis'.[121] Alexander F., a 58-year-old single ship's carpenter, admitted in March 1909, 'lived a fast life, was markedly alcoholic, and 14 years ago contracted syphilis.'[122] James D., a 31-year-old single ship's draughtsman, admitted in December 1911, was 'apparently accustomed to sexual intercourse and even after he had contracted syphilis would return to his former habits, having heard that he could not be reinfected.'[123] Finally, and without debating the patient's version of events, the case notes of Robert C., a 53-year-old married physician and surgeon, admitted in June 1920, note that his wife deserted him, having been a 'restless, bad-tempered creature' who 'had time only for eating, drinking and pleasure'. As a result, the patient blamed her for his contracting venereal disease.[124]

Others denied syphilitic infection if it was suggested to them as a possible explanation for their illness. Alexander Y., a 34-year-old single watchmaker, admitted to Gartnavel in March 1919, claimed that he had 'never had sexual intercourse in his life. He had several rubber preventatives in his pocket – says a man gave him them a week ago but he had no use for them.'[125] James C., a 53-year-old married physician, admitted in June 1920, when asked if he knew what GPI was, replied 'General Paralysis, I should think so.' However, on suggesting that he apply the diagnosis to himself, the patient denied all possibility, but then conceded '[w]ell I may have got it since I came in here: its damnable.'[126]

A history of miscarriage or poor health in the patient's existing children were also considered to be indicative of GPI, particularly once the syphilitic aetiology had been more widely accepted. The family history of Elizabeth N., a 48-year-old married housewife, admitted to Gartnavel in November 1923, records that she had been married twice but 'had no children by her second husband; and she had a miscarriage during the first year following her second marriage.'[127] This appears to be taken by the admitting physicians as proof of syphilis. The wife of William H., a 43-year-old married blacksmith, admitted to Rosslynlee in August 1917, 'does not admit having had any miscarriages – it is probable all the same that [her husband] has had syphilis'.[128] Likewise, John D., a 41-year-old married marine engineer, admitted to Gartnavel in July 1917, had no children but his wife was 'careful to explain' that this was 'not due to disease or other defect' but 'to her stumbling as she hurried off a train after her husband'.[129] Alternatively, Alexander N., a 49-year-old widowed wine and spirit merchant, admitted in November 1917, was noted to have 'six healthy children all alive, wife had no miscarriages'.[130] Similarly, James D., a 43-year-old married wholesale supply agent, admitted in March 1928, was said to have 'three children all alive. No still births or miscarriages.'[131]

For some, syphilis does not even appear to have been considered as the cause of insanity. As one example, Robert N., a clergyman, was admitted to Gartnavel in 1901 with GPI caused by 'anxiety and brain work' and with no mention of less respectable lifestyle factors such as alcohol or syphilis in his case notes. His cause of insanity was elaborated upon further within his case notes, that 'for some years' he 'had a good deal of worry in connection with his church owing to the numbers diminishing through no fault of his own, but due to the migration of the population'.[132] Alienists may simply not have conceived of such causes as excessive alcohol consumption being applicable where the social characteristics of a patient such as Robert N. did not fit their construction of the disease.

Alternatively, it might be the case that physicians were aware of such socially unacceptable factors in some of their middle-class or female patients but did not note them, or at least did not inform the patient's friends or relatives of this, because it might embarrass and stigmatise those concerned. For example, Susan B., a 26-year-old married ropeworker, admitted in April 1930, did not pay to reside in Gartnavel but was registered as a private patient. Even though her GPI was deemed to be congenital, it was noted that her positive Wassermann test would place her in a shameful position, so that the patient's sister-in-law was not informed of the patient's full state but merely that 'her blood... [was] in a bad condition – I [the physician] did not go into any details'.[133]

There was less sensitivity in the description of working-class male patients. James T., a 31-year-old married carter, admitted to Woodilee in October 1922, was admitted with GPI caused by 'women and drink'. It was noted that he 'would spend all his money on drink', 'pawned everything he could lay his hands on', 'smoked heavily', and was 'believed to have had venereal disease'.[134] James C., a 33-year-old single plain net manufacturer, admitted to the REA in July 1911, was simply described as 'alcoholic and erotic'.[135] Few females were so described, but exceptions included Jane U., a 34-year-old single lodging house-keeper, who was noted to have contracted GPI because she had been 'leading a fast life', while Susan D., a 36-year-old married housewife, was described as being 'intemperate, immoral'.[136] Margaret L., a 42-year-old single domestic servant, admitted to Rosslynlee in August 1891, was '[h]appy go lucky – a rover – fond of men'.[137]

It is clear that the case-note evidence very closely mirrors the general debate in a number of respects. Alienists tended to conceive of GPI's aetiology in a fairly broad way, rather than to look for one single, specific cause, a possible reason why the syphilitic hypothesis was slow to be accepted. The strains and debauched excesses of civilisation played an integral part in such multi-causal theories, encouraging alienists to adopt a wider role as moral guardians to their patient populations. However, there are also several diverging aspects worthy of note. By the 1920s, as alienists were beginning publicly to embrace the importance – if not necessity – of syphilis as an aetiological factor, the REA physicians were still attributing less than ten per cent of their GPI cases directly to syphilis. Indeed, the case-note causes for GPI patients admitted to the four Scottish asylums continued to include such diverse single factors as 'bereavement', 'overwork', 'lowness of system', and 'kick from a horse'. We also find a surprising number of patients whose GPI was said to be of 'unknown origin' during this decade, with alienists seemingly unable to attribute the disease to any cause whatsoever.

The social epidemiology of GPI in the four Scottish asylums

Throughout its history, GPI was consistently portrayed as afflicting a noticeably tight and well-defined patient population. Its epidemiology is thus fairly significant, as discussed above. It was perceived to be a disease of the city. It was also perceived to be a disease largely of the working classes. Ford Robertson was in the minority of medical commentators when he stated that GPI was 'a disease of the rich and the great as well as of the poor', and that it was 'by no means confined to the lower social strata'.[138] The majority of British writers do not in fact appear to have accepted this characterisation of the disease.[139] On the whole, physicians claimed that they found GPI to be much more frequent in the lower classes, at a ratio of at least 1.5 pauper males to one private, and twice as many pauper females as private. Although cerebral strain was often cited as one potential cause, as it was noted in the *Glasgow Medical Journal*, 'members of the learned professions' did not appear to be 'especially susceptible', nor did 'intellectual work or any other special kind of occupation seem to predispose the individual to paresis'.[140]

The REA was the only one of the four Scottish asylums to admit a sizeable number of both pauper and private patients in this period, so that any statistically significant analysis of these four institutions by class would prove deeply problematic.[141] However, syphilis does not appear to have been diagnosed in any of the wealthy East House women admitted to the REA in this period, and the physicians of this institution observed that GPI was extremely rare in gentlewomen. The majority of general paralytics admitted to the Scottish asylums had an occupational label suggesting working-class status, and were mainly butchers, carters, clerks, domestic servants, housewives, labourers, miners and soldiers. Those few private patients who were diagnosed with GPI tended to attract an unusually respectable aetiological explanation for their affliction. Thus, Mary O., a teacher admitted to Rosslynlee in October 1903, was described as 'steady and sober', the causes of her illness noted to be worry and a potential breakdown.[142] Similarly, when a 56-year-old married teacher, Robert N., was admitted to Woodilee in February 1907, his wife gave an account of the history of the patient and his illness which weaved his regular church attendance and status as a caring father into an explanation of his poor health:

> Mr [N.] has been failing very much in health for a good while. Often when going to church, which is four and a half miles from us, he would have to stand on the road for want of breath. He always said to me his heart was affected and he has taken our little boy's illnesses (accident to eyes) very much to heart.[143]

Syphilis was only occasionally mentioned in such private patients admitted with a diagnosis of GPI.

The age of those diagnosed with GPI was commonly between thirty and fifty years, according to the published medical literature. It was noted that the disease could occur outside these ages, but apart from some cases of juvenile GPI, the published literature and my patient samples reveal GPI to be a disease very much of middle age, as Table 6.7 displays overleaf. In fact the average age of the general paralytic population in each asylum is strikingly similar: 40 in Woodilee, 42 in Gartnavel and the REA, and 43 in Rosslynlee. The final common social characteristic of GPI-diagnosed patients was held to be their potential history of reported excess or

Table 6.7

Age Range of Scottish General Paralytics, 1880–1930

Age Range	Number	%
0-20	14	2
21-30	75	8
31-40	341	37
41-50	320	35
51-	161	18

n=911

Source: *Four Asylum Case Notes,* 1880–1930, LHSA LHB7/51/34–120, LHSA LHB33/12/5–36, NHSGGCA13/5/62–67 and 123–48, NHSGGCA13/5/98–122 and 149–194, NHSGGCA30/4/1–63, and NHSGGCA30/5/1–61.

'debauchery', as discussed above, so that alienists appear to have been extremely interested in establishing whether or not the patient had ever over-indulged in alcohol, tobacco or sexual intercourse. Thus, GPI was popularly perceived to be a disease associated with middle-aged, working-class urban dwellers with an alcoholic or promiscuous past, a belief that the annual reports and case notes of all four Scottish asylums reflect clearly.

The gendering of the disease was equally significant. If we look more generally at admissions to British asylums, female admissions began to outnumber male admissions from at least the 1890s onwards. Female longevity and vulnerability to modern living were generally believed to account for this trend. Yet, males were deemed much more prone to GPI than females, in the ratio of as many as eleven to one. In the more conservative estimate of the Scottish Commissioners in Lunacy, the disease affected four times more men than women.[144] The four Scottish asylums had an average gender ratio of five to one, although Gartnavel's gender divide was more extreme, with only eight per cent female to ninety-two per cent male general paralytics.[145]

Such a disproportion in gender might seem likely to us for several reasons. Firstly, more men were diagnosed with venereal disease and would thus be expected to go on to acquire GPI. Secondly, shame might discourage more women than men from seeking medical attention despite knowing that they suffered from this dreadful affliction. In addition, confinement for treatment might be more urgent for a male where he was the breadwinner of the family. However, medical commentators attempted to explain GPI's epidemiology rather differently. Its marked sexual disproportion was often claimed to be because men were subjected to 'greater moral shocks and mental strain', as well as the 'greater frequency' with which they indulged in 'excess, especially alcoholic'.[146] There was only one type of woman in whom it was considered appropriate to diagnose GPI – prostitutes and those morally-dubious lower-class women who could be easily associated with promiscuity and vice.

This gendered epidemiological trend is clearly reflected within the Scottish asylum case notes. The majority of women admitted to the four asylums with GPI had factors like 'bereavement', 'menopause', 'paralysis', 'senility', 'worry' or 'unknown' noted as their cause of insanity. Only in a handful of female cases is syphilis mentioned, and usually with a question mark after it, or it is occasionally called 'acquired syphilis' or 'syphilis contracted from husband', thus displacing any blame from the women themselves. Susan C., a 50-year-old widowed dressmaker, admitted to Rosslynlee in March 1921, had syphilis '(got from her first husband)'.[147] On the other hand, Margaret E., a 35-year-old prostitute, admitted to the REA in October 1880, had syphilis given as the cause of her GPI, openly and without qualification.[148] Unusually, from 1914 onwards, the female general paralytics admitted to Woodilee commonly had syphilis listed as an exciting cause. However, as a parochial asylum, these women were relatively poor and of a fairly low status in society. As noted above, the Woodilee records also exhibited a much greater tendency than the other Scottish asylums to attribute the cause of insanity in their general paralytics to syphilis.

Yet, from the close of the nineteenth century, various Scottish sources began to document a changing trend in the gendering of the disease. In 1890, the Dundee Asylum annual report stated it 'worthy of notice' that of the twenty-two deaths recorded from GPI and organic brain disease in that year, 'no fewer than thirteen were females, which would indicate a remarkable increase of late years of such affections in the female sex'.[149] By 1905, the Gartnavel physicians were noting a similar trend, although they were careful to distance themselves from it, given the social standing of their clientèle. It was remarked that, whilst all eight of their GPI admissions in that year were male, this contrasted 'very markedly' with other asylums 'drawing their patients from the lower and lowest strata of the population, and in one of which the number of female cases of general paralysis admitted [in the previous year] was actually in excess of the males.'[150] This comment in fact referred to the REA. In that same year, Clouston noted that the comparative increase of GPI in females was 'striking' among the poorer classes.[151] As an assistant physician at the REA in the 1860s, he recalled, 'it was so uncommon a thing to have a woman admitted suffering from general paralysis that the medical staff would all go to see such a case when it did come.' Whilst during the early years of his Physician-Superintendency in the

1870s, only a handful of female admissions were diagnosed with GPI, by 1905, Clouston recorded thirty-eight female admissions with this disease, though he qualified that 'all of them but one [were] of the rate-paid class'. The physician noted with alarm the fact that this was the first time in the REA's history that the number of female general paralytic admissions exceeded that of the men, a 'unique and unprecedented fact'.[152] Nonetheless, he reassured readers that GPI was still very much a class-based disease, due to the fact that 'our better-off people live more cleanly'.[153]

The social construction of GPI

At this point it is important explicitly to differentiate incidence and diagnosis. It might be the case that, rather than naturally occurring predominantly in urban males, alienists simply diagnosed GPI more often in this group because they fitted the social characteristics of the disease as well as, or rather than, the medical characteristics. For example, there was an average of only two GPI admissions per year at Inverness District Asylum between 1889 and 1908, with no more than five such admissions in any one year.[154] Indeed the alienists of that institution seemed proud of this lack of cases, presumably due to the immoral associations of the disease. However, in 1893, their Physician-Superintendent wrote that, while GPI appeared to be 'almost unknown' in his institution, Irish asylums and 'among savage races' his recent observations gave him 'every reason to believe that it [was] not at all so rare here as [was] generally alleged by authorities on the subject'.[155] To believe that the aetiology of GPI was based purely upon epidemiological observations assumes a straightforward relationship between the disease's 'natural' appearance and doctors' interpretations of it. Another, perhaps less naïve, reading of the evidence might suggest that the epidemiology and aetiology of GPI were in fact mutually constructing and reinforcing.

Types of explanation were needed to account for the fact that more men than women, more poor than rich, and more urban than country residents, were being diagnosed with GPI. The profile and identity of this disease – particularly its aetiology and strong associations with alcoholism, vice and stress – fitted with a masculine model of disease. Thus, we see an easy fit, in the late nineteenth century, between dominant Victorian social ideologies and the widespread medical belief that lower-class males and 'unsavoury' women were most likely to contract this disease. Clouston's explanation of the preponderance of male general paralytics was that 'if women drank bad liquor and lived riotous existences, they also might become general paralytics'.[156] There was clearly a moral judgement going on in such cases. Women were not expected to behave in ways that led to their contracting GPI, dabbling in the excesses and strains of modern civilisation. It was perhaps only with changing social perceptions of a woman's place in society that it became gradually more acceptable, or at least more common, for women to indulge in such forms of behaviour, and an increased diagnostic rate of GPI in women was subsequently charted.

It is very possible that alienists were more efficient at diagnosing GPI in those who fitted the social characteristics of the disease precisely because they were looking for such a disease in these patients. That is, diagnosis did not reflect incidence but merely measured the ability of alienists to recognise the disease in those who fitted the social as well as the medical profile of the disease. If a patient was male, working class, and an urban resident, particularly with a history that exhibited a connection with excessive alcohol consumption or promiscuous sexual intercourse, the disease may have been more easily recognised. Female and middle-class patients might display similar symptoms yet receive an alternative diagnosis, due to the social construction of the disease and the fact that their social profile did not appear to fit the prevailing image of GPI. As one example, William E., a 59-year-old married general manager, admitted to the REA in August 1918, was noted to be a: 'Total abstainer; habits said to be correct', who was not exposed to any particular stresses in his life.[157] This patient was diagnosed initially with organic confusional insanity, and not until post mortem was the GPI diagnosis arrived at. A relatively small but nonetheless significant number of such 'steady' patients received a diagnosis of mania, melancholia, acute excitement or organic brain disease upon admission to these asylums, and their GPI diagnosis was given only at post mortem. Perhaps such patients were simply not considered for that diagnosis because they did not fit the social profile of the disease. However, such a hypothesis would be difficult to prove or quantify and would almost certainly require recourse to the historically dubious art of retrospective diagnosis in a statistically significant number of both GPI and non-GPI diagnosed patients in this period.

Notes

1. A. Hurd, 'Etiology of Paresis', *American Journal of Insanity*, 58 (1902), 564–9: 565.
2. T. Clouston, *Clinical Lectures on Mental Diseases*, 5th edn (London: J. and A. Churchill, 1898), 377–418.
3. G. Wilson 'The Diathesis of General Paralysis', 1892, Lothian Health Services Archive (LHSA), GD16, 3.
4. *Ibid.*, 6.
5. T. Clouston, *Unsoundness of Mind* (London: Methuen, 1911), 109.
6. A minority of observers chose to differ. Obersteiner, Hirschl, and Fournier found only a low percentage of alcoholics among their neurosyphilitic cases.

See J. Moore, 'The Syphilis–General Paralysis Question', *Review of Neurology and Psychiatry*, 8 (1910), 259–71: 266.

7. D. Leigh in C. Thompson (ed.), *The Origins of Modern Psychiatry* (Chichester: John Wiley and Sons, 1987), 219.

8. Cited in G. Zilboorg and W. Henry, *A History of Medical Psychology* (New York: Norton, 1941), 538.

9. Clouston, *op. cit.* (note 2), 379.

10. M. Thompson, 'The Wages of Sin: The Problem of Alcoholism and General Paralysis in Nineteenth-Century Edinburgh', in W. Bynum, R. Porter and M. Shepherd (eds), *The Anatomy of Madness: Essays in the History of Psychiatry*, Vol. III (London: Routledge, 1988), 329, 335.

11. A. Beveridge, 'Madness in Victorian Edinburgh: A Study of Patients Admitted to the Royal Edinburgh Asylum under Thomas Clouston, 1873–1908', Part 2, *History of Psychiatry*, 6 (1995), 133–56: 139.

12. Cited in W. Ford Robertson, 'Discussion on the Pathology of General Paralysis of the Insane', *British Medical Journal*, 2 (1903), 1065–9: 1068.

13. *Ibid.*, 1069.

14. A. Fournier, *Les Affections Parasyphilitiques* (Paris: Rueff et Cie Editeurs, 1894), 225, cited in E. Lomax, 'Infantile Syphilis as an Example of Nineteenth Century Belief in the Inheritance of Acquired Characteristics', *Journal of the History of Medicine*, 34 (1979), 23–39: 36; Moore, *op. cit.* (note 6), 268.

15. Ford Robertson, *op. cit.* (note 12), 1066.

16. T. Clouston, 'How the Scientific Way of Looking at Things Helps Us in Our Work', 1908, LHSA LHB7/14/8, 9.

17. *64th Crichton Royal Institution, Dumfries, Annual Report*, 1903, LHSA GD17/1/39, 11–12.

18. 'Discussion', *Journal of Mental Science*, 53 (1907), 605–15: 609.

19. 'Insanity and Degeneration', *Royal Edinburgh Asylum Presscuttings Book*, Vol. VI, 1906, LHSA LHB7/12/6, 76/20.

20. 'Discussion', *op. cit.* (note 18), 609.

21. Ford Robertson, *op. cit.* (note 12), 1069.

22. 'The Bacillus of Paralysis: Medical Opinion', *Royal Edinburgh Asylum Presscuttings Book*, Vol. VI, 1906, LHSA LHB7/12/6, 76/20.

23. Ford Robertson was involved in a similar failed venture in relation to his work on carcinogenesis in the same decade. In collaboration with Henry Wade, he directed a search for an infective cause of cancer, using a similar staining technique to that used in GPI brains. See W. Ford Robertson and H. Wade, 'Cancer and Plasmodiaphorae', *Lancet*, 2 (1904), 469; Editorial, 'The Etiology of Carcinoma', *Lancet*, 1 (1905), 244–5. As Ford Robertson had done for the toxin theory of GPI, he advanced bold claims, many of which he was later obliged to retract. See D. Gardner, 'Henry Wade

(1876–1955) and Cancer Research: Early Years in the Life of a Pioneer of Urological Surgery', *Journal of Medical Biography*, 11 (2003), 81–6.

24. G. Zilboorg and W. Henry, *A History of Medical Psychology* (New York: Norton, 1941), 543.

25. H. Noguchi and J. Moore, 'A Demonstration of Treponema Pallidum in the Brain in Cases of General Paralysis', *Journal of Experimental Medicine*, 17 (1913), 232–9.

26. V. Fisher, *An Introduction to Abnormal Psychology* (New York: Macmillan, 1937), 368.

27. A. Diefendorf, 'Etiology of Dementia Paralytica', *British Medical Journal*, 2 (1906), 744–8: 747.

28. D. Henderson and R. Gillespie, *A Textbook of Psychiatry for Students and Practitioners* (London: Oxford University Press, 1927), 290.

29. 'The Physically Deteriorating Influences of Civilisation', *Lancet*, 1 (1887), 1248: 1248.

30. R. Porter, 'Diseases of Civilization', in W. Bynum and R. Porter (eds), *Companion Encyclopedia of the History of Medicine*, Vol. I (London: Routledge, 1993), 592.

31. *Ibid.*

32. C. Rosenberg, 'Pathologies of Progress: The Idea of Civilization as Risk', *Bulletin of the History of Medicine*, 72 (1998), 714–30: 715.

33. A. Hurd, 'Etiology of Paresis', *American Journal of Insanity*, 58 (1902), 566.

34. T. Clouston, 'The Developmental Aspects of Criminal Anthropology', 1894, LHSA GD16, 221.

35. T. Clouston, 'Health of Body and Soundness of Mind: A Lay Sermon', 1903, LHSA GD16, 18.

36. *74th Royal Edinburgh Asylum Annual Report*, 1886, LHSA LHB7/7/9, 16.

37. *80th Royal Edinburgh Asylum Annual Report*, 1882, LHSA LHB7/7/8, 23.

38. The American neurologist, George Miller Beard (1839–83), coined the term 'neurasthenia' and was the first to postulate an aetiological link between it and modern life. For a detailed history of this disorder in America and Western Europe, see M. Gijswijt-Hofstra and R. Porter, *Cultures of Neurasthenia from Beard to the First World War* (Amsterdam: Rodopi, 2001).

39. *80th Royal Edinburgh Asylum Annual Report*, 1892, LHSA LHB7/7/10, 14.

40. T. Clouston, *Clinical Lectures on Mental Diseases*, 5th edn (London: J. and A. Churchill, 1898), 379.

41. 'Insanity and Degeneration', *Royal Edinburgh Asylum Presscuttings Book*, Vol. VI, 1906, LHSA LHB7/12/6, 76/20.

42. *71st Royal Edinburgh Asylum Annual Report*, 1883, LHSA LHB7/7/9, 20.

43. *38th Commissioners of Lunacy for Scotland Annual Report*, 1896, NHS Greater Glasgow and Clyde Archives, NHSGGCA13B/14/64, liii.

44. *89th Royal Edinburgh Asylum Annual Report*, 1901, LHSA LHB7/7/10, 14.

45. *24th Inverness District Asylum Annual Report*, 1888, Northern Health Services Archives (NHSA), HHB3/8/10, 12.

46. *38th Report of the General Board of Commissioners in Lunacy for Scotland*, 1906, NHSGGCA13B/14/c.65, lxi.

47. *83rd Royal Edinburgh Asylum Annual Report*, 1885, LHSA LHB7/7/9, 13.

48. *91st Royal Edinburgh Asylum Annual Report*, 1903, LHSA LHB7/7/11, 18.

49. Cited in R. Nye, 'Degeneration, Neurasthenia and the Culture of Sport in Belle Epoque France', *Journal of Contemporary History*, 17 (1982), 51–68: 56.

50. H. Rimke and A. Hunt, 'From Sinners to Degenerates: The Medicalization of Morality in the 19th Century', *History of the Human Sciences*, 15:1 (2002), 59–88: 74.

51. R. Nye, 'Sociology and Degeneration: The Irony of Progress', in J. Chamberlin and S. Gilman (eds), *Degeneration: The Dark Side of Progress* (New York: Columbia University Press, 1985), 67.

52. B. Luckin, 'Revisiting the Idea of Degeneration in Urban Britain, 1830–1900', *Urban History*, 33:2 (2006), 234–52: 234.

53. Nye, *op. cit.* (note 51), 51–2; Nye, *op. cit.* (note 49), 53.

54. D. Pick, *Faces of Degeneration: A European Disorder, c.1848–c.1918* (Cambridge: Cambridge University Press, 1989), 7.

55. Degenerationism appears to have reached its zenith between 1880 and 1914, although Luckin asserts that more historiographical attention should be paid to the earlier period, where a combination of economic, medico-environmental and epidemiological developments – as documented by historians such as Gareth Stedman Jones and Anne Hardy in relation to the metropolis of London – transformed early nineteenth-century racial pre-occupations into this more mature *fin-de-siècle* degenerationist style of thought. See Luckin, *op. cit.* (note 52), 238–41. See, also, G. Stedman Jones, *Outcast London: A Study in the Relationship between Classes in Victorian Society* (Oxford: Clarendon Press, 1971); A. Hardy, *The Epidemic Streets: The Rise of Preventive Medicine 1856–1900* (Oxford: Clarendon Press, 1993).

56. I. Dowbiggin, 'Review of D. Pick, "Faces of Degeneration: A European Disorder, c.1848–c.1918"', *Bulletin of the History of Medicine*, 64 (1990), 488–9.

57. N. Stepan, 'Biological Degeneration: Races and Proper Places', in Chamberlin and Gilman, *op. cit.* (note 51), 112.

58. G. Jones, *Social Hygiene in Twentieth-Century Britain* (London: Croom Helm, 1986), 18. See, also, M. Hawkins, *Social Darwinism in European and American Thought, 1860-1945: Nature as Model and Nature as Threat* (Cambridge: Cambridge University Press, 1997).

59. See, for example, R. Soloway, 'Counting the Degenerates: The Statistics of Race Deterioration in Edwardian England', *Journal of Contemporary History*, 17:1 (1982), 137–64: 153–4.
60. Porter, *op. cit.* (note 30), 593.
61. The formation and struggles of the eugenics movement have received considerable academic scrutiny. For a good recent example, see D. Stone, *Breeding Superman: Nietzsche, Race and Eugenics in Edwardian and Interwar Britain* (Liverpool: Liverpool University Press, 2002).
62. Wilson, *op. cit.* (note 3), 3.
63. *Ibid.*, 5.
64. Cited in *ibid.*, 7.
65. Cited in M. Spongberg, *Feminizing Venereal Disease: The Body of the Prostitute in Nineteenth-Century Medical Discourse* (London: Macmillan, 1997), 158.
66. R. Stewart, 'The Increase of General Paralysis in England and Wales: Its Causation and Significance', *Journal of Mental Science*, 42 (1896), 760–77: 774.
67. *Ibid.*, 776.
68. See, for example, E. Showalter, *The Female Malady: Women, Madness and English Culture, 1830–1980* (London: Virago, 1996), 111.
69. G. Berrios and R. Porter (eds), *A History of Clinical Psychiatry* (London: Athlone, 1995), 59.
70. Thompson, *op. cit.* (note 10), 326, 331.
71. *89th Royal Edinburgh Asylum Annual Report*, 1901, LHSA LHB7/7/10, 14.
72. M. Craig, *Psychological Medicine: A Manual on Mental Diseases for Practitioners and Students* (London: J. and A. Churchill, 1917), 223.
73. *Barony Parochial Asylum Annual Report*, 1902, NHSGGCA30/2/12A, 21.
74. See, for example, J. Cassel, *The Secret Plague: Venereal Disease in Canada, 1838–1939* (Toronto: University of Toronto Press, 1987), 100.
75. J. Walkowitz, *Prostitution and Victorian Society: Women, Class and the State* (Cambridge: Cambridge University Press, 1980), 55.
76. *87th Royal Edinburgh Asylum Annual Report*, 1899, LHSA LHB7/7/10, 15.
77. Clouston, *op. cit.* (note 16), 16.
78. *90th Royal Edinburgh Asylum Annual Report*, 1902, LHSA LHB7/7/11, 11.
79. However, this might be seen as ironic, given the statistical breakdown of the four asylum general paralytic populations – 1 per cent divorced, 7 per cent widowed, 28 per cent single, and a significant 64 per cent married.
80. T. Clouston, *Before I Wed, Or Young Men and Marriage* (London: Cassell and Company, 1913).
81. Thompson, *op. cit.* (note 10), 335–6.
82. Showalter, *op. cit.* (note 68), 195.

83. Yet, as he himself was only too well aware, marriage provided little protection from the disease. In fact, Fournier's chief mission in life was said to be to promote an understanding of the dangers syphilis posed, especially within marriage. See A. Fournier, *Syphilis and Marriage* (Paris: Masson, 1880).

84. J. Thornley, 'Syphilis', MD thesis, University of Glasgow (1886), 42.

85. See A. Beveridge, 'Thomas Clouston and the Edinburgh School of Psychiatry', in G. Berrios and H. Freeman (eds), *150 Years of British Psychiatry, 1841–1991* (London: Royal College of Physicians, 1991), 378.

86. *92nd Royal Edinburgh Asylum Annual Report*, 1904, LHSA LHB7/7/11, 19.

87. C. Rosenberg, *Explaining Epidemics and Other Studies in the History of Medicine* (Cambridge: Cambridge University Press, 1992), 268–9.

88. Water damage to some REA admission registers does not permit this asylum to be included in the comparison. While the total sample patient population in Table 6.4 is actually 546, the number of admission and case-note causes included in this table is 551 and 576 respectively. This is because a small number of patients had numerous causes assigned to them rather than a single cause, so that percentages in themselves are slightly misleading.

89. *Barony Parochial Asylum Case Book*, NHSGGCA30/4/52/64.

90. *Ibid.*, NHSGGCA30/4/30/12.

91. *Midlothian and Peebles District Asylum Case Books*, LHSA LHB33/12/12/15 and LHB33/12/12/118.

92. *Glasgow Royal Asylum Case Book*, NHSGGCA13/5/145/233.

93. *Ibid.*, NHSGGCA13/5/138/148.

94. *Ibid.*, NHSGGCA13/5/190/839.

95. As it later transpires in the case notes, the 'misconducting himself' refers specifically to sexual intercourse. See *ibid.*, NHSGGCA13/5/139/530.

96. *Midlothian and Peebles District Asylum Case Book*, LHSA LHB33/12/11/196.

97. *Royal Edinburgh Asylum Case Book*, LHSA LHB7/51/71/829.

98. *Ibid.*, LHSA LHB7/51/54/603.

99. *Midlothian and Peebles District Asylum Case Book*, LHSA LHB33/12/9/33.

100. *Barony Parochial Asylum Case Book*, NHSGGCA30/4/36/10.

101. *Glasgow Royal Asylum Case Book*, NHSGGCA13/5/186/595.

102. *88th Royal Edinburgh Asylum Annual Report*, 1900, LHSA LHB7/7/10, 29-30.

103. *Midlothian and Peebles District Asylum Case Book*, LHSA LHB33/12/14/61.

104. *Glasgow Royal Asylum Case Book*, NHSGGCA13/5/145/593.

105. *Royal Edinburgh Asylum Case Books*, LHSA LHB7/51/40/550 and LHB7/51/50/251.

106. *Barony Parochial Asylum Case Book*, NHSGGCA30/5/34/40.

107. *Midlothian and Peebles District Asylum Case Book*, LHSA LHB33/12/16/325.

108. *Glasgow Royal Asylum Case Book*, NHSGGCA13/5/186/573.

109. *Royal Edinburgh Asylum Case Book*, LHSA LHB7/51/63/441.
110. *Ibid.*, LHSA LHB7/51/71/481.
111. *Barony Parochial Asylum Case Book*, NHSGGCA30/4/4/341.
112. *Royal Edinburgh Asylum Case Book*, LHSA LHB7/51/20/69.
113. *Barony Parochial Asylum Case Book*, NHSGGCA30/4/16/45.
114. *Ibid.*, NHSGGCA30/4/31/33.
115. D. Skae and T. Clouston, 'The Morisonian Lectures on Insanity for 1873', *Journal of Mental Science*, 21 (1875), 1–20: 14.
116. *Royal Edinburgh Asylum Case Book*, LHSA LHB7/51/80/473.
117. *Glasgow Royal Asylum Case Book*, NHSGGCA13/5/127/298.
118. See, for example, L. Churchill and S. Churchill, 'Storytelling in Medical Arenas: The Art of Self-Determination', *Soundings*, 1 (1982), 73–9; A. Kleinman, *The Illness Narratives: Suffering, Healing, and the Human Condition* (New York: Basic Books, 1988).
119. For an excellent introduction to narratives within psychiatry, see S. Swartz, 'Shrinking: A Postmodern Perspective on Psychiatric Case Histories', *South African Journal of Psychology*, 26 (1996), 150–6.
120. *Royal Edinburgh Asylum Case Book*, LHSA LHB7/51/81/61.
121. *Glasgow Royal Asylum Case Book*, NHSGGCA13/5/190/844.
122. *Ibid.*, NHSGGCA13/5/139/54.
123. *Ibid.*, NHSGGCA13/5/141/72.
124. *Ibid.*, NHSGGCA13/5/147/149.
125. *Ibid.*, NHSGGCA13/5/146/241.
126. *Ibid.*, NHSGGCA13/5/147/149.
127. *Ibid.*, NHSGGCA13/5/184/420.
128. *Midlothian and Peebles District Asylum Case Book*, LHSA LHB33/12/30/64.
129. *Glasgow Royal Asylum Case Book*, NHSGGCA13/5/144/534.
130. *Ibid.*, NHSGGCA13/5/145/54.
131. *Ibid.*, NHSGGCA13/5/186/573.
132. *Ibid.*, NHSGGCA13/5/134/77.
133. *Glasgow Royal Asylum Case Book*, NHSGGCA13/5/190/817.
134. *Barony Parochial Asylum Case Book*, NHSGGCA30/4/53/100.
135. *Royal Edinburgh Asylum Case Book*, LHSA LHB7/51/91/757.
136. *Ibid.*, LHSA LHB7/51/41/333 and LHB7/51/68/541.
137. *Midlothian and Peebles District Asylum Case Book*, LHSA LHB33/12/20/365.
138. W. Ford Robertson, 'The Pathology of General Paralysis of the Insane', *Review of Neurology and Psychiatry*, 4 (1906), 72–85: 74.
139. In Germany, on the other hand, GPI was 'seen to be chiefly a disease of the upper and middle classes'. See E. Engstrom, *Clinical Psychiatry in Imperial Germany: A History of Psychiatric Practice* (Ithaca: Cornell University Press, 2003), 108.

140. C. Wagner, 'Comparative Frequency of General Paralysis', *Glasgow Medical Journal*, 8 (1902), 230: 230.

141. It should be remembered that only pauper patients were admitted to Woodilee; while in 1897, the last of Gartnavel's pauper admissions were removed to the newly built district asylums. Rosslynlee was similarly intended for pauper patients, and only 29 private GPI patients (against 152 paupers) were admitted in the period under study, in order to fill vacant beds and generate profit for the institution.

142. *Midlothian and Peebles District Asylum Case Book*, LHSA LHB33/12/19/177.

143. *Barony Parochial Asylum Case Book*, NHSGGCA30/4/16/45.

144. *55th Commissioners of Lunacy for Scotland Annual Report*, 1913, NHSGGCA13B/14/69, lxv.

145. The percentage of male paralytics for the other three Scottish asylums was 77 per cent in the REA, 80 per cent in Woodilee and 82 per cent in Rosslynlee.

146. See, for example, W. Mickle, *General Paralysis of the Insane*, 2nd edn (London: H.K. Lewis, 1886), 247; and 'Discussion', *Journal of Mental Science*, 20 (1874), 320–4: 320.

147. *Midlothian and Peebles District Asylum Case Book*, LHSA LHB33/12/32/69.

148. *Royal Edinburgh Asylum Case Book*, LHSA LHB7/51/35/799.

149. *70th Dundee Royal Asylum Annual Report*, 1890, LHSA GD17/1/26, 31.

150. *92nd Glasgow Royal Asylum Annual Report*, 1905, NHSGGCA13B/2/223, 13.

151. *93rd Royal Edinburgh Asylum Annual Report*, 1905, LHSA LHB7/7/11, 12.

152. *Ibid.*

153. *94th Royal Edinburgh Asylum Annual Report*, 1906, LHSA LHB7/7/11, 13.

154. The total asylum admissions for this period were between 100 and 200 per year.

155. *29th Inverness District Asylum Annual Report*, 1893, NHSA HHB3/8/10, 12.

156. Cited in R. Lees, 'The Treatment of General Paralysis of the Insane', MD thesis, University of Edinburgh (1938), 5.

157. *Royal Edinburgh Asylum Case Book*, LHSA LHB7/51/106B/37.

7

Conclusions

During the nineteenth century, GPI emerged as a new and devastating psychiatric disorder with regard both to the severity of its symptoms and to the high number of patients diagnosed. By 1902, a staggering twenty-one per cent of male admissions to the Royal Edinburgh Asylum (REA) were said to be general paralytics,[1] and this figure appears to have been fairly representative of Britain as a whole.[2] Worse still, over twenty-eight per cent of REA deaths were attributed to this condition.[3] Moreover, the vast majority of these admissions and deaths were middle-aged men, in the words of one nineteenth-century alienist 'arrested suddenly in the height of prosperity', and doomed to degenerate 'into a state of hopeless fatuity' before dying 'far beyond the reach of friendly consolation'.[4] GPI constituted the most statistically significant and feared of the diseases which came to be grouped as 'neurosyphilis' in the early twentieth century.

The overriding aim of this volume was to provide a detailed and geographically localised account of this disease category. Four institutions – two royal and two parochial asylums – were selected from lowland Scotland which were held to be broadly representative of Scottish provision for the insane during the late nineteenth and early twentieth centuries. Crucially, a complete run of case notes and admission registers exist for each of these institutions, furnishing an exceptionally rich set of insights into the social background and medical experience of their neurosyphilitic patients. However, the findings of this study suggest that, in relation to this particular diagnostic group, the history of the Scottish asylums, their alienists and patients, also form part of a much wider British story.

In exploring the shaping of GPI, considerations have centred around its diagnosis, treatment and aetiology, although some observations have also been offered with respect to how alienists used this disease to advance their own professional status in late-Victorian and early Edwardian society. By focusing in depth upon a local context, we gain insight into the variety of roles the physician assumed simultaneously: as individual practitioners who confronted the versatility of disease; as members of a professional group whose collective behaviour defined diagnosis, treatment and aetiological explanation, and who collectively ascribed meaning or importance to such actions; and as members of a much wider societal group whose deeply-rooted fears and impressions were embedded within their medical practice.

An examination of the clinical diagnosis of GPI before the introduction of laboratory methods reveals that it was not the stable and easily identified disease category that contemporary physicians and subsequent historians have frequently portrayed it to be. A detailed analysis of the case notes shows that a significant number of patients in the Scottish sample were diagnosed initially with another mental condition, most commonly mania or melancholia. Indeed, GPI was not confirmed in some patients until post mortem revealed its morbid appearances, only death clinching the diagnosis. Chapter 3 attributes this to the polymorphous symptomatology, clinical 'imitations' and 'stadial' nature of GPI. The last of these appears to have been the most significant factor in initial misdiagnoses, for patients entering the asylum in a relatively early stage of the disease might not yet have exhibited the more characteristic physical symptoms. Perhaps additionally, as Chapter 6 suggests, GPI was not recognised initially in some patients because they did not fit the 'social' profile of the disease.

In short, it appears to have been extremely difficult to diagnose GPI in the earlier stages of the disease, and very often a clear diagnosis could not be given until its final stages. Scottish evidence supports in some way the clinician-historian German Berrios, who argues that GPI was not a conceptually stable disease during the nineteenth century because definitions of the disorder were broad and open to vast disagreement.[5] Yet, the Scottish data also show that such 'misdiagnoses' were ultimately corrected by reference to the specific and tangible cluster of textbook symptoms associated with GPI throughout the 1880 to 1930 period. In many instances, a 'degrees of fit' argument was probably applied by practising clinicians who were only too aware that the physical symptoms often took longer to develop. Thus, whilst the admission certificates lack much reference to physical symptoms, the vast majority of those Scottish patients who received a final diagnosis of GPI exhibited a common set of characteristic mental and physical symptoms by the end of their asylum stay.

This study then turned to examine the impact of laboratory methods upon diagnosis. Most historical accounts of GPI offer a fairly superficial interpretation, based upon the assumption that the laboratory's sophisticated technical tools led to unequivocal advances in understanding and managing the disease.[6] Such assumptions may be unduly influenced by widespread claims in the published medical literature that the Wassermann test played an immediate and central role in the diagnosis and treatment of GPI, and in the developing identity of the neurosyphilis disease group more generally. Certainly, good rhetorical use was made of the laboratory model within psychiatry. The Wassermann test was portrayed as central to the scientific investigation of the insane and as psychiatry's most potent symbol of the laboratory era. However, this study argues that it is important to balance alienists' words with an assessment of what appeared to be happening in actual daily asylum practice, and we find significant disparities when we turn to the clinical records.

Despite the high incidence of general paralytics who were Wassermann tested in the four Scottish asylums, detailed study using patient case notes indicates that the relationship between testing and the diagnosis of GPI was irregular rather than uniform. If there was disagreement between the judgement of the clinician and the findings of the laboratory, the former appears to have taken precedence. Despite their published comments on the power of the laboratory, most alienists seem to have felt that their clinical diagnostic skills were at best aided, not replaced, by this new serological tool. As L.S. Jacyna notes in his influential study of the impact of pathology upon surgery in the Glasgow Western Infirmary, by the end of the nineteenth century laboratory medicine had by no means triumphed over the skepticism of clinicians in the sphere of routine diagnosis.[7] It seems that this finding can be extended to psychiatry, where the diagnosing of GPI using the Wassermann test was mediated by a range of institutional, professional and social factors as well as the scientific, technical and instrumental features of the procedure.

One might argue that the position of clinical alienists is to be understood in terms of a professional claim to knowledge of particular diseases. While psychiatry had more need than most medical specialties to reinforce its scientific legitimacy, we cannot take at face value claims that the Wassermann test revolutionised the management of GPI, or was seized upon indiscriminately simply because it represented the excitement of laboratory medicine. In fact, on an individual level, alienists appear to have been deeply ambivalent over how they should incorporate such new laboratory diagnostic tools into their practice. It short, it seems fair to say that the greatest importance of the Wassermann test lay in its symbolic or rhetorical, rather than its practical, utility. The laboratory was possibly most valuable to alienists as a way to advance their professional interests, enabling them publicly to present their specialty as 'scientific' by being seen to make use of laboratory-based techniques.

Edward Hare, the clinician–historian and epidemiologist, claims that the diagnosis of GPI 'became objective' in the first decade of the twentieth century, once the specific reactions of the CSF had been elucidated.[8] However, as pointed out in Chapter 4, not everyone was tested, only those already suspected of having the disease. Laboratory testing was still reliant on judgements made about the individual patient, thus the diagnostic process continued to be socially mediated. Furthermore, the results of testing were often disregarded if they contradicted other clinical assessments. Socially sustained judgements relating to the prevailing alienist mindset were not abandoned at the laboratory door.

The clinician–historian Juliet Hurn asserts that GPI maintained relative conceptual stability over this period, even as physicians' images and interpretations of it changed over the first half of the twentieth century.[9] The medical historian should distinguish between two issues here: the diagnosis of the disease and wider conceptualisations of the diagnosed disease. Within the Scottish context, information gathered from sampled case notes over the period from 1880 to 1930 indicates that the clinical symptoms associated with GPI remained static, despite the supposed impact of laboratory-based diagnostic methods. Indeed, when George Robertson, Physician-Superintendent of the REA, gave a 'Clinique' presentation to an audience of medical students in 1920 in order to demonstrate the key physical and mental symptoms physicians should use to diagnose GPI, these symptoms were identical to those cited half a century earlier by his predecessors, Thomas Clouston and David Skae.[10]

However, in certain key respects, the wider conceptualisation of GPI as a disease category appears to have undergone a fundamental transformation in the early twentieth century. Within the published literature at least, the advent of the laboratory transformed GPI from a clinical classification – or even a 'somato–aetiological' classification as advanced by Skae – to a pathological classification based principally on the presence of the syphilitic spirochaete. Moreover, given that pronounced difficulties persisted with regard to the diagnosis of GPI, for the same reasons as in the pre-Wassermann period and with the addition of competitive rivalry between lab and clinic, this study extends Berrios' findings on the nineteenth-century conceptual instability of GPI into the twentieth-century laboratory era.

How, then, do we reconcile such instability with contemporary and historiographic claims that alienists considered GPI a paradigm disease, and in particular that the organic basis of GPI was believed to hold the key to the physical causation of insanity more widely? The nineteenth-century published literature suggests that alienists were fascinated and frustrated by GPI in equal measure, especially by its complex blend of the mental and physical, but there is little in the case notes to suggest that they saw it as the Rosetta Stone of psychiatry, a key to unlocking the mysteries of the mind. In particular, evidence would suggest that, at a practical level, alienists were far from united behind the syphilitic hypothesis and accommodated themselves only gradually to such organic theories. As Berrios asks, if nineteenth-century alienists were inherently organic in their approach, why not accept the syphilitic hypothesis as 'a gift from the gods'?[11] Such claims must therefore be considered rhetoric on a par with the reception of the laboratory within psychiatry.

Treatment is another area within the history of GPI that has been illuminated by the comparing and contrasting of case notes, annual reports and published literature. Triumphalist accounts were common in the years after the introduction of malarial therapy, and have persisted in historical accounts to the present day.[12] Accounts in the British literature quickly captured the optimism of the Continental experience in portraying a 'remarkable discovery' that could 'revolutionise' the treatment of GPI.[13] However, as with the effectiveness of the laboratory in diagnosis, the published comments of physicians on both the practicalities and efficacy of malarial therapy lie in stark contrast to the case-note findings. The supposed successes of the Wassermann reaction and malarial therapy have been taken directly from annual reports, whereas what we might term the 'clinical reality' of diagnosis and treatment as revealed in the case notes proves very different. As with the laboratory, there appears to have been great complexity in doctors' attitudes towards the 'friendly fever'.[14]

With the deliberate infection of patients with malaria, GPI became one of the first psychiatric disorders to be treated 'heroically' by a somatic therapy. It could be contended that this section of the patient population was exploited for experimental reasons when this new and seemingly bizarre form of therapy was introduced to the asylum. The American epidemiologists Stephanie Austin, Paul Strolley, and Tamar Lasky have commented bluntly that: 'Ethical considerations did not constrain researchers from injecting known pathogens into mental patients.'[15] However, the eventually unanimous decision to award the Nobel Prize for malarial therapy demonstrates that its mainstream endorsement was not dampened by ethical misgivings. Indeed, the award of the Prize to Wagner-Jauregg may, in turn, have hastened the spread of malarial therapy by conferring great prestige upon it.

It must be remembered that GPI was portrayed as constituting one of the most hopeless and cruel diseases met in asylum practice for much of the period under study. Anti-syphilitic treatments appear to have been minimally effective in cases of late syphilis, arresting the disease at best. Thus Colonel L.W. Harrison, Director of the Venereal Disease Department at St Thomas's Hospital and Special Adviser on Venereal Diseases to the Ministry of Health, bemoaned the fact that: 'We may put out the fire but we can do nothing towards rebuilding the house'.[16] Given the invariably fatal prognosis of GPI, desperate remedies were in all likelihood embraced enthusiastically. Indeed, as one clinician argued, 'to contemplate with arms folded a patient with general paralysis, is to enter into a compact with Death.'[17] Under these circumstances, the Scottish general paralytic *non-treatment* statistics could arguably be interpreted more dramatically than the malarial statistics, as the deliberate refusal to treat patients, thereby sentencing them to almost certain death.

Given the ways in which medical and social processes have been shown to intermingle in the diagnosis and treatment of GPI between 1880 and 1930, it is unsurprising that historical ideas surrounding its causation share the same characteristics. Despite the fact that the discovery of the spirochaete was a significant step towards establishing syphilis as the cause of GPI, there was in fact substantial resistance to the syphilitic hypothesis of GPI, as is evidenced in the Scottish asylum case notes. Thomas Clouston and David Yellowlees seem merely to have reflected the general view of British alienists in being unconvinced of the syphilitic basis of GPI. Even with mounting evidence in support of the syphilis hypothesis, alienists at first resisted and then accommodated themselves gradually to this aetiology by incorporating it into pre-existing theories. The 'parasyphilis' and 'pseudo-GPI' diagnoses became an especially neat way to entertain the syphilis theory without having to accept it fully, and physicians were slow to move to the more rigorously aetiological 'neurosyphilis' as an umbrella term which denoted unequivocal syphilis of the nervous system.

We can only fully understand alienists' perceptions of GPI during the period of this study by locating the multi-causal theories that surrounded it within broader social concerns, medical ideologies and sexual politics of the late nineteenth and early twentieth centuries. During the *fin-de-siècle* period, Britain was haunted by fantasies of decay and degeneration,[18] and, to some extent, those fears relating to urban degeneration and diseases of civilization were epitomised by GPI. Indeed, one might argue that the medical ideologies relating syphilis and GPI were used to legitimise and lend scientific validity to the concepts of civilisation and degeneration as sources of illness. Alienists conceptualised GPI as a result of the complex interplay between the temptations and excesses of urbanisation. This stance entailed a social predisposition to characterise the disease as one which affected city dwelling, middle-aged, working-class males. This study has shown that the social characteristics of most general paralytics in the four asylums fit this profile.

Disease has historically been construed as both indicator and product of adverse social conditions, and theories of causation and pathology used as vehicles to articulate and legitimate wider cultural criticisms.[19] Hypotheses proposed to account for the causation of GPI tell us much about the concerns of alienists in this period. Contemporaries framed a picture of GPI that sought to reduce the threat posed by the randomness of disease whilst simultaneously articulating their own social and cultural values. Smoking and alcohol were woven into the identity of GPI as a disease associated with immorality, promiscuity and excess, while the level of church attendance was one device employed as a measure of respectability. Thus, the act of diagnosis assumed a joint medical–moral agenda and became a form of moral regulation. Within the diagnostic and curative processes, as alienists judged and regulated the behaviour of their patients, they assumed an additional role. Propelled into acting as moral guardians and 'priests of the body' to their urban populations, they taught prudent adherence to the Victorian moral values of continence, monogamy, and racial hygiene as an integral part of their medical practice.

Coda

No neurosyphilitic patients are known to reside in any Scottish asylum in the early twenty-first century. The antibiotic era has witnessed a dramatic drop in the neurosyphilis rate, so that the condition has become widely regarded as simply a disease of the past that modern physicians need not familiarise themselves with. Yet, there are several aspects of current medical debate which suggest that this diagnostic label should not be confined to the medical dustbin just yet.

First, we have seen a significant rise in worldwide rates of primary and secondary syphilis in the last decade. Figures have risen dramatically throughout the United Kingdom since 1998. In Scotland alone, a total of 246 cases of infectious syphilis were reported during 2006, the highest number for more than fifty years.[20] Incidentally, the vast majority of these cases were diagnosed in Edinburgh, Glasgow and Aberdeen, the major Scottish cities, syphilis thus continuing to be conceived by the medical profession as very much an urban disease. Medical commentators suggest that there may be an eventual corresponding upsurge in cases of tertiary syphilis in the light of this recent resurgence of early syphilis if patients are not adequately treated.[21] This has encouraged a number of physicians to attempt to 'remind the medical community of this forgotten entity' so that cases can be recognised and treated efficiently.[22] Since most psychiatrists rarely, if ever, see a case of the neurosyphilitic diseases, they might otherwise be unlikely to consider this differential diagnosis.

Secondly, there is the limited impact of treatment upon this disease group. Despite the efficacy of penicillin in treating early syphilis, indiscriminate or inadequate antibiotic treatment – including its use as a treatment for unrelated disorders – has allegedly contributed to a recent rise in cases of neurosyphilis, particularly atypical presentations such as asymptomatic, pure neuro-ophthalmological or psychosis-related neurosyphilis.[23] Such incidences of syphilis 'incognito' complicate the recognition of neurosyphilis still further, as the 'great imitator' continues to outmanoeuvre clinicians. Thus, not only is the incidence of syphilis rising, but its manifestations appear to be evolving, which again complicates diagnosis of this, it seems, persistently unstable diagnostic group. Furthermore, the early recognition of neurosyphilis is imperative since antibiotic therapy in the later stages tends merely to arrest the various types of the disease, particularly tabes dorsalis and GPI. Thus, patients who are not diagnosed early enough are unlikely to regain previous cognitive performance.[24] Pencillin shares this notable drawback with its precursor, malarial therapy.

Finally, we must consider the relationship between neurosyphilis and human immunodeficiency virus (HIV). Over the past two decades, there has been a striking increase in the prevalence, or at least recognition, of concurrent syphilis and HIV infection.[25] In fact, a specific relationship has been found to exist between HIV and neurosyphilis, leading physicians to assert that, while neurosyphilis is unusual in immunocompromised patients, it is not exceptional within the context of HIV infection.[26] Such studies have fuelled recent suggestions that syphilis might impact upon the course of HIV – syphilis alleged to facilitate both the transmission and acquisition of HIV – and in particular create an increased risk of neurological complications.[27] Most notably, physicians have begun to recognise a form of HIV-associated dementia as constituting 'one of the most devastating complications of HIV infection', a disorder characterised by substantial memory and intellectual decline, marked psychomotor slowing and motor abnormalities.[28] Such neuropsychological impairment as a result of HIV infection has been well documented since the early days of the epidemic,[29] although the mechanism by which HIV causes such cognitive-motor impairment is as yet unresolved.[30] Estimates of the prevalence of this dementia range from seven to thirty-three per cent, rising to as much as sixty-six per cent in those with advanced HIV disease.[31] Such data serves to illustrate the continuing relevance of the neurosyphilis disease group within twenty-first-century medicine, and the enduring threat that 'the cruel madness of love' may yet again pose to society.

Notes

1. W. Ford Robertson, 'Discussion on the Pathology of General Paralysis of the Insane', *British Medical Journal*, 2 (1903), 1065–9: 1067.
2. See J. Hurn, 'The Changing Fortunes of the General Paralytic', *Wellcome History*, 4 (1997), 5–6: 5, which estimates that up to twenty per cent of late nineteenth-century British male asylum admissions were due to GPI.
3. *38th Commissioners of Lunacy for Scotland Annual Report*, 1896, NHS Greater Glasgow and Clyde Archives, NHSGGCA13B/14/64, liii.
4. D. Skae, 'Contributions to the Natural History of General Paralysis', *Edinburgh Medical Journal*, 5 (1859–60), 885–905: 905.

5. See G. Berrios, '"Depressive Pseudodementia" or "Melancholic Dementia": A Nineteenth Century View', *Journal of Neurology, Neurosurgery, and Psychiatry*, 48:5 (1985), 393–400.

6. Such accounts stretch at least from G. Zilboorg and W. Henry, *A History of Medical Psychology* (New York: Norton, 1941) onwards.

7. L. Jacyna, 'The Laboratory and the Clinic: The Impact of Pathology on Surgical Diagnosis in the Glasgow Western Infirmary, 1875–1910', *Bulletin of the History of Medicine*, 62:3 (1988), 384–406.

8. E. Hare, 'The Origin and Spread of Dementia Paralytica', *Journal of Mental Science*, 105 (1959), 594–626: 612.

9. J. Hurn, 'The History of General Paralysis of the Insane in Britain, 1830 to 1950', PhD thesis, University of London (1998), 16.

10. G. Robertson, 'Clinique on GPI', 25 February 1920, Lothian Health Services Archive (LHSA), GD16, 5–15. Using a 37-year-old man as a typical example of the disease, Robertson drew attention to the man's mental symptoms of elated and grandiose mood, mental inco-ordination and deterioration of intellect, loss of memory and impairment of judgement, before turning to the physical signs of Argyll–Robertson phenomenon of the eyes, staggering gait, tremor of hands, tongue and lips, and affected speech.

11. Berrios, *op. cit.* (note 5), 398.

12. While Whitrow's biography of Wagner-Jauregg considers the Austrian alienist's development of malaria therapy in some detail, her prime concern seems to be to eulogise her subject. See M. Whitrow, *Julius Wagner-Jauregg, 1857–1940* (London: Smith-Gordon, 1993).

13. 'Diseases that Cure Diseases: The Newest Wonder in Medical Science', *Royal Edinburgh Asylum Presscuttings Book*, Vol. VII, 1923, LHSA LHB7/12/7, 176.

14. This was an informal term adopted in North America. See, for example, F. Cross, 'Friendly Fever', *Good Housekeeping*, 100:2 (1935), 46–7.

15. S. Austin, P. Strolley and T. Lasky, 'The History of Malariotherapy for Neurosyphilis', *Journal of the American Medical Association*, 268:4 (1992), 516–19: 518.

16. L. Harrison, 'An Address on the Treatment of Syphilis, with Special Relation to its Later Manifestations', *Lancet*, 1 (1923), 4–8: 4.

17. Cited in J. Robb, 'Review of Balado and Esteves', *Journal of Mental Science*, 76 (1930), 358: 358.

18. S. Ledger and R. Luckhurst (eds), *The Fin de Siècle: A Reader in Cultural History, c.1880–1900* (Oxford: Oxford University Press, 2000), xiii.

19. C. Rosenberg, 'Pathologies of Progress: The Idea of Civilization as Risk', *Bulletin of the History of Medicine*, 72 (1998), 714–30: 716.

20. K. Bussey, 'Number of Syphilis Cases is Highest in 50 Years', *Glasgow Herald*, 28 November 2007.

21. See, for example, M. Thompson and S. Samuels, 'Neurosyphilis: Is it Still a Clinically Relevant Form of Dementia?', *Expert Review of Neurotherapeutics*, 2 (2002), 665–8.

22. See R. Gilad, *et al.*, 'Neurosyphilis: The Reemergence of an Historical Disease', *Israel Medical Association Journal*, 9:2 (2007), 117–18, whose article is said to have been written in light of the fifty-fold increase in the incidence of syphilis documented in the former Soviet Union since the early 1990s.

23. See, for instance, M. Jacob, *et al.*, 'Beware of Neuro-Syphilis', *Journal of Neurology*, 252:5 (2005), 609–10; E. Kararizou, *et al.*, 'Psychosis or Simply a New Manifestation of Neurosyphilis', *The Journal of International Medical Research*, 34:3 (2006), 335–7.

24. See, for example, R. Nitrini, 'The Cure of One of the Most Frequent Types of Dementia: A Historical Parallel', *Alzheimer Disease and Associated Disorders*, 19:3 (2005), 156–8: 156.

25. See, for instance, B. Stoner, 'Current Controveries in the Management of Adult Syphilis', *Clinical Infectious Diseases*, 44: Supplement 3 (2007), 130–46; N. Zetola and J. Klausner, 'Syphilis and HIV Infection: An Update', *Clinical Infectious Diseases*, 44 (2007), 1222–8. The latter stresses the 'disproportionate burden' of syphilis upon 'men who have sex with men', which might be seen as a further twist on the diagnostic 'medico–moral judgement' discussed in Chapter 6.

26. See, for example, S. Saik, *et al.*, 'Neurosyphilis in Newly Admitted Psychiatric Patients: Three Case Reports', *Journal of Clinical Psychiatry*, 65:7 (2004), 919–21.

27. S. Letendre, *et al.*, 'Neurologic Complications of HIV Disease and their Treatment', *Topics in HIV Medicine*, 15:2 (2007), 32–9.

28. M. Török, 'Neurological Infections: Clinical Advances and Emerging Threats', *Lancet Neurology*, 6:1 (2007), 16–18: 17. The conundrum as to why only some patients afflicted with primary syphilis progressed to the neurosyphilitic stage is echoed here, Török acknowledging that 'the reason why only some HIV-infected patients develop this disorder is not clear'.

29. See, for instance, B. Navia, B. Jordan and R. Price, 'The AIDS Dementia Complex: 1. Clinical Features', *Annals of Neurology*, 19 (1986), 525–35.

30. See, for example, I. Grant, T. Marcotte and R. Heaton, 'Neurocognitive Complications of HIV Disease', *Psychological Science*, 10:3 (1999), 191–5; E. Koutsilieri, *et al.*, 'The Pathogenesis of HIV-Induced Dementia', *Mechanisms of Ageing and Development*, 123:8 (2002), 1047–53.

31. J. Dilley, *et al.*, 'The Decline of Incident Cases of HIV-Associated Neurological Disorders in San Francisco, 1991–2003', *AIDS*, 19 (2005), 634–5.

Appendices

Appendix 1

Table Contents for the Royal Edinburgh Asylum Database

LETTERS
ID *
Letter ID ^*
Writer
Receiver
Date
Letter content

CERTIFICATE
SYMPTOMS
ID *
Symptom ID ^*
Symptom
Symptom
coded *

ADMISSION
CERTIFICATES
ID *
East or West House
Voluntary/certified
Date 1
Doctor 1
1st Certificate
contents
Date 2
Doctor 2
2nd Certificate contents
Extra facts
Relative(s) mentioned
By whose authority sent

HISTORY:
CAUSATION
ID *
Disposition
Habits
Prev bodily illnesses
Previous attacks?
PA details
Hereditary propensity?
HP details
Predisposing cause(s)
Exciting cause(s)

HISTORY:
SYMPTOMS
ID *
1st mental
1st bodily
Recent mental
Recent bodily
Insane habits
Suicidal?
Dangerous?
Epileptic?
Duration
Other facts

MENTAL STATE
ID *
Exaltation
Depression
Excitement
Enfeeblement
Memory
Coherence
Can answer questions
Delusions/hallucinations
Other abnormalities

BODILY STATE
ID *
Appearance
Skin
Hair
Eyes
Pupils
Muscularity
Fatness
Nervous system
Reflex action
Special senses
Retina

Lungs
Heart
Tongue
Bowels
Other organs
Appetite
Palate
Urine
Menstruation
Pulse
Temperature
Height

Weight
Bodily state
Lab tests
Blood tests?
Amount
Date(s)
Result(s)
CSF tests?
Amount
Date(s)
Result(s)
Abnormalities

SOCIAL DETAILS	PROGRESS	
ID *	ID *	Length of stay *
Case note reference *	Form	Number of progress entries *
General register ref *	Disease	Post-mortem?
Forename	Skae's classification	Cause(s) of death
Surname	Prognosis	Mental symptoms
Gender	Diagnosis	Delusions
Age	Result of treatment	Bodily symptoms
Marital status	Asylum transfers	Work in asylum
Occupation	Admission date	Which ward(s)
Occupation coded	Discharge date	Remarks
Education		
Religion		
Private/pauper		
Address of patient	TREATMENT	
Address of relative	ID *	Treatments
Previous admissions	Treatment ID ^*	Treatments coded *
Photographs?	Order of treatments*	Comments
Remarks	Date of treatments	

ID = Primary Key; ^ = Foreign Key;
*= A Derived Variable; ? = Yes/No Response

Appendix 2

Scottish Asylum Physician-Superintendents

REA		WOODILEE	
W. McKinnon	**1839–1846**	**J. Rutherford**	**1874–1883**
D. Skae	1846–1873	R. Blair	1883–1902
T. Clouston	1873–1908	H. Marr	1902–1910
G.M. Robertson	1908–1932	H. Carre	1910–1936
D.K. Henderson	1932–1955		

GARTNAVEL		ROSSLYNLEE	
W. Hutcheson	**1841–1849**	**T. Anderson**	**1874–1880**
A. McIntosh	1849–1874	R. Cameron	1880–1888
D. Yellowlees	1874–1901	R.B. Mitchell	1888–1916
L. Oswald	1901–1921	J.H.C. Orr	1916–1942
D.K. Henderson	1921–1932		

Sources
and Select Bibliography

Primary Sources

Archival Material

Edinburgh Central Library:

XRA 242, *1st–10th Annual Reports of the Scottish Board of Health,* 1919–28.

XRA 244 H1, *Dundee Public Health Department Reports of the Medical Officer of Health,* 1919–30.

qXRA 244 H1, *Glasgow Corporation Reports of the Medical Officer of Health,* 1899–1930.

NHS Greater Glasgow and Clyde Archives, Mitchell Library, Glasgow:

GARTNAVEL

NHSGGCA13B/2/221–225, *Glasgow Royal Asylum Annual Reports,* 1874–1940.

NHSGGCA13/5/62–67 & 123–148, *Glasgow Royal Asylum Male Case Books,* 1876–1921.

NHSGGCA13/5/98–122 & 149–177, *Glasgow Royal Asylum Female Case Books,* 1877–1921.

NHSGGCA13/5/178–194, *Glasgow Royal Asylum Case Records,* 1921–31.

NHSGGCA13/6/78–80, *Glasgow Royal Asylum Register of Lunatics,* 1871–1963.

NHSGGCA13/7/87–137, *Glasgow Royal Asylum Admission Documents,* 1880–1930.

WOODILEE

NHSGGCA30/1/1–7, *Printed Minutes of Glasgow Lunacy District Board and Committees (Woodilee and Gartloch)*, 1898–1923.

NHSGGCA30/2/9, *Barony Parochial Asylum Annual Report*, 1883.

NHSGGCA30/2/10, *Barony Parochial Asylum Annual Report*, 1897.

NHSGGCA30/2/11–20, *Barony Parochial Asylum Annual Reports*, 1900–19.

NHSGGCA30/4/1–63, *Barony Parochial Asylum Male Case Books*, 1875–1931.

NHSGGCA30/5/1–61, *Barony Parochial Asylum Female Case Books*, 1875–1931.

NHSGGCA30/8/3, *6 Pamphlets containing Regulations for Management of Glasgow District Asylums at Woodilee and Gartloch and Rules for Guidance of Attendants*, 1900–9.

NHSGGCA30/10/1–4, *Barony Parochial Asylum Register of Admissions*, 1875–1957.

OTHER

NHSGGCA13B/14/52–72, *Commissioners of Lunacy for Scotland Annual Reports*, 1859–1938.

NHSGGCA21/1/1, *Scottish Western Asylums' Research Institute, Minutes of the Board of Management*, 1931–45.

NHSGGCA21/2/1, *20th Scottish Western Asylums' Research Institute Annual Report*, 1929.

NHSGGCA21/2/2, *West of Scotland Neuro-Psychiatric Research Institute 2nd Annual Report*, 1933.

NHSGGCA21/2/3, *33rd Scottish Asylums' Pathological Scheme Annual Report*, 1929.

NHSGGCA21/2/4, *34th Scottish Mental Hospitals' Pathological Scheme Annual Report*, 1930.

NHSGGCA21/2/5, *39th Scottish Mental Hospitals' Pathological Scheme Annual Report*, 1936.

48th and 50th Scottish Mental Hospitals' Pathological Scheme Annual Report, 1945 and 1947, courtesy of Alex Gordon.

NHSGGCA21/3/1, *Correspondence and Papers relating to the Reorganisation of the Scottish Western Asylums' Research Institute*, 1931.

Lothian Health Services Archive, Edinburgh University Library:

REA

LHB7/1/5–10, *Royal Edinburgh Asylum Manager's Minute Books*, 1871–1937.

LHB7/7/5–15, *Royal Edinburgh Asylum Annual Reports*, 1813–1939.

LHB7/11/2, 'An Outline of the History of the Royal Edinburgh Hospital', taken from *The Morningside Mirror*, 1942.

LHB7/11/4, Catford, E., 'The Royal Edinburgh Asylum: A Hospital with a Great Tradition'.

LHB7/11/7, Catford, E., 'A Hospital Comes of Age: The Story of the Royal Edinburgh Hospital, 1813–1963'.

LHB7/12/1–8, *Royal Edinburgh Asylum Presscuttings Books*, 1862–1938.

LHB7/14/2, *Royal Edinburgh Asylum Pamphlets*, 1863–79.

LHB7/19/18, Mitchell, A., 'Memorandum on the Position of the Royal Edinburgh Asylum for the Insane', 1883.

LHB7/35/5–13, *Royal Edinburgh Asylum General Register of Patients*, 1876–1933.

LHB7/51/34–120, *Royal Edinburgh Asylum Case Books*, 1879–1931.

GD12/1, Catford, E., 'Draft History of the Royal Edinburgh Hospital, 1774 to 1856', written in the late-1950s.

GD16, Robertson, G., 'Cliniques', 1917–20.

GD16, Ritchie, D., 'Reports of Leith Cases', 1913–15.

ROSSLYNLEE

LHB33/1/1–8, *Minutes of the Midlothian and Peebles District Board of Lunacy*, 1870–1924.

LHB33/2/1–3, *Midlothian and Peebles District Asylum Annual Reports,* 1871–1939.

LHB33/4/12, *Register of Chronic Cases,* 1897–1937.

LHB33/5/1–2, *Register of Discharges and Removals,* 1874–1942.

LHB33/12/5–36, *Midlothian and Peebles District Asylum Case Books,* 1880–1931.

LHB33/16/10, *Rules and Regulations for Staff,* 1915.

OTHER

LHB16/2/2–13, *Annual Reports of the City of Edinburgh Public Health Department,* 1920–31.

GD16, *Edinburgh University Calendar,* 1911–12.

GD17/1/20–5, *Annual Reports of the Asylums of Scotland,* 1882–8.

GD17/1/36–44, *Annual Reports of the Asylums of Scotland,* 1900–8.

GD17/5/1–35, *Reports of the General Board of Commissioners in Lunacy for Scotland,* 1857–1938.

Northern Health Services Archives, Aberdeen and Inverness:

GRHB2/8/6–10, *Royal Lunatic Asylum of Aberdeen Annual Reports,* 1881–1930.

HHB3/8/8–14, *Inverness District Asylum Annual Reports,* 1866–1931.

HHB3/8/42, *Report on Commissioners 'Notes': The Inverness District Asylum – Notes by Sir Arthur Mitchell on the Deaths Occurring in the Asylum.*

The National Archives, Public Record Office, London:

FD1/1401, *Committee on Mental Disorders: Pathological Work for the Laboratory of the Scottish Asylums (Reports and Correspondence),* 1921–5.

FD4/14, *Medical Research Committee and Medical Research Council: Reports of the Special Committee upon the Standardisation of Pathological Methods: The Wassermann Test,* 1918.

FD4/21, *Medical Research Committee and Medical Research Council: Report of the Special Committee upon the Standardisation of Pathological Methods and Diagnostic Value of the Wassermann Test,* 1918.

FD4/23, *Medical Research Council Special Report: An Analysis of the Results of Wassermann Reactions in 1,435 Cases of Syphilis or Suspected Syphilis,* 1919.

MH51/537, *Lunacy Commission and Board of Control: Correspondence on Malarial Treatment,* 1928–43.

MH51/538, *Lunacy Commission and Board of Control: Correspondence on Malarial Treatment,* 1927–44.

MH51/697, *Lunacy Commission and Board of Control Correspondence and Papers: Treatment of General Paralysis of the Insane by Induced Mild Malaria,* 1924.

MH51/698, *Lunacy Commission and Board of Control: Treatment of General Paralysis of the Insane by Induced Mild Malaria,* 1924–55.

Pamphlets

Clouston, T., 'Concerning Drink and Insanity', 1900, LHSA GD16.

Clouston, T., 'The Developmental Aspects of Criminal Anthropology', 1894, LHSA GD16.

Clouston, T., 'Health of Body and Soundness of Mind: A Lay Sermon', 1903, LHSA GD16.

Clouston, T., 'How the Scientific Way of Looking at Things Helps Us in Our Work', 1908, LHSA LHB7/14/8.

Clouston, T., 'On the Use of Hypnotics, Sedatives and Motor Depressants in the Treatment of Mental Diseases', 1889, LHSA GD16.

Clouston, T., 'Sulphonal – Its Advantages and Disadvantages', 1895, LHSA GD16.

'Glasgow District Asylum, Woodilee, Lenzie: General Management of the Asylum, and General Rules for the Guidance of Attendants', 1900, NHSGGCA30/8/3.

Greenlees, T., 'The Circulatory Apparatus in General Paralysis of the Insane', 1904, LHSA GD16.

Henderson, D., 'Cerebral Syphilis – A Clinical Analysis of Twenty-Six Cases – Seven with Autopsy', 1913, LHSA GD16.

Henderson, D., 'Tabes Dorsalis and Mental Disease', 1911, LHSA GD16.

MacPherson, J., 'Surgical Treatment of Insanity', 1895, LHSA GD16.

Robertson, G., 'Clinique on General Paralysis', 1918, LHSA GD16.

Robertson, G., 'The Discovery of General Paralysis', 1923, LHSA GD16.

Robertson, G., 'General Paralysis of the Insane: The Morison Lectures', 1913, LHSA GD16.

Robertson, G., 'The Hospitalisation of the Scottish Asylum System', 1922, LHSA LHB7/14/10.

Robertson, W., 'The Pathology of General Paralysis of the Insane: The Morison Lectures', 1906, LHSA GD16.

Robertson, W., McRae, G. and Jeffrey, J., 'Bacteriological Investigations into the Pathology of General Paralysis of the Insane', 1903, LHSA GD16.

Social and Sanitary Society of Edinburgh, 'Too Early and Imprudent Marriages', LHSA GD16.

Wilson, G., 'The Diathesis of General Paralysis', 1892, LHSA GD16.

Books

Austin, T., *A Practical Account of General Paralysis, its Mental and Physical Symptoms, Statistics, Causes, Seat and Treatment* (London: John Churchill, 1859).

Barker, W., *Mental Diseases: A Manual for Students* (London: Cassell and Co., 1902).

Blandford, G., *Insanity and its Treatment* (Edinburgh: Oliver and Boyd, 1871).

Browning, C. and MacKenzie, I., *Recent Methods in the Diagnosis and Treatment of Syphilis* (London: Constable and Company, 1911).

Bucknill, J. and Tuke, D., *A Manual of Psychological Medicine* (London: John Churchill, 1858, 1862 and 1874).

Clouston, T., *Before I Wed, or Young Men and Marriage* (London: Cassell and Company, 1913).

Clouston, T., *Clinical Lectures on Mental Diseases* (London: J. and A. Churchill, 1883).

Clouston, T., *Clinical Lectures on Mental Diseases,* 5th edn (London: J. and A. Churchill, 1898).

Clouston, T., *The Hygiene of Mind* (London: Methuen and Co., 1906).

Clouston, T., *Unsoundness of Mind* (London: Methuen, 1911).

Craig, M., *Psychological Medicine: A Manual on Mental Diseases for Practitioners and Students* (London: J. and A. Churchill, 1917).

Dowse, T., *The Brain and its Diseases, Volume I: Syphilis of the Brain and Spinal Cord* (London: Baillière, Tindall and Cox, 1879).

Fisher, V., *An Introduction to Abnormal Psychology* (New York: Macmillan, 1937).

Fournier, A., *Syphilis and Marriage* (Paris: Masson, 1880).

Gowers, W., *A Manual of Diseases of the Nervous System, Volume 1: Diseases of the Nerves and Spinal Cord,* 2nd edn (London: J. and A. Churchill, 1892).

Harrison, L., *The Diagnosis and Treatment of Venereal Diseases in General Practice* (London: Hodder and Stoughton, 1919).

Henderson, D. and Gillespie, R., *A Textbook of Psychiatry for Students and Practitioners* (London: Oxford University Press, 1927).

Hunt, E., *Mental Maladies: A Treatise on Insanity* (Philadelphia: Lea and Blanchard, 1845).

Kellogg, T., *A Textbook of Mental Diseases for the Use of Students and Practitioners of Medicine* (London: J. and A. Churchill, 1897).

Lavater, J., *Essays on Physiognomy, Designed to Promote the Knowledge and Love of Mankind* (London: John Stockdale, 1810).

Lees, D., *Practical Methods in the Diagnosis and Treatment of Venereal Diseases for Medical Practitioners and Students* (Edinburgh: E. and S. Livingstone, 1927).

Mickle, W., *General Paralysis of the Insane,* 2nd edn (London: H.K. Lewis, 1886).

Power, D. and Murphy, J., *A System of Syphilis,* Vol. VI (London: Oxford University Press, 1910).

Prichard, J., *A Treatise on Insanity and Other Disorders Affecting the Mind* (London: Sherwood, Gilbert and Piper, 1835).

Robertson, W., *A Textbook of Pathology in Relation to Mental Diseases* (Edinburgh: William Clay, 1900).

Romberg, M., *A Manual of Nervous Diseases of Man*, 2 vols (London: Sydenham Society, 1853).

Southard, E. and Jarrett, M., *The Kingdom of Evils: Psychiatric Social Work Presented in One Hundred Case Histories, Together with a Classification of Social Divisions of Evil* (London: Allen and Unwin, 1922).

Tuke, D. H., *Chapters in the History of the Insane in the British Isles* (London: Kegan Paul, 1882).

Medical Journals

References to specific articles appearing in these journals are given in the notes.

American Journal of Insanity

Archives of Neurology

Archives of Neurology and Psychiatry

British Journal of Psychiatry

British Journal of Venereal Diseases

British Medical Journal

Edinburgh Medical Journal

Glasgow Medical Journal

Journal of the American Medical Association

Journal of Mental Science

Journal of Nervous and Mental Diseases

Lancet

Review of Neurology and Psychiatry

The Hospital

The Practitioner

Theses

Duff, E., 'Modern Conceptions in Syphilology with Special Reference to Serological Diagnosis and Treatment by the Arylarsonates and Bismuth', MD thesis, University of Edinburgh (1935).

Dymock, T., 'A Review of the Treatment of General Paralysis', MD thesis, University of Glasgow (1933).

Gibb, W., 'On Some of the Features of General Paralysis of the Insane', MD thesis, University of Glasgow (1885).

Lees, R., 'The Treatment of General Paralysis of the Insane', MD thesis, University of Edinburgh (1938).

Mackenzie, D., 'The Evaluation and Differentiation of Mental Disorders Associated with Syphilis of the Nervous System', MD thesis, University of Glasgow (1950).

McCully, J., 'Non-Specific Therapy in the Treatment of Neurosyphilis', MD thesis, University of Glasgow (1930).

McLeod, N, 'General Paralysis of the Insane with Special Reference to its Treatment by Malaria', MD thesis, University of Edinburgh (1928).

Paton, T., 'Therapeutic Malaria in General Paralysis of the Insane, with a Clinical Survey of 32 Cases so Treated', MD thesis, University of Glasgow (1933).

Raffan, G., 'A Treatise on the Aetiology, Pathology, Diagnosis and Treatment of Syphilis', MD thesis, University of Edinburgh (1913).

Reid, B., 'Malarial Therapy in General Paralysis', MD thesis, University of Glasgow (1932).

Steel, J., 'Malarial Therapy in General Paralysis of the Insane', MD thesis, University of Edinburgh (1926).

Tennent, T., 'An Investigation into the Value of Tryparsamide in the Treatment of General Paralysis of the Insane, with Special Consideration of the Clinical and Serological Factors which may Affect the Prognosis', MD thesis, University of Glasgow (1930).

Thornley, J., 'Syphilis', MD thesis, University of Glasgow (1886).

Secondary Sources

Ackerknecht, E., *Medicine at the Paris Hospital, 1794–1848* (Baltimore: The Johns Hopkins Press, 1967).

Ackerknecht, E., 'A Plea for a "Behaviourist" Approach in Writing the History of Medicine', *Journal of Medicine and Allied Sciences*, 22 (1967), 211–14.

Andrews, J., 'Case Notes, Case Histories, and the Patient's Experience of Insanity at Gartnavel Royal Asylum, Glasgow, in the Nineteenth Century', *Social History of Medicine*, 11:2 (1998), 255–81.

Andrews, J., 'A Failure to Flourish? David Yellowlees and the Glasgow School of Psychiatry', parts 1 and 2, *History of Psychiatry*, 8 (1997), 177–212 and 333–60.

Andrews, J., *'They're in the Trade ... of Lunacy, They "Cannot Interfere" – They Say': The Scottish Lunacy Commissioners and Lunacy Reform in Nineteenth-Century Scotland* (London: Wellcome Institute for the History of Medicine, 1998).

Andrews, J., *et al.*, *The History of Bethlem* (London: Routledge, 1997).

Andrews, J. and Smith, I. (eds), *'Let There be Light Again': A History of Gartnavel Royal Hospital from its Beginnings to the Present Day* (Glasgow: Gartnavel, 1993).

Anon, 'A Final Curtain', *British Medical Journal*, 1 (1975), 578.

Austin, S., Strolley, P. and Lasky, T., 'The History of Malariotherapy for Neurosyphilis', *Journal of the American Medical Association*, 268:4 (1992), 516–19.

Baldamus, W., 'Ludwig Fleck and the Development of the Sociology of Science', in Elias, N. (ed.), *Human Figurations* (Amsterdam: Amsterdams Sociologisch Tijdschrift, 1977), 135–56.

Barfoot, M. and Beveridge, A., 'Madness at the Crossroads: John Home's Letters from the Royal Edinburgh Asylum, 1886–1887', *Psychological Medicine*, 20 (1990), 263–84.

Barfoot, M. and Beveridge, A., '"Our Most Notable Inmate": John Willis Mason at the Royal Edinburgh Asylum, 1864–1901', *History of Psychiatry*, 4 (1993), 159–208.

Barfoot, M. and Morrison-Low, A., 'W.C. McIntosh and A.J. Macfarlan: Early Clinical Photography in Scotland', *History of Photography*, 23:3 (1999), 1–9.

Bartlett, P. and Wright, D., *Outside the Walls of the Asylum: The History of Care in the Community 1750–2000* (London and New Brunswick: Athlone, 1999).

Beach, T., 'The History of Alzheimer's Disease: Three Debates', *Journal of the History of Medicine and Allied Sciences*, 42 (1987), 327–49.

Berridge, V., *AIDS in the UK: The Making of Policy, 1981–1994* (Oxford: Oxford University Press, 1986).

Berrios, G., '"Depressive Pseudodementia" or "Melancholic Dementia": A Nineteenth Century View', *Journal of Neurology, Neurosurgery, and Psychiatry*, 48:5 (1985), 393–400.

Berrios, G., *The History of Mental Symptoms: Descriptive Psychopathology since the Nineteenth Century* (Cambridge: Cambridge University Press, 1996).

Berrios, G., 'Memory and the Cognitive Paradigm of Dementia During the Nineteenth Century: A Conceptual History', in Murray, R. and Turner, T. (eds), *Lectures on the History of Psychiatry: The Squibb Series* (London: Gaskell, 1990), 194–211.

Berrios, G. and Freeman, H. (eds), *150 Years of British Psychiatry, 1841–1991* (London: Gaskell, 1991).

Berrios, G. and Porter, R. (eds), *A History of Clinical Psychiatry: The Origin and History of Psychiatry Disorders* (London: Athlone, 1995).

Beveridge, A., 'Life in the Asylum: Patients' Letters from Morningside, 1873–1908', *History of Psychiatry*, 9 (1998), 431–69.

Beveridge, A., 'Madness in Victorian Edinburgh: A Study of Patients Admitted to the Royal Edinburgh Asylum under Thomas Clouston, 1873–1908', parts 1 and 2, *History of Psychiatry*, 6 (1995), 21–54 and 133–56.

Beveridge, A. and Williams, M., 'Inside "The Lunatic Manufacturing Company": The Persecuted World of John Gilmour', *History of Psychiatry*, 13 (2002), 19–49.

Boyle, M., 'Is Schizophrenia What it Was? A Re-Analysis of Kraepelin's and Bleuler's Population', *Journal of the History of the Behavioral Sciences*, 26 (1990), 323–33.

Brandt, A., *No Magic Bullet: A Social History of Venereal Disease in the United States since 1880* (New York and Oxford: Oxford University Press, 1985).

Brandt, A., 'Sexually Transmitted Diseases', in Bynum, W. and Porter, R. (eds), *Companion Encyclopedia of the History of Medicine*, Vol. I (London: Routledge, 1993), 562–84.

Brandt, A., 'The Syphilis Epidemic and its Relation to AIDS', *Science*, 239 (1988), 375–80.

Braslow, J., 'Effect of Therapeutic Innovation on Perception of Disease and the Doctor–Patient Relationship: A History of General Paralysis of the Insane and Malarial Fever Therapy, 1910–1950', *American Journal of Psychiatry*, 152:1 (1995), 660–5.

Braslow, J., *Mental Ills and Bodily Cures: Psychiatric Treatment in the First Half of the Twentieth Century* (Berkeley, Los Angeles and London: University of California Press, 1997).

Brown, E., 'French Psychiatry's Initial Reception of Bayle's Discovery of General Paresis of the Insane', *Bulletin of the History of Medicine*, 68:2 (1994), 235–53.

Bruetsch, W., 'Neurosyphilitic Conditions: General Paralysis, General Paresis, Dementia Paralytica', in Arieti, S. (ed.), *American Handbook of Psychiatry* (New York: Basic Books, 1974), 134–51.

Burns, S., *Early Medical Photography in America, 1839–1883* (New York: The Burns Archive, 1983).

Burrows, A. and Schumacher, I., *Portraits of the Insane: The Case of Dr Diamond* (London and New York: Quartet Books, 1990).

Bynum, W. and Porter, R., *Medicine and the Five Senses* (Cambridge and New York: Cambridge University Press, 1993).

Bynum, W., Porter, R. and Shepherd, M. (eds), *The Anatomy of Madness: Essays in the History of Psychiatry*, Vol. I (London and New York: Tavistock, 1985).

Bynum, W., Porter, R. and Shepherd, M. (eds), *The Anatomy of Madness: Institutions and Society*, Vol. II (London and New York: Routledge, 1985).

Bynum, W., Porter, R. and Shepherd, M. (eds), *The Anatomy of Madness: The Asylum and Psychiatry*, Vol. III (London and New York: Routledge, 1988).

Callahan, C. and Berrios, G., *Reinventing Depression: A History of the Treatment of Depression in Primary Care, 1940–2004* (Oxford and New York: Oxford University Press, 2005).

Carter, K. Codell, *The Rise of Causal Concepts of Disease: Case Histories* (Aldershot: Ashgate, 2003).

Cassel, J., *The Secret Plague: Venereal Disease in Canada, 1838–1939* (Toronto, Buffalo and London: University of Toronto Press, 1987).

Chamberlin, J. and Gilman, S. (eds), *Degeneration: The Dark Side of Progress* (New York: Columbia University Press, 1985).

Churchill, L. and Churchill, S., 'Storytelling in Medical Arenas: The Art of Self-Determination', *Soundings*, 1 (1982), 73–9.

Coleborne, C., 'Families, Patients and Emotions: Asylums for the Insane in Colonial Australia and New Zealand, c.1880–1910', *Social History of Medicine*, 19 (2006), 425–44.

Condrau, F., 'The Patient's View Meets the Clinical Gaze', *Social History of Medicine*, 20 (2007), 525–40.

Cunningham, A. and Williams, P. (eds), *The Laboratory Revolution in Medicine* (Cambridge: Cambridge University Press, 1992).

Davidson, R., *Dangerous Liaisons: A Social History of Venereal Disease in Twentieth-Century Scotland* (Amsterdam: Rodopi, 2001).

Davidson, R. and Hall, L. (eds), *Sex, Sin and Suffering: Venereal Disease and European Society since 1870* (London and New York: Routledge, 2001).

Davies, K., '"Sexing the Mind?": Women, Gender and Madness in Nineteenth Century Welsh Asylums', *Llafur*, 7:1 (1996), 29–40.

Davis, G. and Davidson, R., '"The Fifth Freedom" or "Hideous Atheistic Expediency": The Medical Community and Abortion Law Reform in Scotland, c.1960–75', *Medical History*, 50:1 (2006), 29–48.

Digby, A., *Madness, Morality and Medicine: A Study of the York Retreat, 1796–1914* (Cambridge: Cambridge University Press, 1985).

Dilley, J., *et al.*, 'The Decline of Incident Cases of HIV-Associated Neurological Disorders in San Francisco, 1991–2003', *AIDS*, 19:6 (2005), 634–5.

Doody, G., Beveridge, A. and Johnstone, E., 'Poor and Mad: A Study of Patients Admitted to the Fife and Kinross District Asylum between 1874 and 1899', *Psychological Medicine*, 26 (1996), 887–97.

Dowbiggin, I., '"An Exodus of Enthusiasm": G. Alder Blumer, Eugenics, and US Psychiatry, 1890–1920', *Medical History*, 36 (1992), 379–402.

Dowbiggin, I., 'Review of D. Pick, "Faces of Degeneration: A European Disorder, *c.*1848–*c.*1918"', *Bulletin of the History of Medicine*, 64 (1990), 488–9.

Duffin, J., *Lovers and Livers: Disease Concepts in History* (Toronto: Toronto University Press, 2005).

Engstrom, E., *Clinical Psychiatry in Imperial Germany: A History of Psychiatric Practice* (Ithaca and London: Cornell University Press, 2003).

Fennell, P., *Treatment without Consent: Law, Psychiatry and the Treatment of Mentally Disordered People since 1845* (London and New York: Routledge, 1996).

Fish, F., 'David Skae, MD, FRCS, Founder of the Edinburgh School of Psychiatry', *Medical History*, 9 (1965), 36–53.

Fleck, L., *The Genesis and Development of a Scientific Fact* (Chicago: University of Chicago Press, 1979).

Foucault, M., *The Birth of the Clinic* (London: Tavistock, 1973).

Foucault, M., *The History of Sexuality*, 3 vols (London: Penguin, 1990).

Foucault, M., *Madness and Civilization: A History of Insanity in the Age of Reason* (London: Routledge, 1995).

Fox, D. and Lawrence, C., *Photographing Medicine: Images and Power in Britain and America since 1840* (New York and London: Greenwood, 1988).

Freedman, D., *et al.*, *Statistics*, 2nd edn (New York and London: W.W. Norton and Company, 1991).

Freeman, H. and Berrios, G. (eds), *150 Years of British Psychiatry, Vol. II: The Aftermath* (London: Athlone Press, 1996).

Gardner, D., 'Henry Wade (1876–1955) and Cancer Research: Early Years in the Life of a Pioneer of Urological Surgery', *Journal of Medical Biography*, 11 (2003), 81–6.

Gardner, D., *Surgeon, Scientist, Soldier: The Life and Times of Henry Wade, 1876–1955* (London: Royal Society of Medicine, 2005).

Garfinkel, H., *Studies in Ethnomethodology* (New Jersey: Prentice-Hall, 1976).

Gijswijt-Hofstra, M. and Porter, R., *Cultures of Neurasthenia from Beard to the First World War* (Amsterdam and New York: Rodopi, 2001).

Gilad, R., *et al.*, 'Neurosyphilis: The Reemergence of an Historical Disease', *Israel Medical Association Journal*, 9:2 (2007), 117–18.

Grant, I., Marcotte, T. and Heaton, R., 'Neurocognitive Complications of HIV Disease', *Psychological Science*, 10:3 (1999), 191–5.

Green-Lewis, J., *Framing the Victorians: Photography and the Culture of Realism* (Cornell: Ithaca, 1996).

Hardy, A., *The Epidemic Streets: The Rise of Preventive Medicine 1856–1900* (Oxford: Clarendon Press, 1993).

Hare, E., 'The Origin and Spread of Dementia Paralytica', *Journal of Mental Science*, 105 (1959), 594–626.

Hare, E., 'The Two Manias: A Study of the Evolution of the Modern Concept of Mania', *British Journal of Psychiatry*, 138 (1981), 89–99.

Harrison, G., *Mosquitoes, Malaria and Man: A History of the Hostilities since 1880* (New York: Dutton, 1978).

Harvey, C. and Press, J., *Databases in Historical Research: Theory, Methods and Applications* (London: Macmillan Press, 1996).

Hawkins, M., *Social Darwinism in European and American Thought, 1860–1945: Nature as Model and Nature as Threat* (Cambridge: Cambridge University Press, 1997).

Henderson, D., *The Evolution of Psychiatry in Scotland* (Edinburgh and London: E. and S. Livingstone, 1964).

Higgs, E. and Melling, J., 'Chasing the Ambulance: The Emerging Crisis in the Preservation of Modern Health Records', *Social History of Medicine*, 10 (1997), 127–36.

Horwitz, A. and Wakefield, J., *The Loss of Sadness: How Psychiatry Transformed Normal Sorrow into Depressive Disorder* (Oxford: Oxford University Press, 2007).

Houston, R., 'Institutional Care for the Insane and Idiots in Scotland before 1820', parts 1 and 2, *History of Psychiatry*, 12 (2001), 3–31 and 177–97.

Houston, R., *Madness and Society in Eighteenth-Century Scotland* (Oxford: Clarendon Press, 2000).

Howell, J., 'Early Use of X-Ray Machines and Electrocardiographs at the Pennsylvania Hospital', *Journal of the American Medical Association*, 255:17 (1986), 2320–3.

Howell, J., 'Machines and Medicine: Technology Transforms the American Hospital', in Long, D. and Golden, J. (eds), *The American General Hospital: Communities and Social Contexts* (Ithaca and London: Cornell University Press, 1989), 109–34.

Howell, J., *Technology in the Hospital: Transforming Patient Care in the Early Twentieth Century* (Baltimore and London: John Hopkins University Press, 1995).

Howell, J., 'Trust and the Tuskegee Experiments', in Duffin, J. (ed.), *Clio in the Clinic: History in Medical Practice* (Oxford: Oxford University Press, 2005), 213–25.

Hull, A., 'Teamwork, Clinical Research, and the Development of Scientific Medicines in Interwar Britain: The "Glasgow School" Revisited', *Bulletin of the History of Medicine*, 81 (2007), 569–93.

Hunter, K., *Doctors' Stories: The Narrative Structure of Medical Knowledge* (Princeton: Princeton University Press, 1991).

Hurn, J., 'The Changing Fortunes of the General Paralytic', *Wellcome History*, 4 (1997), 5–6.

Hutton, G., *Woodilee Hospital, 125 Years* (Glasgow: Greater Glasgow Health Board, 1997).

Ion, R. and Beer, M., 'The British Reaction to Dementia Praecox, 1893-1913', parts 1 and 2, *History of Psychiatry*, 13 (2002), 285–304 and 419–31.

Jacob, M., *et al.*, 'Beware of Neuro-Syphilis', *Journal of Neurology*, 252:5 (2005), 609–10.

Jacyna, L.S., 'Construing Silence: Narratives of Language Loss in Early Nineteenth-Century France', *Journal of the History of Medicine and Allied Sciences*, 49 (1994), 333–61.

Jacyna, L.S., 'The Laboratory and the Clinic: The Impact of Pathology on Surgical Diagnosis in the Glasgow Western Infirmary, 1875–1910', *Bulletin of the History of Medicine*, 69:3 (1988), 384–406.

Jones, E., Rahman, S., and Woolven, R., 'The Maudsley Hospital: Design and Strategic Direction, 1923–1939', *Medical History*, 51 (2007), 357–78.

Jones, G., *Social Hygiene in Twentieth-Century Britain* (London: Croom Helm, 1986).

Jones, J., *Bad Blood: The Tuskegee Syphilis Experiment* (New York: The Free Press, 1993).

Jordanova, L., 'The Social Construction of Medical Knowledge', *Social History of Medicine*, 8:2 (1995), 361–81.

Kararizou, E., *et al.*, 'Psychosis or Simply a New Manifestation of Neurosyphilis', *The Journal of International Medical Research*, 34:3 (2006), 335–7.

Kleinman, A., *The Illness Narratives: Suffering, Healing, and the Human Condition* (New York: Basic Books, 1988).

Koutsilieri, E., *et al.*, 'The Pathogenesis of HIV-Induced Dementia', *Mechanisms of Ageing and Development*, 123:8 (2002), 1047–53.

Lawrence, C., 'Incommunicable Knowledge: Science, Technology, and the Clinical Art in Britain, 1850–1914', *Journal of Contemporary History*, 20 (1985), 503–20.

Lawrence, C., *Rockefeller Money, The Laboratory, and Medicine in Edinburgh, 1919–1930: New Science in an Old Country* (Rochester: University of Rochester Press, 2005).

Lawrence, C., 'A Tale of Two Sciences: Bedside and Bench in Twentieth-Century Britain', *Medical History*, 43 (1999), 421–49.

Ledger, S. and Luckhurst, R. (eds), *The Fin de Siècle: A Reader in Cultural History, c.1880–1900* (Oxford: Oxford University Press, 2000).

Leese, P., *Shell Shock: Traumatic Neurosis and the British Soldiers of the First World War* (Basingstoke and New York: Palgrave Macmillan, 2002).

Leigh, D., *The Historical Development of British Psychiatry*, Vol. I (Oxford, London, New York and Paris: Pergamon Press, 1961).

Letendre, S., *et al.*, 'Neurologic Complications of HIV Disease and their Treatment', *Topics in HIV Medicine*, 15:2 (2007), 32–9.

Lomax, E., 'Infantile Syphilis as an Example of Nineteenth Century Belief in the Inheritance of Acquired Characteristics', *Journal of the History of Medicine*, 34 (1979), 23–39.

Luckin, B., 'Revisiting the Idea of Degeneration in Urban Britain, 1830–1900', *Urban History*, 33:2 (2006), 234–52.

MacKenzie, C., *Psychiatry for the Rich: A History of Ticehurst Private Asylum, 1792–1917* (London: Routledge, 1992).

Marland, H., *Dangerous Motherhood: Insanity and Childbirth in Victorian Britain* (Basingstoke and New York: Palgrave Macmillan, 2004).

Mazumdar, P., '"In the Silence of the Laboratory": The League of Nations Standardizes Syphilis Tests', *Social History of Medicine*, 16:3 (2003), 437–59.

McCandless, P., 'A Female Malady?: Women at the South Carolina Lunatic Asylum, 1828–1915', *Journal of the History of Medicine and Allied Sciences*, 54 (1999), 543–71.

Melling, J. and Forsythe, B. (eds), *Insanity, Institutions and Society, 1800–1914: A Social History of Madness in Comparative Perspective* (London and New York: Routledge, 1999).

Merskey, H., 'Somatic Treatments, Ignorance, and the Historiography of Psychiatry', *History of Psychiatry*, 5 (1994), 387–91.

Meyer, A., 'Frederick Mott, Founder of the Maudsley Laboratories', *British Journal of Psychiatry*, 122 (1973), 497–516.

Micale, M., *Approaching Hysteria: Disease and its Interpretations* (Princeton: Princeton University Press, 1995).

Morton, R. and Rashid, S., 'Role of Fever in Infection: Has Induced Fever Any Therapeutic Potential in HIV Infection?', *Genitourinary Medicine*, 73:3 (1997), 212–15.

Navia, B., Jordan, B. and Price, R., 'The AIDS Dementia Complex: 1. Clinical Features', *Annals of Neurology*, 19 (1986), 525–35.

Nicol, A. and Sheppard, J., 'Hospital Clinical Records', *British Medical Journal*, 291 (1985), 614–15.

Nicol, A. and Sheppard, J., 'Why Keep Hospital Clinical Records?', *British Medical Journal*, 290 (1985), 263–4.

Nicol, W., 'General Paralysis of the Insane', *British Journal of Venereal Disease*, 32 (1956), 9–16.

Nitrini, R., 'The Cure of One of the Most Frequent Types of Dementia: A Historical Parallel', *Alzheimer Disease and Associated Disorders*, 19:3 (2005), 156–8.

Nowell-Smith, H., 'Nineteenth-Century Narrative Case Histories: An Inquiry into Stylistics and History', *Canadian Bulletin of Medical History*, 12 (1995), 47–67.

Nye, R., *Crime, Madness, and Politics in Modern France: The Medical Concept of National Decline* (Princeton: Princeton University Press, 1984).

Nye, R., 'Degeneration, Neurasthenia and the Culture of Sport in Belle Epoque France', *Journal of Contemporary History*, 17 (1982), 51–68.

Oppenheim, J., *"Shattered Nerves": Doctors, Patients, and Depression in Victorian England* (New York and Oxford: Oxford University Press, 1991).

Oriel, J., *The Scars of Venus: A History of Venereology* (London: Springer-Verlag, 1994).

Petrie, J. and McIntyre, N. (eds), *The Problem Oriented Medical Record: Its Use in Hospitals, General Practice and Medical Education* (Edinburgh: Churchill Livingstone, 1979).

Pick, D., *Faces of Degeneration: A European Disorder, c.1848–c.1918* (Cambridge: Cambridge University Press, 1989).

Pickstone, J., 'Medicine in Industrial Britain: The Uses of Local Studies', *Social History of Medicine*, 2:2 (1989), 197–203.

Porter, R., 'Diseases of Civilization', in Bynum, W. and Porter, R. (eds), *Companion Encyclopedia of the History of Medicine*, Vol. I (London: Routledge, 1993), 585–600.

Porter, R., *Mind-Forg'd Manacles: A History of Madness in England from the Restoration to the Regency* (London: Athlone Press, 1987).

Porter, R., *A Social History of Madness: Stories of the Insane* (London: Weidenfeld and Nicolson, 1987).

Porter, R., and Wright, D. (eds), *The Confinement of the Insane: International Perspectives, 1800–1965* (Cambridge: Cambridge University Press, 2003).

Quétel, C., *History of Syphilis* (Cambridge: Polity Press, 1990).

Ray, L., 'Models of Madness in Victorian Asylum Practice', *European Journal of Sociology*, 22 (1981), 229–64.

Reiser, S., 'Creating Form Out of Mass: The Development of the Medical Record', in Mendelsohn, E. (ed.), *Transformation and Tradition in the Sciences: Essays in Honor of I. Bernard Cohen* (Cambridge: Cambridge University Press, 1984), 303–16.

Reverby, S. (ed.), *Tuskegee's Truths: Rethinking the Tuskegee Syphilis Study* (Chapel Hill and London: University of North Carolina Press, 2000).

Rimke, H. and Hunt, A., 'From Sinners to Degenerates: The Medicalization of Morality in the 19th Century', *History of the Human Sciences*, 15:1 (2002), 59–88.

Risse, G. and Warner, J., 'Reconstructing Clinical Activities: Patient Records in Medical History', *Social History of Medicine*, 5 (1992), 183–205.

Rollin, H., 'The Horton Malaria Laboratory, Epsom, Surrey (1925–1975)', *Journal of Medical Biography*, 2 (1994), 94–7.

Rosebury, T., *Microbes and Morals: The Strange Story of Venereal Disease* (London: Secker and Warburg, 1972).

Rosenberg, C., *The Cholera Years: The United States in 1832, 1849, and 1866* (Chicago: Chicago University Press, 1962).

Rosenberg, C., 'Erwin H. Ackerknecht, Social Medicine, and the History of Medicine', *Bulletin of the History of Medicine*, 81 (2007), 511–32.

Rosenberg, C., *Explaining Epidemics and Other Studies in the History of Medicine* (Cambridge: Cambridge University Press, 1992).

Rosenberg, C., 'Pathologies of Progress: The Idea of Civilization as Risk', *Bulletin of the History of Medicine*, 72 (1998), 714–30.

Rosenberg, C., 'What is Disease? In Memory of Owsei Temkin', *Bulletin of the History of Medicine*, 77 (2003), 491–505.

Rosenberg, C. and Golden, J. (eds), *Framing Disease: Studies in Cultural History* (New Brunswick and New Jersey: Rutgers University Press, 1992).

Rousseau, G., *et. al.* (eds), *Framing and Imagining Disease in Cultural History* (Basingstoke and New York: Palgrave Macmillan, 2003).

Sadler, W., *Practice of Psychiatry* (London: Henry Kimpton, 1953).

Saik, S., *et al.*, 'Neurosyphilis in Newly Admitted Psychiatric Patients: Three Case Reports', *Journal of Clinical Psychiatry*, 65:7 (2004), 919–21.

Scull, A., *The Insanity of Place, The Place of Insanity: Essays on the History of Psychiatry* (London and New York: Routledge, 2006).

Scull, A., *Museums of Madness: The Social Organization of Insanity in Nineteenth-Century England* (London: Allen Lane, 1979).

Scull, A., 'Somatic Treatments and the Historiography of Psychiatry', *History of Psychiatry*, 5 (1994), 1–12.

Shephard, B., *A War of Nerves* (London: Jonathan Cape, 2000).

Showalter, E., *The Female Malady: Women, Madness and English Culture, 1830–1980* (London: Virago, 1996).

Soloway, R., 'Counting the Degenerates: The Statistics of Race Deterioration in Edwardian England', *Journal of Contemporary History*, 17:1 (1982), 137–64.

Spongberg, M., *Feminizing Venereal Disease: The Body of the Prostitute in Nineteenth-Century Medical Discourse* (London: Macmillan, 1997).

Stedman Jones, G., *Outcast London: A Study in the Relationship between Classes in Victorian Society* (Oxford: Clarendon Press, 1971).

Stone, D., *Breeding Superman: Nietzsche, Race and Eugenics in Edwardian and Interwar Britain* (Liverpool: Liverpool University Press, 2002).

Stoner, B., 'Current Controveries in the Management of Adult Syphilis', *Clinical Infectious Diseases*, 44: Supplement 3 (2007), 130–46.

Sturdy, S. and Cooter, R., 'Science, Scientific Management, and the Transformation of Medicine in Britain, *c.*1870–1950', *History of Science*, 36 (1998), 421–66.

Suzuki, A., *Madness at Home: The Psychiatrist, the Patient, and the Family in England, 1820–1860* (Berkeley and London: University of California Press, 2006).

Swartz, S., 'Shrinking: A Postmodern Perspective on Psychiatric Case Histories', *South African Journal of Psychology*, 26:3 (1996), 150–6.

Thompson, C. (ed.), *The Origins of Modern Psychiatry* (Chicester: John Wiley and Sons, 1987).

Thompson, M. and Samuels, S., 'Neurosyphilis: Is it Still a Clinically Relevant Form of Dementia?', *Expert Review of Neurotherapeutics*, 2 (2002), 665–8.

Thomson, M., *The Problem of Mental Deficiency: Eugenics, Democracy, and Social Policy in Britain, c.1870–1959* (Oxford: Clarendon Press, 1998).

Török, M., 'Neurological Infections: Clinical Advances and Emerging Threats', *Lancet Neurology*, 6:1 (2007), 16–18.

Valenstein, E., *Great and Desperate Cures: The Rise and Decline of Psychosurgery and Other Radical Treatments for Mental Illness* (New York: Basic Books, 1986).

Vogel, M. and Rosenberg, C. (eds), *The Therapeutic Revolution* (Philadelphia: University of Pennsylvania Press, 1979).

Wailoo, K., *Drawing Blood: Technology and Disease Identity in Twentieth-Century America* (Baltimore and London: John Hopkins University Press, 1997).

Walkowitz, J., *Prostitution and Victorian Society: Women, Class and the State* (Cambridge: Cambridge University Press, 1980).

Waugh, M., 'Alfred Fournier, 1832–1914: His Influence on Venereology', *British Journal of Venereal Disease*, 50 (1974), 232–6.

Whitrow, M., *Julius Wagner-Jauregg, 1857–1940* (London: Smith-Gordon, 1993).

Whitrow, M., 'Wagner-Jauregg and Fever Therapy', *Medical History*, 34 (1990), 294–310.

Wright, D., 'Getting Out of the Asylum: Understanding the Confinement of the Insane in the Nineteenth Century', *Social History of Medicine*, 10 (1997), 137–55.

Zetola, N. and Klausner, J., 'Syphilis and HIV Infection: An Update', *Clinical Infectious Diseases*, 44 (2007), 1222–8.

Zilboorg, G. and Henry, W., *A History of Medical Psychology* (New York: Norton, 1941).

Theses (Secondary Sources) and Unpublished Papers

Barfoot, M., 'Love's Labours Lost: The Work, Exercise and Health of Pauper Inmates of Nineteenth Century Scottish Asylums', Scottish Labour History Society, Edinburgh, 1997, unpublished conference paper.

Belt, H. van den, 'Spirochaetes, Serology and Salvarsan: Ludwik Fleck and the Construction of Medical Knowledge about Syphilis', PhD thesis, Wageningen Agricultural University, The Netherlands (1997).

Clark, M., '"The Data of Alienism": Evolutionary Neurology, Physiological Psychology, and the Reconstruction of British Psychiatric Theory, *c.*1850–*c.*1900', PhD thesis, University of Oxford (1982).

Davis, G., '"Lovers and Madmen have such Seething Brains": Historical Aspects of Neurosyphilis in Four Scottish Asylums, *c.*1880–1930', PhD thesis, University of Edinburgh (2001).

Halliday, E., 'Themes in Scottish Asylum Culture: The Hospitalisation of the Scottish Asylum, 1880-1914', PhD thesis, University of Stirling (2003).

Hurn, J., 'The History of General Paralysis of the Insane in Britain, 1830 to 1950', PhD thesis, University of London (1998).

Mathews, S., 'Matter of Mind? The Contributions of Neuropathologist Sir Frederick Walker Mott (1853–1926) to British Psychiatry *c.*1895–1923', PhD thesis, University of Manchester (2006).

Nicolson, M. and Smith, D., 'Science and Clinical Scepticism: The Case of Ralph Stockman and the Glasgow Medical Faculty', Science and Technology Dynamics Internal Progress Conference, Amsterdam, 1997, unpublished conference paper.

Rice, F., 'Madness and Industrial Society: A Study of the Origins and Early Growth of the Organisation of Insanity in Nineteenth-Century Scotland, *c.*1830–1870', PhD thesis, 2 vols, University of Strathclyde (1981).

Sturdy, H., 'Boarding-Out the Insane, 1857–1913: A Study of the Scottish System', PhD thesis, University of Glasgow (1996).

Summerly, P., 'Visual Pathology: A Case Study in Late Nineteenth Century Clinical Photography in Glasgow', PhD thesis, University of Glasgow (2003).

Thompson, M., 'The Mad, the Bad and the Sad: Psychiatric Care in the Royal Edinburgh Asylum (Morningside), 1813–1894', PhD thesis, Boston University Graduate School (1984).

Wall, R., 'Using Bacteriology in the Hospital and Society: England, 1880–1939', PhD thesis, Imperial College London (2007).

Index

Page numbers in bold text indicate an illustration.

275